The Difficult Airway

David B. Glick, MD, MBA
Richard M. Cooper, B.Sc, M.Sc, MD, FRCPC
Andranik Ovassapian, MD
Editors

The Difficult Airway

An Atlas of Tools and Techniques for Clinical Management

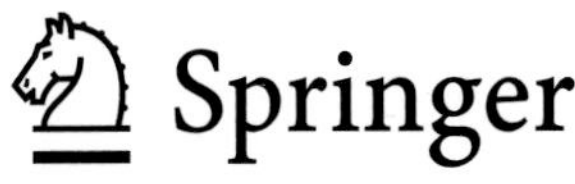
Springer

Editors
David B. Glick, MD, MBA
Department of Anesthesia & Critical Care
The University of Chicago
Chicago, IL, USA

Andranik Ovassapian, MD (*deceased*)
Department of Anesthesia & Critical Care
The University of Chicago
Chicago, IL, USA

Richard M. Cooper, B.Sc, M.Sc, MD, FRCPC
Department of Anesthesia
University of Toronto
Department of Anesthesia and Pain Management
Toronto General Hospital
Toronto, ON, Canada

ISBN 978-0-387-92848-7 ISBN 978-0-387-92849-4 (eBook)
DOI 10.1007/978-0-387-92849-4
Springer New York Heidelberg Dordrecht London

Library of Congress Control Number: 2012951846

Printed on acid-free paper

Springer is part of Springer Science+Business Media (www.springer.com)

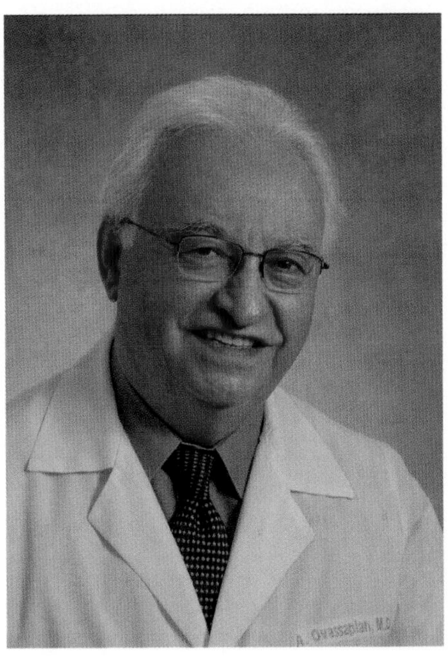

To our loving wives and wonderful children,
and to the memory of Dr. Andranik Ovassapian—pioneer,
mentor, colleague, and friend to a generation of physicians
and nurses the world over.

David B. Glick
Richard M. Cooper

Preface

Few challenges can sour faster or lead to more devastating outcomes than failed attempts to control a difficult airway. Things can go from calm to catastrophic in little more than the time that you are able to hold your breath, and death or profound neurologic injury are the possible results. The concerns regarding the management of difficult airways are shouldered by many in the healthcare field as anesthesiologists, intensive care physicians, emergency room physicians, as well as nurses in many different venues, and out-of-hospital first responders may all be tasked with providing airway support and/or definitive airway control to a wide range of patients. Unfortunately, the majority of patients with airways that are difficult to manage are either unsuspected difficult airways or require urgent airway management. Either way, there is often precious little time to develop a plan for how best to approach the problem. The American Society of Anesthesiologists' Difficult Airway Algorithm, and algorithms like it, were developed in large part to offer a pre-planned approach to the difficult airway to streamline the efforts from the time of identifying the difficult airway to successful management of the airway. The advantage of the ASA algorithm is that it includes many different techniques and tools to help the provider overcome the entire gamut of airway challenges. The drawback to the wide range of approaches is that it poses a significant experiential challenge to the airway manager who wants to become familiar with the many options available to manage a difficult airway. This problem has been exacerbated by the rapid evolution in airway management tools and the techniques for their use that have occurred in the past 10–15 years. Our purpose in writing *The Difficult Airway* was to provide the necessary background and instructions in the many techniques listed in the ASA algorithm so that any practitioner, from the novice to the seasoned veteran, will feel comfortable in selecting and practicing unfamiliar techniques and devices or better appreciate the role that familiar ones might play. To this end, we have benefitted greatly from the experiences and expertise of an international collection of practitioners who have each written and illustrated a chapter covering techniques that they, in many cases, have pioneered.

Much of the inspiration for this work as well as the selection of the authors for each of the chapters came from Dr. Andranik Ovassapian. Dr. Ovassapian's groundbreaking work with fiberoptic bronchoscopy and his involvement in the founding and early leadership of the Society for Airway Management has served as the foundation for much of the work that has followed regarding the management of the expected and unexpected difficult airway. For that, a generation of clinicians and their patients owe him a tremendous debt. We were all deeply saddened by his death during the writing of this book, but trust that the lessons he taught us will continue to improve patient safety and satisfaction for many years to come.

Acknowledgements

First and foremost, we would like to thank all the authors who generously shared their time and their experience in preparing the chapters for *The Difficult Airway*. We would also like to thank Joni Fraser, our developmental editor, who tirelessly pursued all the loose ends that any project of this kind inevitably has and made sure that everything came together properly; our assistant editor, Joanna Perey, who managed the communications with the artists and editors at Springer; and Shelley Reinhardt, our senior editor, who took over the project while it was still in its earliest stages and navigated us through a string of challenges and changes that made it possible for our vision for this book to become a reality.

Contents

Contributors

Richard M. Cooper, B.Sc, M.Sc, MD, FRCPC
Department of Anesthesia, University of Toronto, Toronto, ON, Canada
Department of Anesthesia and Pain Management, Toronto General Hospital, Toronto, ON, Canada

Julio Cortiñas-Diaz, MD, PhD
Department of Surgery, University of Santiago de Compostela School of Medicine, Hospital Clinico Universitario, Santiago de Compostela, Spain

Martin H. Dauber, MD
Department of Anesthesia & Critical Care, The University of Chicago, Chicago, IL, USA

Louise Ellard, MBBS, FANZCA
Department of Anesthesia and Pain Management, Toronto General Hospital, Toronto, ON, Canada

David B. Glick, MD, MBA
Department of Anesthesia & Critical Care, University of Chicago Hospitals, Chicago, IL, USA

Corina Lee, MB ChB, FRCA, MRCP
Department of Anesthesia and Pain Management, Toronto General Hospital, Toronto, ON, Canada

Michael R. Hernandez, MD
Department of Anesthesia & Critical Care, University of Chicago Medical Center, Chicago, IL, USA

Richard M. Levitan, MD
Department of Emergency Medicine, Thomas Jefferson University Hospital, Philadelphia, PA, USA

Sachin Kheterpal, MD, MBA
Department of Anesthesiology, University of Michigan Hospital System, Ann Arbor, MI, USA

P. Allan Klock, Jr., MD

Department of Anesthesiology and Critical Care, University of Chicago Hospitals, Chicago, IL, USA

Seth Manoach, MD
Department of Anesthesiology and Emergency Medicine, SUNY Downstate Medical Center and Kings County Hospital, Brooklyn, NY, USA

Mark E. Nunnally, MD, FCCM
Department of Anesthesiology and Critical Care, University of Chicago Medical Center, Chicago, IL, USA

Michael F. O'Connor, MD
Department of Anesthesia & Critical Care, The University of Chicago, Chicago, IL, USA

Irene P. Osborn, MD
Department of Anesthesiology, Mount Sinai Medical Center, New York, NY, USA

Satya Krishna Ramachandran, MD, FRCA
Department of Anesthesiology, University of Michigan Hospital System, Ann Arbor, MI, USA

Kerstin M. Stenson, MD, FACS
Section of Otolaryngology–Head and Neck Surgery, Department of Surgery, The University of Chicago, Chicago, IL, USA

Avery Tung, MD
Department of Anesthesia & Critical Care, The University of Chicago, Chicago, IL, USA

Janis P. Tupesis, MD
Department of Emergency Medicine, University of Wisconsin School of Medicine and Public Health, Madison, WI, USA

Nathan T. Van Dyk, MD
Emergency Department, Vista East Medical Center, Waukegan, IL, USA

Ashutosh Wali, MD, FFARCSI
Departments of Anesthesiology, Obstetrics and Gynecology, Baylor College of Medicine, Houston, TX, USA

Advanced Airway Management, Baylor College of Medicine, Houston, TX, USA

Michael Woo, MD
Department of Anesthesia & Critical Care, The University of Chicago, Chicago, IL, USA

Zdravka Zafirova, MD
Department of Anesthesia & Critical Care, The University of Chicago, Chicago, IL, USA

1

The Difficult Airway: Definitions and Algorithms

Zdravka Zafirova and Avery Tung

Introduction

Maintaining a stable, patent airway is a fundamental element of acute care medical practice. While airway management is conceptually straightforward, the wide variety of clinical circumstances, patients, and tools can make the task of ensuring a stable, open airway under all clinical conditions extremely challenging. Care providers involved in airway management must therefore not only be technically skilled but also sufficiently flexible to adjust to changing conditions, risk/benefit balances, and goals. One aspect of airway management that requires particular attention is the airway that is difficult to secure or keep patent. For clinical or anatomic reasons, both bag mask ventilation and

Z. Zafirova (✉)
Department of Anesthesia & Critical Care, The University of Chicago,
5841 S. Maryland Ave. MC 4028, Chicago, IL 60637, USA
e-mail: zzafirova@dacc.uchicago.edu

A. Tung
Department of Anesthesia & Critical Care, The University of Chicago,
Chicago, IL 60637, USA

D.B. Glick et al. (eds.), *The Difficult Airway: An Atlas of Tools and Techniques for Clinical Management*,
DOI 10.1007/978-0-387-92849-4_1, © Springer Science+Business Media New York 2013

tracheal intubation in such a patient population may be difficult without specialized expertise or tools. Because adequate oxygen delivery through a patent airway is critical to life support and resuscitative efforts, the risks of inadequate airway management are high, adding to the challenge.

One significant advance in difficult airway management is the development of algorithms to standardize the technical approach to successful endotracheal intubation in a patient with a difficult airway. Such algorithms are relatively recent (The American Society of Anesthesiologists difficult airway algorithm originated in 1993), and integrate clinical experience, evidence, and technical expertise into a stepwise approach to anticipated and unanticipated airway challenges. This chapter will focus on current concepts regarding the definition of a difficult airway, the incidence of difficult airways in and out of the operating room, and current algorithms for management of the difficult airway.

Definitions

Considerable variability exists in the literature definition of the difficult airway (DA) has not been clearly established in the literature. Differences in study design, assessment tools, operator skill, and relevant metrics for defining difficulty have contributed to this lack of consensus. Most studies have divided the difficult airway into two components: difficult mask ventilation (DMV) and difficult intubation. A difficult airway may then involve either component or both. Definitions for DMV, for example, may range from subjective anesthesiologist assessment to a need for four-hand ventilation[1] or alternative intervention and additional personnel[1]. Other metrics have included the presence of a clinically relevant gas leak during ventilation, a need for increased fresh gas flows above 15 L/min or use of oxygen flush valve more than twice[2], lack of perceptible chest movement[2], $SpO_2 < 92$ %[2], and need for a different operator[2]. One recent classification of mask ventilation has been developed by Han and consists of 5 grades (Table 1.1).

Similarly, published metrics for difficult intubation include requiring more than two attempts or more than 10 min with conventional laryngoscopy, requiring more than three or four attempts to successfully intubate, a perceived need for a stylet, and inability to intubate the trachea after at least three unsuccessful attempts with stylet or by an experienced staff anesthesiologist[2]. Adnet and coworkers proposed a continuum of difficulty based upon several parameters referred to as the Intubation Difficulty Scale (IDS), assigning numerical values to parameters such as number of attempts, number of operators, number of alternative techniques, Cormack and Lehane laryngoscopic grade, increased lifting force, application of laryngeal pressure, and vocal cord mobility[3].

In the 1993 American Society of the Anesthesiologists (ASA) guidelines for difficult airway management[4] DMV was defined as present when an unassisted anesthesiologist is unable to maintain $SpO_2 > 90$ % using positive pressure ventilation with 100 % oxygen in a patient with $SpO_2 > 90$ % before the anesthetic intervention. In addition, these guidelines considered mask ventilation to be difficult if the anesthesiologist is unable to prevent or reverse signs of inadequate ventilation[4]. An intubation sequence was defined as difficult if insertion of the endotracheal tube required more than three attempts or more than 10 min with conventional laryngoscopy[4]. Obviously, an experienced laryngoscopist might

Table 1.1. Classification of difficulty of mask ventilation.[25]

Grade 0	Ventilation by mask not attempted
Grade 1	Readily able to ventilate by mask
Grade 2	Able to ventilate by mask with oral airway or other adjuvant
Grade 3	Difficult mask ventilation (inadequate, unstable, or requiring two practitioners)
Grade 4	Unable to mask ventilate

recognize a difficult or impossible laryngoscopy on the first attempt and not engage in multiple time-wasting, unproductive efforts.

A more recent version of the ASA guidelines used criteria more clinically relevant to anesthesia practitioners. In the 2003 revision, the Task Force defined a difficult airway as a clinical situation where a conventionally trained anesthesiologist experiences difficulty with face mask ventilation of the upper airway, difficulty with tracheal intubation, or both [5]. DMV was defined as the inability to provide adequate ventilation with a mask as evidenced by the absence or the inadequacy of breath sounds, chest movement, spirometric measures of exhaled gas flow, exhaled carbon dioxide ($ETCO_2$) as well as inadequate oxygen saturation (SpO_2), cyanosis, the auscultatory signs of severe obstruction, gastric air entry or dilatation and hemodynamic changes associated with hypoxemia or hypercarbia. Difficult intubation was defined as the inability to visualize the vocal cords during multiple attempts at direct laryngoscopy, and difficulty or failure to place the endotracheal tube despite multiple attempts.

Most published definitions of the difficult airway center on the ability of the practitioner to perform *face mask* ventilation within specific parameters or intubate *by direct laryngoscopy* within a specific time or number of attempts. It is easy to see that defining the difficult airway is itself difficult. Changing technologies, variability in operator skill, and the use of alternate airway techniques may result in an ongoing reexamination of these definitions. Familiarity with alternate airway devices is an example. Failed face mask ventilation may be easily managed with a supraglottic airway device. A skilled bronchoscopist may choose that technique rather than direct laryngoscopy in a patient with risk factors for difficult direct laryngoscopy. Similarly, an intubation easily performed by video laryngoscopy or a lightwand is difficult to classify via standard "visualize the cords" metrics. Some direct laryngoscopies fail to reveal the larynx but a patient may still be easily intubated, while video laryngoscopy may provide complete laryngeal exposure but intubation is difficult. In addition, variability in operator skill may cause an airway to be difficult for one provider, but not for another. Literature assessments of incidence, complication rate, and success rate for difficult intubation should thus be interpreted with these caveats in mind.

Incidence

As noted above, the incidence of difficult airway management clearly depends on the definition used and the patient population studied. For DMV, reported incidences range between 0.07 and 5 %. Several prospective studies demonstrated the incidence to be 0.08 % [6], 0.9[7], 1.4 %[8], 4.9 %[9], and 5 %[2]. The largest prospective study was performed in 2006 and included 22,660 MV attempts identified by electronic database review. Kheterpal et al. defined mask ventilation as difficult if it was inadequate, unstable, or required two providers with or without muscle relaxant and found that the rate of DMV was 1.4 % and the rate of impossible mask ventilation was 0.16 %[10]. In a 2009 follow-up study focusing on impossible mask ventilation, the same authors evaluated 53,041 attempts at mask ventilation and found a 0.15 % incidence of IMV[1].

Published estimates of the incidence of difficult intubation (DI) range from 0.1 to 13 %, with the incidence of impossible intubation (ImI) between 0.3 and 0.5 %. Difficult or impossible mask ventilation can occur by itself or in association with difficult (direct) laryngoscopy and/or intubation. In the retrospective study by Kheterpal et al. in 2009, 19/77 (25 %) patients had a combination of impossible mask ventilation and difficult intubation by direct laryngoscopy, defined as a grade III or IV Cormack-Lehane laryngoscopy view or more than three attempts at intubation by an anesthesiology attending[1]. The combination of impossible mask ventilation and impossible intubation is encountered much less frequently with incidences of 0.01–2 per 10,000 patients in some studies and 0.3–1.5 % in others. Because the study by Kheterpal et al. was retrospective, these numbers are low estimates as many patients with known difficult airways may have been intubated by other means.

Several associated conditions can alter the risk of difficult intubation or ventilation. Morbid obesity (MO) and obstructive sleep apnea (OSA) have both been implicated as risk factors for DI. One recent prospective study found a DI rate of 3.3 % in MO patients undergoing bariatric surgery, but no correlation between OSA and DI, and no ImI[11].

Acromegaly also increases the incidence of DI. Older retrospective studies estimate the incidence at 12–30 %, and a more recent prospective study found an incidence of 26 % [12]. In thyroid surgery patients, the reported incidence of DI is also increased relative to normal patients (5.3–13 %). One prospective study in 324 patients undergoing thyroid surgery observed similar risks of DI in patients with or without goiter in 11.7 % vs. 9.9 %, respectively[13]. A similar study by Bouaggad reported an incidence of DI of 5.3 %[14]. A study evaluating the risk of DI in patients with known or newly found goiter scheduled for any nonemergency surgery found a higher incidence of ImI than the general population[15].

Obstetric patients also have a higher incidence of DI. A study by Djabatey reviewed 3,430 general anesthetics in obstetric patients and found the incidence of DMV to be 0, and the incidence of DI 0.67 %, with no failed intubations[16]. Out of the 23 DI, 9 were anticipated and 3 awake fiberoptic intubations were performed. Another prospective study of 1,095 general anesthetics for cesarean section reported a rate of DI of 3.3 %, with failed intubation incidence of 0.4 % and successful laryngeal mask airway (LMA) management in all failed intubations[17].

Algorithms for Addressing the Difficult Airway

To facilitate a uniform approach to the challenge of the difficult airway, several national anesthesiology societies have developed algorithms for difficult airway management. The American Society of Anesthesiologists guidelines were introduced in 1993 and updated in 2003 [4,5]. These guidelines, developed using literature evidence, expert opinion, and input from ASA members, address the issues of preoperative evaluation, definition and predictors of DMV and DI, basic preparation for difficult airway management, specific airway strategies, and step-by-step algorithms for securing and extubating the difficult airway.

The ASA guidelines begin with the preoperative evaluation, and suggest that such evaluation should include a history of prior difficult airway management and conditions that may predispose to a difficult airway. Assessment of the likelihood of difficulty with patient cooperation or consent and difficulty with surgical airway establishment should also be performed. No specific diagnostic tests beyond assessment of history and physical are recommended.

The ASA guidelines then make several basic recommendations about the approach to the difficult airway. These include informing the patient, ensuring the presence of an additional capable assistant, and pre-oxygenation by face mask. In addition, the ready availability of a basic set of airway instruments is recommended to assist with anticipated and unanticipated DMV/DI scenarios. Such a setup should be accessible at all anesthetizing locations and other areas where acute difficult airway management may be encountered. It is also essential that those likely to use such carts be familiar with the contents and their proper use. The ASA guidelines provide suggestions regarding the items to be included in the basic setup and their modification depending on the location and the preoperative evaluation (Table 1.2).

Finally, the 2003 ASA guidelines recommend that clinicians develop specific strategies for facilitating intubation of the difficult airway. The linking of such strategies into sequences then generates algorithms analogous to those used for life-threatening cardiac events. The difficult airway algorithm is depicted in Figure 1.1, and is categorized into five parts.

The first part focuses on assessment of the likelihood and clinical impact of four basic management problems: difficult ventilation, difficult intubation, difficulty with patient

Table 1.2. Suggested equipment for a difficult airway cart (American Society of Anesthesiologists).
Rigid laryngoscope blades of alternate design and size (may include video laryngoscopy)
Tracheal tubes of assorted sizes
Tracheal tube guides
Supraglottic airway devices
Flexible bronchoscopic intubation equipment
Retrograde intubation equipment
At least one device suitable for emergency noninvasive airway ventilation (Combitube®, jet ventilation stylet, transtracheal jet ventilator)
Equipment suitable for emergency invasive airway access
Exhaled CO_2 detector

consent or cooperation, and difficult tracheostomy. The second part focuses on delivering supplemental oxygen throughout the process of difficult airway management. The third part identifies three specific decisions that must be made during the course of difficult airway management. These are awake vs. asleep intubation, noninvasive vs. invasive technique for initial intubation, and preservation vs. ablation of spontaneous ventilation. The fourth part is a recommendation to identify an alternative approach. Finally, the fifth part explicitly recommends the use of exhaled carbon dioxide to confirm tracheal intubation.

Other national societies have also created difficult airway algorithms in recent years. Several prominent examples include the French Society of Anaesthesia and Critical Care (SFAR) in 1996[18] (which was updated in 2008 and published in the form of a series of questions and expert opinions[19, 20]), the Canadian Airway Focus Group (CAFG) in 1998 [21], the Italian Society of Anaesthesia, Resuscitation and Intensive Therapy (SIAARTI) in 1998 with an update on adult airway management in 2005 and pediatric airway management in 2006[22], the German Society of Anaesthesiology and Intensive Care Medicine[23], and the Difficult Airway Society (DAS) in United Kingdom in 2004[24].

A significant difference between guidelines is their definition of difficult intubation. Both the threshold number of intubation attempts and need for specific intubating conditions differ with respect to what constitutes difficult intubation. To address this issue, more recent recommendations have shifted emphasis from the absolute number of attempts or the time involved to include the experience of the laryngoscopist, the optimal position, and the use of alternative devices.

Adequate pre-intervention airway evaluation using various airway characteristics, maintenance of predetermined airway equipment array, planning in case of unanticipated difficult airway, maintenance of oxygenation during attempts, and calling early for help are among other principles consistently emphasized in the various algorithms. In contrast, although the recommendation for availability of alternative airway devices occurs in most guidelines, recommendations as to specific devices and when they should be deployed vary among the difficult airway algorithms. Table 1.3 depicts some relevant differences between airway management algorithms produced by different societies. Table 1.4 presents highlights of difficult airway management (DAM) scenarios in different guidelines and recommendations.

Taken together these strategies and algorithms provide a comprehensive roadmap for addressing the known and unknown difficult airway. Because airway strategies continuously evolve, it is likely that this framework will also change with changing practice. Indeed the ASA algorithms and those of the CAFG are currently undergoing revisions. Three recent developments in airway management suggest that difficult airway management may continue to evolve.

Recent large-scale retrospective analyses suggest that true DMV is rare, and that nearly all cases of DMV are eventually intubated, even when muscle relaxant is given. These data indicate that the practice of withholding muscle relaxant until effective mask ventilation is verified may be unnecessary. If such data change clinical practice, the incidence and subsequent management options for the difficult airway may also change. Perhaps of even

DIFFICULT AIRWAY ALGORITHM

1. Assess the likelihood and clinical impact of basic management problems:
   - A. Difficult Ventilation
   - B. Difficult Intubation
   - C. Difficulty with Patient Cooperation or Consent
   - D. Difficult Tracheostomy
2. Actively pursue opportunities to deliver supplemental oxygen throughout the process of difficult airway management
3. Consider the relative merits and feasibility of basic management choices:

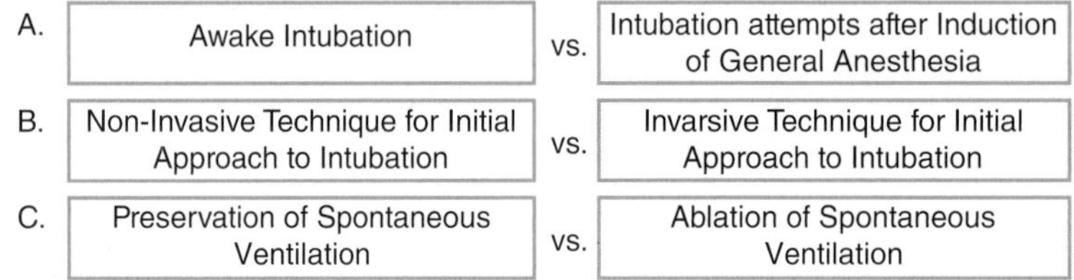

4. Develop primary and alternative strategies:

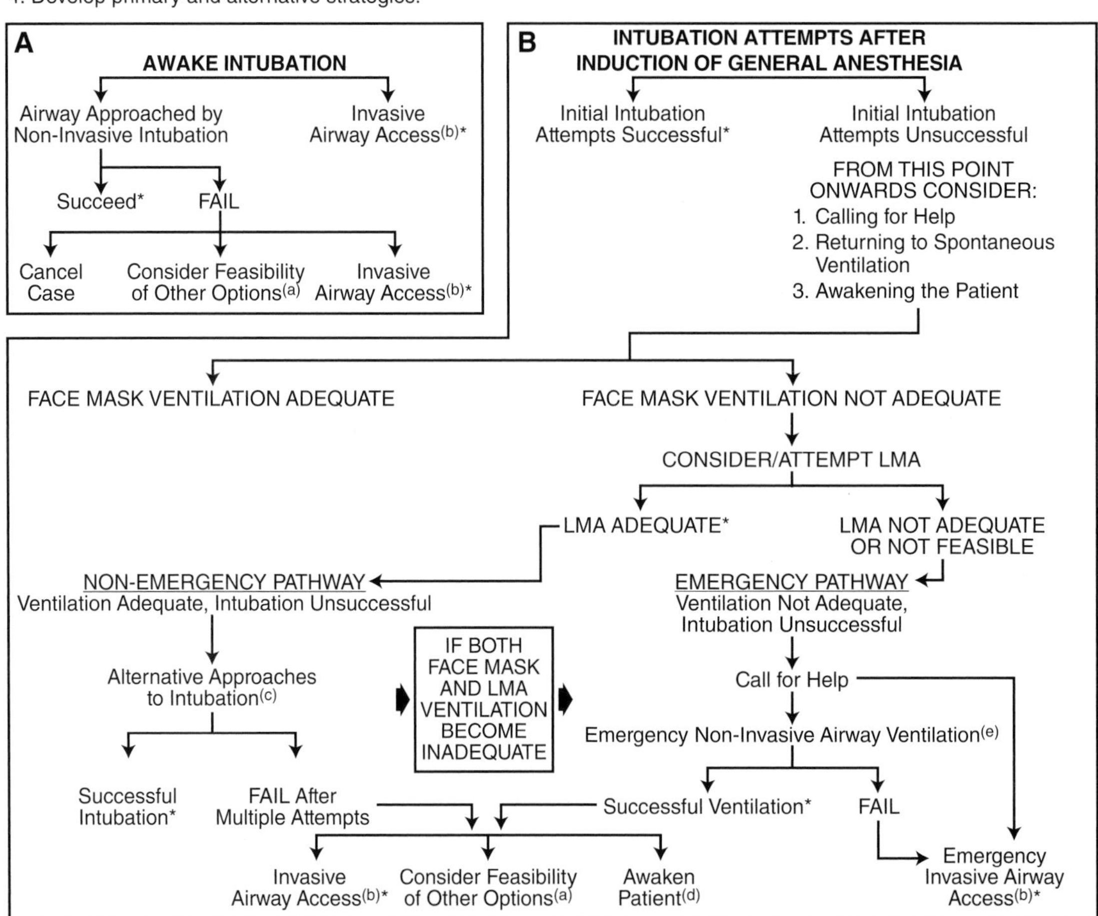

***Confirm ventilation, tracheal intubation, or LMA placement with exhaled CO_2**

a. Other options include (but are not limited to): surgery utilizing face mask or LMA anesthesia, local anesthesia infiltration or regional nerve blockage. Pursuit of these options usually implies that mask ventilation will not be problematic. Therefore, these options may be of limited value if this step in the algorithm has been reached via the Emergency Pathway.

b. Invasive airway access includes: surgical or perculaneous tracheostomy or cricothyrotomy.

c. Alternative non-invasive approaches to difficult intubation include (but are not limited to): use of different laryngoscope blades, LMA as an intubation conduit (with or without fiberoptic guidance), fiberoptic intubation, intubating stylet or tube changer, light wand, retrograde intubation, and blind oral or nasal intubation.

d. Consider re-preparation of the patient for awake intubation or canceling surgery.

e. Options for emergency non-invasive airway ventilation include (but are not limited to): rigid bronchoscope, esophageal-tracheal combitube ventilation, or transtracheal jet ventilation.

Figure 1.1. ASA difficult airway algorithm. Reprinted with permission from Practice Guidelines for Management of the Difficult Airway. An Updated Report by the American Society of Anesthesiologists Task Force on Management of the Difficult Airway. Anesthesiology 2003; 98:1269–77.

Table 1.3. Summary of difficult airway management algorithms.

Airway issue / Algorithm	Definition of difficult ventilation and intubation (laryngoscopy attempts)	Anticipated difficult airway, preoperative evaluation	Recommendations on specific devices
ASA 2003	Absent/inadequate chest movement, breath sounds, auscultatory signs of severe obstruction, exhaled CO_2, spirometric measures of exhaled gas flow; cyanosis, gastric air entry/dilatation, inadequate SpO_2; hemodynamic changes associated with hypoxemia or hypercarbia inadequate mask seal, excessive gas leak, excessive resistance to the ingress or egress of gas	Evaluation—length of upper incisors, relation of maxillary and mandibular incisors during normal jaw closure and voluntary protrusion, interincisor distance, visibility of uvula, shape of palate, compliance of mandibular space, thyromental distance, length, thickness, and angle of motion of neck	Suggested Contents of the Portable Storage Unit for DAM: rigid laryngoscope blades of alternate design and size, rigid FOB/laryngoscope, ETT of assorted sizes and guides (semirigid stylets, ventilating tube changer, light wands, Magill forceps), LMA of assorted sizes (intubating LMA/*LMA-Proseal*™), flexible FOB intubation equipment, retrograde intubation equipment, at least one device suitable for emergency noninvasive airway ventilation (esophageal tracheal Combitube, a hollow jet ventilation stylet, TTJV), equipment suitable for emergency invasive airway access (e.g., cricothyroidotomy), exhaled CO_2 detector
	Multiple attempts by conventionally trained laryngoscopist, inability to visualize any portion of the vocal cords, failed ETT placement	Inform the patient (or responsible person) of risks and procedures At least one additional individual immediately available to assist in DAM Mask preoxygenation before DAM Actively pursue opportunities to deliver oxygen throughout the DAM	
French conference 2008	Inability to maintain $SpO_2 > 92$ % with mask ventilation, leak around the mask, need for fresh gas flow >15 L/min or use >2 times of the rapid oxygen flush, lack of chest movement, two hand ventilation, change of operator >2 attempts by experienced laryngoscopist, suboptimal exposure, or use of alternative technique	Body weight, cervical mobility, mouth opening, thyromental distance, Mallampati class, comorbidities; formula to calculate a score based on multiple factors	Essential equipment for ventilation, difficult intubation, and emergency airway
CAFG 1998	Difficult ventilation and laryngoscopy definition the same as the ASA guidelines; difficult intubation: >2 attempts by experienced laryngoscopist with the same blade, change of blade or adjunct to laryngoscopy (bougie) or use of alternative device/procedure	Mallampati class, receding chin, short neck, protruding maxillary incisors	Mandatory devices: selection of laryngoscopy blades, malleable bougie, alternative to face mask ventilation, alternative to direct laryngoscope, transtracheal airway kit
DAS 2004	Four attempts or more than 2 attempts with same laryngoscope	Not specified	Not specified
SIAARTI 2005	Failed delivery of adequate tidal volume without airway device, external help, or intubation	Written documentation of the mandatory airway parameters—MP test, interincisor distance, mental-thyroidal distance, maxillary prognathism and correction possibility, neck-flexion-extension degree	Mandatory devices: rigid laryngoscope with medium and long curved blades, cuffed standard and armored ETT 5.5–8 ID, malleable stylet, tracheal introducer, Magill forceps, LMA/EGD, cannula for cricothyroid membrane puncture, percutaneous cricothyroidotomy set
	Repeated attempts (>2) with correct head position, external laryngeal manipulation, experienced laryngoscopist; necessity of nonstandard devices/procedures, withdrawal and replanning	Presence of mandatory devices and availability of secondary devices upon request	Secondary devices: flexible FOB, face mask, and oral airways for FOB, retrograde intubation set

CL Cormack-Lehane grade; *MP* Mallampati grade; *LMA* laryngeal mask airway; *EGD* extraglottic device; *TTJV* transtracheal jet ventilator; *FOB* fiberoptic bronchoscope; *OELM* optimum external laryngeal manipulation; *BURP* backward, upward, and rightward pressure; *DAM* difficult airway management

Table 1.4. Highlights of DAM scenarios in different guidelines and recommendations.

Airway issue / Algorithm	Unanticipated difficult intubation	Cannot intubate, cannot ventilate
ASA 2003	Actively pursue opportunities for supplemental oxygen (mask, LMA, jet ventilation), call for help, return to spontaneous ventilation, awaken patient, alternative intubation approach—different laryngoscope blades, blind intubation (oral or nasal), FOB intubation, intubating stylet or tube changer, LMA/LMA as an intubating conduit, light wand, retrograde intubation, invasive airway access, esophageal tracheal Combitube, intratracheal jet stylet, oral and nasopharyngeal airways, rigid ventilating bronchoscope, two-person mask ventilation	Call for help; emergency noninvasive ventilation—LMA, rigid bronchoscope ventilation, esophageal tracheal Combitube, TTJV; invasive airway access—surgical or percutaneous cricothyroidotomy or tracheostomy
French conference 2008	Introducer, LMA, FOB, special blades, awaken patient	Call for help, LMA, supraglottic device, transtracheal oxygenation, cricothyroidotomy, tracheostomy, awaken patient
CAFG 1998	Sniff position, OELM, BURP, maintain oxygentation, adjunct to laryngoscopy (gum elastic bougie), alternative blade, light stylet, Bullard laryngoscope, FOB, transtracheal airway, awaken patient	Consider immediate direct laryngoscopy or alternative to mask ventilation (Combitube, LMA), transtracheal airway (retrograde, cricothyroidotomy, tracheostomy)
DAS 2004	Maintain oxygenation, call for help, use alternative technique not more than two attempts, introducer ("gum elastic bougie"), different laryngoscope blade, LMA, awaken patient; during rapid sequence induction, use of alternative blades with cricothyroid pressure, followed by mask ventilation and wake up—not recommend LMA unless unable to oxygenate with mask	Maximum head extension, jaw thrust, assistance with mask seal, reduce cricothyroid force, call for help, LMA, Combitube, cannula or surgical cricothyroidotomy, surgical or percutaneous tracheostomy not considered fast enough in emergency
SIAARTI 2005	Oxygenation and reevaluation between attempts, cessation of attempts if re-oxygenation difficult, call for help, head in modified Jackson's position ("sniffing"), laryngeal manipulation maneuver (BURP, Sellick), alternative intubation options—different blade for deeper insertion, stylet to conform the ETT, tracheal introducer for Seldinger technique, Magill forceps, LMA, FOB intubation (not recommended in emergency), define difficulty by CL grade and further steps, immediate withdrawal after third attempt if intubation deemed not manageable with alternative device	LMA/EGD, cricothyroid membrane puncture, TTJV, cricothyroidotomy; *surgical tracheotomy NOT a first choice*

greater importance, most situations involving DMV can and perhaps should be managed by earlier use of a supraglottic airway rather than persistent attempts with a face mask to achieve marginal improvement.

The second recent change is the increasingly widespread use of videolaryngoscopy or optical stylets to facilitate the indirect viewing of the larynx. Although this approach to airway management has existed for several years, recent technological advances have made it more user-friendly. Little data exist to properly evaluate the use of video laryngoscopy in the management of the difficult airway, although early reports suggest an ability to substitute video laryngoscopy for direct laryngoscopy in at least some difficult airway situations. Further work will likely clarify the role of video laryngoscopy relative to direct and flexible bronchoscopic strategies.

Finally, the refinement of supraglottic airway strategies has allowed them to become more widely used as a difficult airway technique as an alternative or a bridge to tracheal intubation. The Aintree catheter for example allows clinicians to intubate the trachea via flexible bronchoscopy through a supraglottic airway using flexible bronchoscopic guidance. As with other strategies, increasing use of this technique may cause clinicians to avoid direct laryngoscopy altogether, particularly in the anticipated difficult airway, redefining the incidence and the severity of difficult laryngoscopy.

Conclusion

Although an extensive literature exists on difficult airway management, defining, measuring, and securing the difficult airway remains an elusive task. Differences among providers and between patients and regional variability in techniques and local strategies have all contributed to the challenge of generating consensus. In general, a difficult airway is characterized either by DMV or difficult intubation. The definition of DMV varies from study to study, but has included clinically relevant gas leak, frequent use of the oxygen flush valve, lack of chest movement, and/or desaturation. Historically, definitions of difficult intubation center on the number of attempts or time required to intubate with conventional laryngoscopy, and/or use of a stylet or alternative approach. The most recent ASA guidelines are more general by comparison, considering a difficult airway any clinical situation where a conventionally trained anesthesiologist has difficulty with ventilation or intubation. Ultimately, any airway algorithm must emphasize the importance of oxygenation, whether delivered by face mask, supraglottic device, or tracheal tube.

The specific incidence of DMV is rare, varying from 0.07 to 5 %. The incidence of difficult intubation (by direct laryngoscopy) is similar, ranging from 0.1 to 13 %. More importantly, although difficult ventilation and intubation correlate, the absolute incidence of combined impossible ventilation AND intubation is extremely rare, with an incidence of 0.01–2 per 10,000 intubations[1].

To address the challenge of difficult intubation, multiple societies have produced guidelines for clinicians. The ASA guidelines, most recently updated in 2003, comprehensively evaluate preoperative preparation and airway strategies, and identify specific decisions that should ideally be made prospectively. Other guidelines target similar objectives, and differ primarily in the specific use of airway devices in their algorithms. Ultimately, these guidelines emphasize preparation, forethought, and the development of directed airway skills to facilitate safe management.

References

1. Kheterpal S, Martin L, Shanks A. Prediction and outcomes of impossible mask ventilation. A review of 50,000 anesthetics. Anesthesiology. 2009;110:891–7.
2. Langeron O, Masso E, Huraux C. Prediction of difficult mask ventilation. Anesthesiology. 2000;92:1229–36.

3. L'Hermite J, Nouvellon E, Cuvillon P. The Simplified Predictive Intubation Difficulty Score: a new weighted score for difficult airway assessment. Eur J Anaesthesiol. 2009;26:1–7.
4. Practice guidelines for management of the difficult airway. A report by the American Society of Anesthesiologists task force on management of the difficult airway. Anesthesiology. 1993;78:597–602.
5. Practice Guidelines for Management of the Difficult Airway. An Updated Report by the American Society of Anesthesiologists Task Force on Management of the Difficult Airway. Anesthesiology. 2003;98:1269–77.
6. El-Ganzouri AR, McCarthy RJ, Tuman KJ. Prospective airway assessment: predictive value of amultivariate risk index. Anesth Analg. 1996;82:1197–204.
7. Rose DK, Cohen MM. The airway: problems and predictions in18,500 patients. Can J Anaesth. 1994;41:372–83.
8. Asai T, Koga K, Vaughan RS. Respiratory complications associated with tracheal intubation and extubation. Br J Anaesth. 1998;80:767–75.
9. Yildiz TS, Korkmaz F, Solak M. Prediction of difficult tracheal intubation in Turkish patients: a multi-center methodological study. Eur J Anaesthesiol. 2007;24:1034–40.
10. Kheterpal S, Han R, Tremper K. Incidence and predictors of difficult and impossible mask ventilation. Anesthesiology. 2006;105:885–91.
11. Neligan P, Porter S, Max B. Obstructive sleep apnea is not a risk factor for difficult intubation in morbidly obese patients. Anesth Analg. 2009;109:1182–6.
12. Schmitt H, Buchfelder M, Radespiel-Trdger M. Difficult intubation in acromegalic patients. Incidence and predictability. Anesthesiology. 2000;93:110–4.
13. Amathieu R, Smail N, Catineau M. Difficult intubation in thyroid surgery: myth or reality? Anesth Analg. 2006;103:965–8.
14. Bouaggad A, Nejmi SE, Bouderka MA. Prediction of difficult tracheal intubation in thyroid surgery. Anesth Analg. 2004;99:603–6.
15. Voyagis GS, Kyriakos KP. The effect of goiter on endotracheal intubation. Anesth Analg. 1997;84:611–2.
16. Djabatey EA, Barclay PM. Difficult and failed intubation in 3430 obstetric general anaesthetics. Anaesthesia. 2009;64(11):1168–71.
17. McDonnell NJ, Paech MJ, Clavisi OM. Difficult and failed intubation in obstetric anaesthesia: an observational study of airway management and complications associated with general anaesthesia for caesarean section. Int J Obstet Anesth. 2008;17(4):292–7.
18. Boisson-Bertrand D, Bourgain JL, Camboulives J, et al. Intubation difficile Societefrancais d'anesthesieet de reanimation. Expertise collective. Annales Francaises D'Anesthesieet de Reanimation. 1996;15:207–14.
19. Diemunsch P, Langeron O, Richard M, Lenfant F. Prediction et definition de la ventilation au masque difficile et de l'intubationdifficile Question 1. Annales Francaises d'Anesthesie et de Reanimation 2008;27:3–14.
20. Langeron O, Bourgain J.-L, Laccoureye O, Legras A, Orliaguet G. Conference d'experts Strategies etalgorithmes de prise en charge d'unedifficultedecontrole des voiesaeriennes Question 5. Annales Francaisesd'Anesthesie et de Reanimation. 2008;27:41–5.
21. Crosby ET, Cooper RM, Douglas MJ, et al. The unanticipated difficult airway with recommendations for management. Can J Anaesth. 1998;45(7):757–76.
22. Frova G, Guarino A, Petrini F, et al. Recommendations for airway control and difficult airway management in paediatric patients. Minerva Anestesiol. 2006;72(9):723–48.
23. Braun U, Goldmann K, Hempel V, Krier C. Airway management. Leitlinie der deutschengesellschaft fur anasthesiologie und intensivmedizin. Anaesthesiol Intensivmed. 2004;45:302–6.
24. Henderson JJ, Popat MT, Latto IT, et al. Difficult Airway Society guidelines for management of the unanticipated difficult intubation. Anaesthesia. 2004;59:675–94.
25. Han R, Tremper KK, Kheterpal S, O'Reilly M. Grading scale for mask ventilation. Anesthesiology. 2004;101:267.

2

The Expected Difficult Airway

Satya Krishna Ramachandran and Sachin Kheterpal

S.K. Ramachandran (✉) • S. Kheterpal
Department of Anesthesiology, University of Michigan
Hospital System, 1500 East Medical Center Drive, Ann Arbor, MI 48109, USA
e-mail: rsatyak@med.umich.edu

D.B. Glick et al. (eds.), *The Difficult Airway: An Atlas of Tools and Techniques for Clinical Management*,
DOI 10.1007/978-0-387-92849-4_2, © Springer Science+Business Media New York 2013

Introduction

The primary purpose of airway management is to oxygenate the patient, as loss of the airway is associated with hypoxemia causing significant morbidity and mortality. Patients need successful airway management as part of a general anesthetic or for resuscitation when a patient is in extremis. Difficulty achieving satisfactory ventilation and oxygenation is a medical emergency, where prevention is better than the cure, and adverse outcomes follow rapidly with unprepared attempts by unskilled practitioners. Since the ASA closed claims studies[1], the critical importance of recognizing the difficult airway and preventing hypoxia has been a primary aspect of airway training. The advent of neuromuscular relaxants in the 1950s ushered in an era of tracheal intubation as this was considered the most effective way to ensure adequate ventilation during surgery. As a result, the vast majority of published literature looks at prediction of difficult tracheal intubation. However, mask ventilation is an equally critical component of successful airway management. Successful mask ventilation provides practitioners with a rescue technique during unsuccessful attempts at laryngoscopy and unanticipated difficult airway situations. Difficulty with both tracheal intubation and mask ventilation is associated with increased risk of patient injury. Several clinical models and tests have been described for the prediction of difficult intubation and mask ventilation. These screening tests use history elements and quantitative or estimated measures of various aspects of the face, upper airway, and neck to ascribe either high or low risk of an expected difficult airway. In order to better understand the performance and accuracy of these tests, a working understanding of the anatomy of the structures of interest is essential. A variety of systemic and local tissue factors impact the ease of tracheal intubation and mask ventilation. While the elective situation permits a rigorous examination of the airway, certain urgent and emergent clinical scenarios preclude a complete and thorough airway examination, making difficult airway situations more likely but less predictable. Irrespective of the urgency of airway instrumentation, clinical suspicion of a difficult airway helps prepare the practitioner for backup airway management strategies that often require additional personnel, equipment, and techniques for successful tracheal intubation. The purpose of this chapter is to describe the clinical features associated with the difficult airway and explore the clinical utility of these features on prediction of difficult mask ventilation and difficult tracheal intubation.

Anatomy of the Difficult Airway

The difficulty of achieving a patent airway varies with several anatomic factors related directly to the upper airway, and these anatomical features can be routinely assessed on patients prior to anesthesia. The upper airway refers to the air space including and above the laryngeal inlet. The upper airway is subdivided into the nasal and oral cavities that lead into the pharynx and down into the laryngeal inlet. The patency and function of these air spaces is maintained by a framework of bony skeleton and several muscles primarily innervated by the vagus, glossopharyngeal, and hypoglossal nerves.

An important contributory factor for upper airway closure relates to alterations in the volume of the tongue in comparison with the effective pharyngeal space. Anatomical factors that increase this incompatibility result in upper airway closure. Additionally, the sharp angle between the oral axis and the pharyngeal axis impacts the ability to visualize the larynx without adequate head extension. In order to better understand the individual components of anatomical variables of interest, these important primary mechanisms are explored in further detail below.

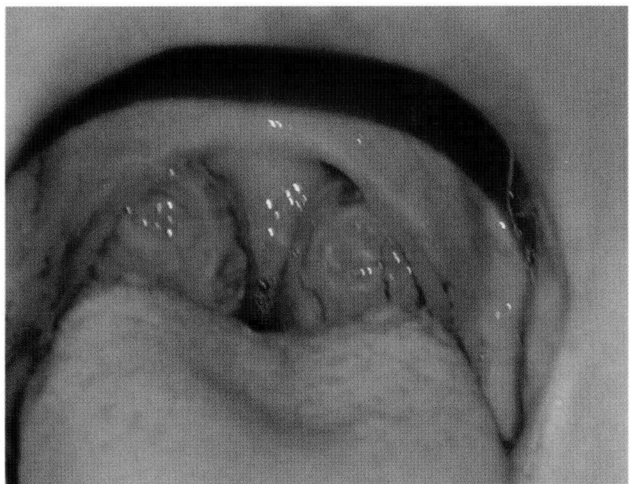

Figure 2.1. (Figs. 3.3.2 pg 129 from "Diagnosis in Otorhinolaryngology" by Matin Onerci) Patients with sleep apnea often present with tonsillar hypertrophy secondary to the increased upper airway fat deposition and Bernoulli effect.

Factors Affecting Tongue-Pharyngeal Volume Disproportion

The anatomical balance of soft tissue and bony framework of the upper airway is affected by conditions that increase tongue size, reduce pharyngeal size, or both. The tongue is attached to the mandible and the hyoid bone through various muscles, thereby limiting the space available for it to be compressed during laryngoscopy. Variations in tongue size are well described in the literature, especially in the presence of coexisting genetic disorders, developmental diseases, obesity and obstructive sleep apnea (OSA). Other congenital and acquired conditions that may result in glossopharyngeal disproportion include macroglossia resulting from hypothyroidism, Beckwith-Wiedemann Syndrome, acromegaly, amyloidosis, angioedema, anaphylaxis, prolonged Trendelenburg positioning, and trauma. The contribution of reduced pharyngeal volume is unclear in the general population, but immediately obvious in patients with upper airway edema, infection, and excessive adipose tissue. The impact of this imbalance on likelihood of airway closure has been explored in cephalometric studies of the upper airway[2]. Patients with OSA were shown to have significantly larger tongues than patients without the disease. The same study also confirmed a more caudal location of the larger tongue in OSA (Figures 2.1 and 2.2).

The contribution of physical forces driven by the Bernoulli Effect[3] on the progression of upper airway narrowing has also been established. Patients with OSA have redundant tissue in the upper airway secondary to the negative pressure caused by orifice flow during obstructive epochs in sleep. The net effect of increased upper airway soft tissue is that the forces that work to maintain airway patency fail during sleep and anesthesia, resulting in total airway collapse[4].

Factors Affecting Access to the Upper Airway

One of the important causes of a difficult airway relates to the physical inability to introduce a laryngoscope into the upper airway with sufficient clearance to allow oral or nasal manipulation of an endotracheal tube. When performing direct laryngoscopy, there must be room for the laryngoscope blade, the endotracheal tube as well as a direct line of sight. Thus, conditions that affect mouth opening all contribute to the difficult airway problem. In addition to fixed limitation of mouth opening, certain conditions such as mandibular trauma and upper airway infection can cause dynamic limitation of mouth opening, primarily related to pain (Figures 2.3 and 2.4).

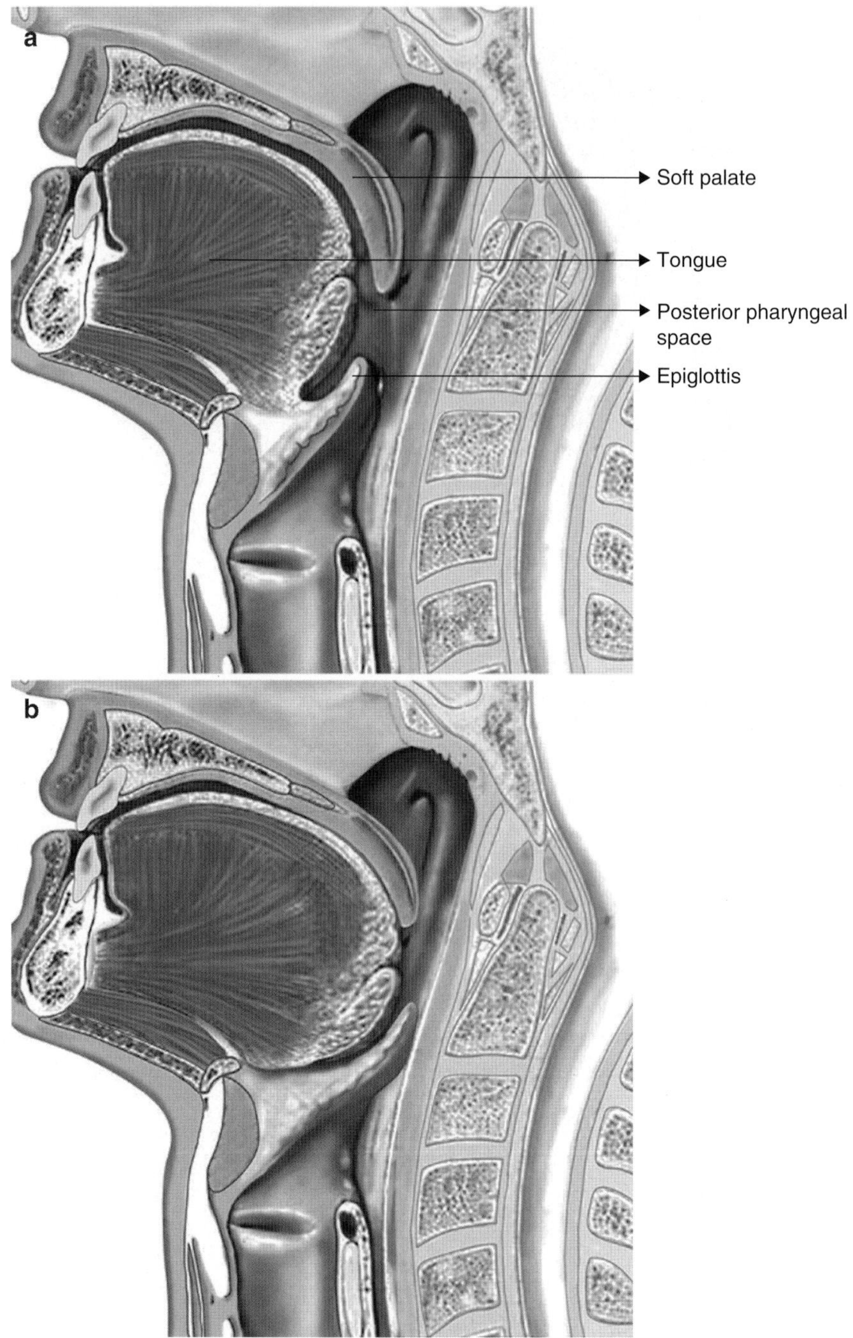

Figure 2.2. (Fig. 3.3.3 (a and b) pg 129 From "Diagnosis in Otorhinolaryngology" by Matin Onerci). Patients with obstructive sleep apnea (**b**) have significantly larger tongues than patients without the condition, predisposing them to airway obstruction.

Factors Affecting Laryngoscopic Visualization Vector

Although the concept of aligning the oropharyngeal axis with the direct laryngoscopy visualization axis is commonly promulgated during didactic airway sessions, this classical concept has not been supported by recent real-time magnetic resonance imagining of the airway. Nevertheless although the exact alignment of the axis is rarely achieved, optimizing the relationship between these axes remains a major goal of direct laryngoscopy. As a result, a focused analysis of the factors limiting this optimization is necessary during discussion of the expected difficult airway.

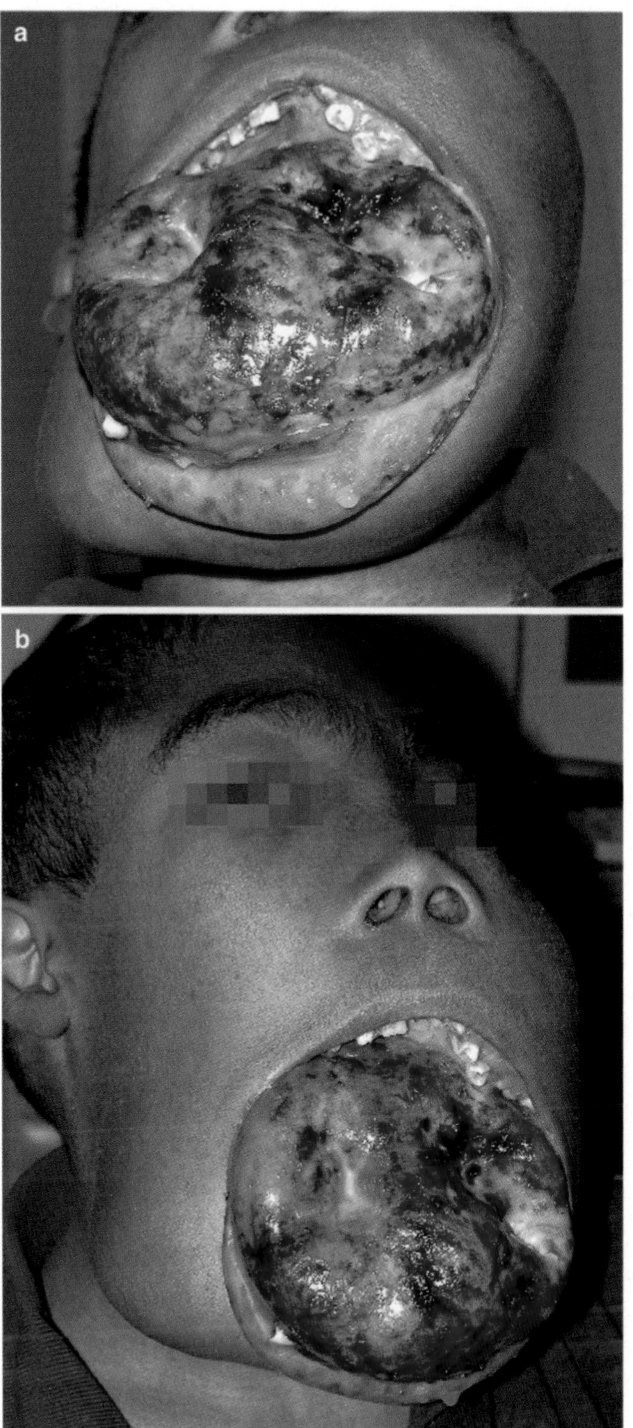

Figure 2.3. (Fig. 3.9.30 (b) pg 158 from "Diagnosis in Otorhinolaryngology" by Matin Onerci) Squamous cell carcinoma which fills the oral cavity and prevents access to the upper airway through the oral route.

Neck Mobility

Optimal laryngoscopic visualization of the larynx is critically dependent on the ability to align the oral and pharyngeal long axes (Fig. 2.5). A direct vector of sight would not be able to reach the larynx if neck mobility is restricted. Although classic teaching suggests

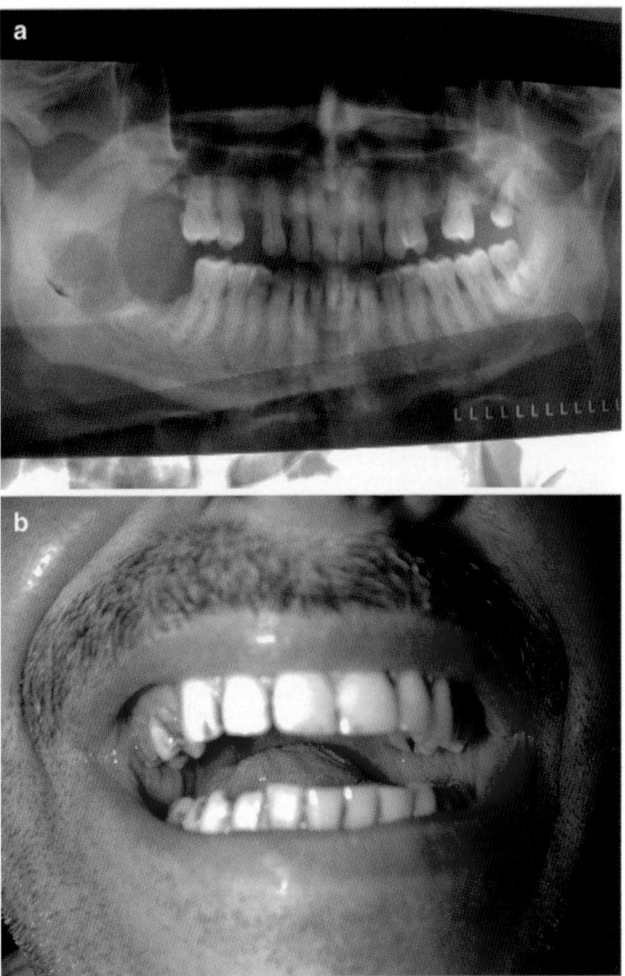

Figure 2.4. (Fig. 3.9.31 (a and b) pg 158 From "Diagnosis in Otorhinolaryngology" by Matin Onerci) (a) Squamous cell carcinoma of the retromolar trigone causing destruction of the mandible. (b) Invasion of the pterygoid muscles causes significant trismus, precluding traditional oral approach to tracheal intubation. Failure to detect this preoperatively could result in an airway emergency after induction of anesthesia.

that the sniffing position is required for optimal laryngoscopic visualization[5], recent literature shows that head extension is the more significant factor in the majority of patients[6,7], except in the presence of obesity, where the sniffing position is advantageous[4]. The caveats to this rule include presence of normal teeth, adequate submental space for tongue compression, normal glottic structure, and position of the larynx. Excessive laryngoscopic force in patients with reduced head extension causes the cervical spine to bow forward, directly pushing the glottis to a more anterior position which is out of reach of the laryngoscopic visualization vector[8].

Dental Factors

Size of the upper incisors has an increasing impact on the visualization vector with progressive limitation of neck mobility. Accordingly, absence of upper incisors permits a better laryngoscopic vector alignment and presence of long upper incisors adversely impacts ease of laryngoscopy and tracheal intubation. It is also important to note that partial loss of upper teeth could cause the laryngoscope blade to get "stuck" between teeth and impede vector alignment[9]. The impact of dental structure on mask ventilation is less clear. Previous studies have indicated that edentulous patients are associated with difficult

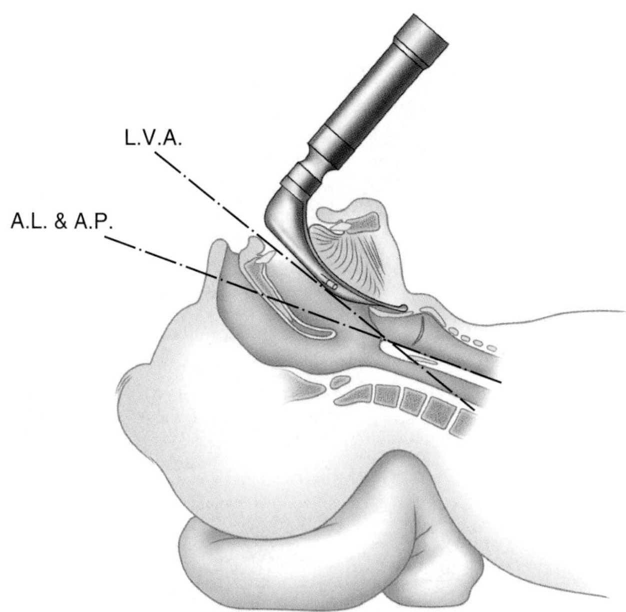

Figure 2.5. (Fig. 7.6 pg 188 From "Principles of airway management" by Finucane and Santora) For the larynoscopic visualization axis (LVA) to permit laryngeal visualization, appropriate positioning of the head and neck is essential. Inability to extend the neck will result in the divergence of line of sight from the laryngeal visualization vector and persistently poor views. Failure to detect limited head extension is commonly associated with difficult intubations.

mask ventilation, but edentulous state was not an independent predictor of difficult or impossible mask ventilation in the largest studies to date[10,11]. Dentures may help maintain upper airway structure and permit a tighter mask fit, but expert opinion on retaining dentures during airway management is unclear.

Submental Factors

The bony cage that makes up the framework of the upper airway is formed by the maxilla, mandible, hard palate forming the "roof," and the cervical vertebral column at the back. Conditions that reduce the anteroposterior distance of the mid-face, mandibular length, and position of the hyoid bone all adversely impact the ease of mask ventilation and tracheal intubation. The floor of the upper airway is formed by soft tissue that is bounded anteriorly and laterally by the mandibular edges and the hyoid bone posteriorly. This virtual space, often referred to as the submentum or the submental space, is of crucial importance to the success or failure of laryngoscopy. The tongue is attached to the mandible and the hyoid bone through upper airway muscles, primarily the genioglossus, the hyoglossus, and the mylohyoid. The mylohyoid extends like a diaphragm across the floor of the submental space. This places a finite limitation to the volume of tongue that can be displaced during laryngoscopy. Tongue volumes in excess of the critical capacity of the submental space influence the laryngoscopic view. Similarly, disease states that reduce the compliance of the submental tissues namely scarring from surgery, burns, or radiation therapy will also impact laryngoscopic view. Correct positioning of the laryngoscopic blade tip in the fold between the tongue and the epiglottis causes the epiglottis to fold upward, bringing the larynx into view. Factors that may interfere with correct placement of the laryngoscope blade include vallecular cysts and lingual tonsillar hypertrophy. The forces that are exerted by the tip of the laryngoscope in this position pull the glosso-epiglottic ligament [12] and cause the hyoid bone to tilt forward. The hyoid bone has ligamentous attachment to the epiglottis, and this forward tilting movement causes the epiglottis to tilt up, opening up the glottic inlet.

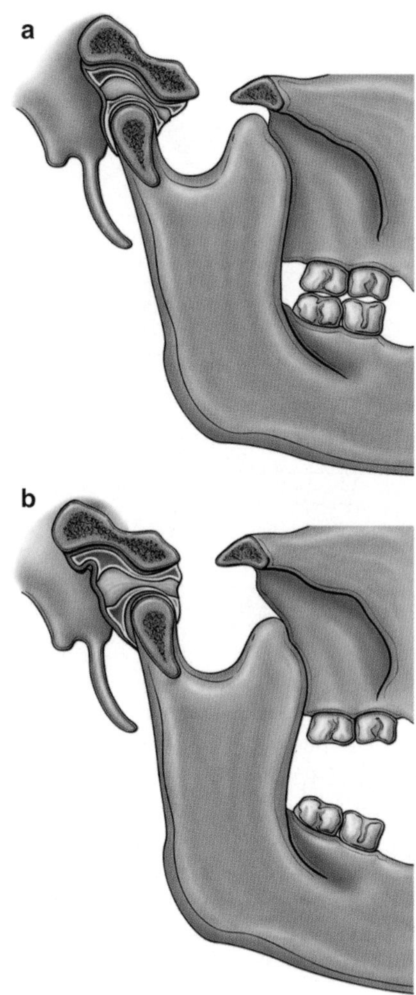

Figure 2.6. (Fig. 5.3 pg 135 From "Principles of airway management" by Finucane and Santora) Temporo-mandibular joint in closed (**a**) and open (**b**) positions. Note the forward sliding and rotation of the mandibular condyle.

The mechanics of the hyoid bone are uniquely different in patients with difficult airways. This was demonstrated in a study where lateral radiography was performed during laryngoscopy in patients with a history of failed tracheal intubation[13]. In these patients the blade tip failed to make contact with the hyoid and instead, the tongue was compressed into a pear shape. This pear-shaped deformity of the tongue pressed down the epiglottis and forced the hyoid to tilt in the opposite direction, with resultant downward folding of the epiglottis onto the posterior pharyngeal wall. This mechanism was confirmed in a subsequent mathematical modeling of osseous factors in difficult intubation[14]. The net effect of this scenario is a persistent epiglottic view on laryngoscopy, because the effective submental volume is critically smaller than the minimum volume displacement of tongue needed to optimally position the laryngoscope tip. Straight laryngoscope blades with smaller displacement volumes than the curved blade offer better laryngeal views based on this mechanistic explanation. The same factors come into play with significant upper incisor overbite, where the effect of a relatively anterior maxilla mimics the effect of a recessed mandible.

Mandibular Subluxation

The process of jaw-thrust causes the mandible to slide forward out of the mandibular socket, resulting in the forward displacement of the tongue and attached submental tissues (Figure 2.6). Disease states associated with a reduction in this mobility have been shown

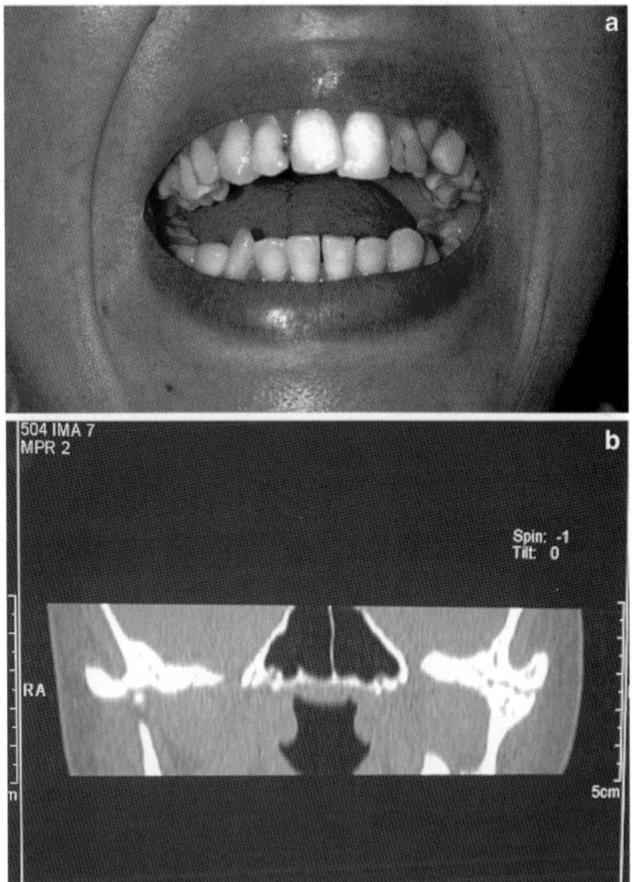

Figure 2.7. (Figs. 3.4.6 (a and b) pg 133 From "Diagnosis in Otorhinolaryngology" by Matin Onerci) Impact of diseased temporomandibular joint on mouth opening. Here *left sided* TMJ ankylosis seen on the coronal CT causes severe trismus and impossible laryngoscopy.

to be associated with difficult mask ventilation and tracheal intubation (Figure 2.7). This component of the laryngoscopic visualization vector has been historically underappreciated and understudied.

Factors Affecting Laryngeal Structures

Successful tracheal intubation is also dependent on the size of the glottic opening and subglottic structures. Fixed or dynamic abnormalities of the laryngeal structures prevent successful tracheal intubation, even in the presence of optimal laryngoscope vector visualization. Several acute and chronic conditions affect laryngeal, subglottic, and tracheal caliber. These conditions typically are associated with clinical signs such as stridor and increasing levels of distress with increasing degrees of airway narrowing.

Anatomy and Physiology of the Compromised and Critical Airway

One way to describe airway narrowing is as follows: occult airway narrowing, stable critically narrowed airway, and compromised airway. Both the latter conditions are associated with a significant risk of difficult mask ventilation, failed tracheal intubation, and the eventual need for surgical airway. Subclinical airway narrowing refers to occult diseases affecting airway caliber with no accompanying signs or symptoms. There is no way to identify these patients prior to laryngoscopy using standard airway physical exam elements. A high index

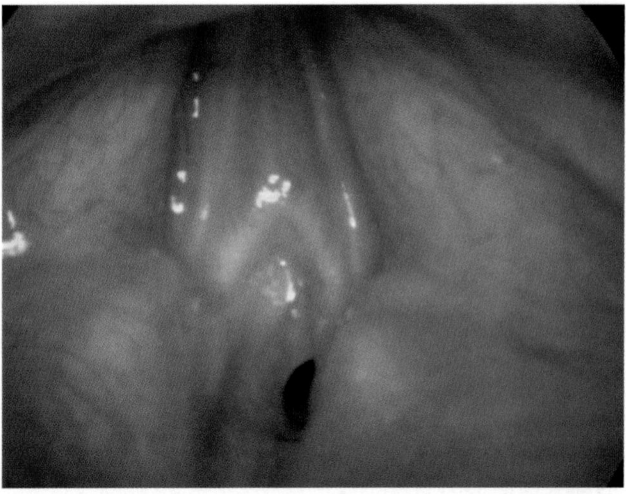

Figure 2.8. (Figs. 3.5.3 pg 135 From "Diagnosis in Otorhinolaryngology" by Matin Onerci) Laryngeal web almost completely occluding the airway. As a rule, presence of hoarseness, stridor, or respiratory distress should alert anesthesiologists to the need for rapid airway management. Such airway pathology requires a great deal of skill as repeated manipulation of the airway could convert a stable airway narrowing to a compromised airway situation.

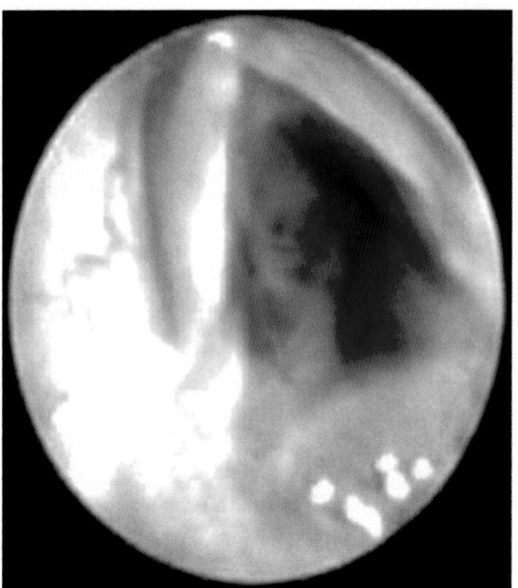

Figure 2.9. (Fig. 3.5.4 pg 135; From "Diagnosis in Otorhinolaryngology" by Matin Onerci) Subglottic hemangiomas are the most common congenital tumors causing stridor. They are generally asymptomatic at birth and may become symptomatic later in life.

of suspicion should be used in certain syndromes and disease conditions that predispose to airway narrowing such as thyroid or anterior mediastinal masses. The stable critically narrowed airway refers to the presence of stridor in the absence of respiratory failure or hypoxia. The implication here is that there is sufficient time to assess the airway thoroughly and plan for successful tracheal intubation, with contingency plans in the event the primary technique fails. However, the margin for error in this class is significantly lower than the subclinical airway narrowing group. The compromised airway refers to stridor in the presence of accompanying respiratory distress or hypoxia. The presence of stridor in an acute setting should alert the practitioner to the presence of a difficult airway, with high likelihood of rapid progression to acute respiratory compromise (Figures 2.8, 2.9, and 2.10).

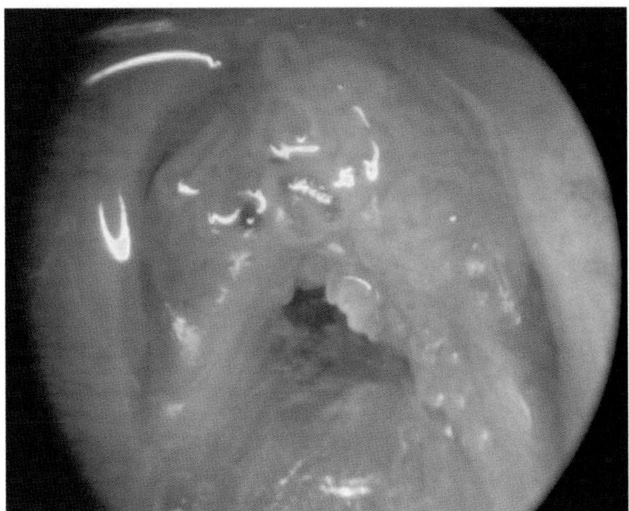

Figure 2.10. (Fig. 3.5.11 pg 136 From "Diagnosis in Otorhinolaryngology" by Matin Onerci) Juvenile laryngeal papillomatosis is the most common benign tumor of the larynx. Patients with this diagnosis often present with increasing degree of stridor and they should be managed with caution.

The upper airway caliber has a great impact on work of breathing as defined by the gas flow equation (for laminar flow [3]):

$$\text{Flow}\,\alpha = \frac{\text{Radius}^4 \times \text{Pressure differential across obstruction}}{\text{Viscosity of inspired air} \times \text{length of upper airway}}$$

Two important clinical implications exist for this equation. Flow is proportional to the fourth power of the radius measured at the narrowest point of the airway. As a result of this fourth power, when the airway caliber is doubled, the flow increases by 16 times and more importantly, when the airway caliber is halved, the flow decreases by 16 times. Thus the pressure differential needed to maintain adequate airflow in the presence of airway narrowing is significantly greater, causing a huge burden on the respiratory muscles. Often, in the presence of chronic airway narrowing, compensatory mechanisms develop resulting in an altered pattern of ventilation with minimum acceptable utilization of respiratory muscle strength. However, this scenario is altered in the presence of acute decompensation. Stridor is associated with turbulent flow[3], where the influence of reduced airway caliber on flow and work of breathing is further exaggerated compared to laminar flow. Turbulent flows need significantly greater pressure differential and increased respiratory effort to achieve satisfactory flow rates. As a result, this is associated with significantly reduced time to secure the airway, introducing an additional time constraint to the difficult airway management and increasing the need for expert airway management.

Clinical Assessment of the Airway

Clinical prediction of the difficult airway follows detailed review of pertinent history, general physical examination, and specific airway-related assessment. The clinical conditions associated with difficult airway can be classified loosely into congenital diseases, traumatic conditions, systemic diseases, airway tumors, and upper airway infections.

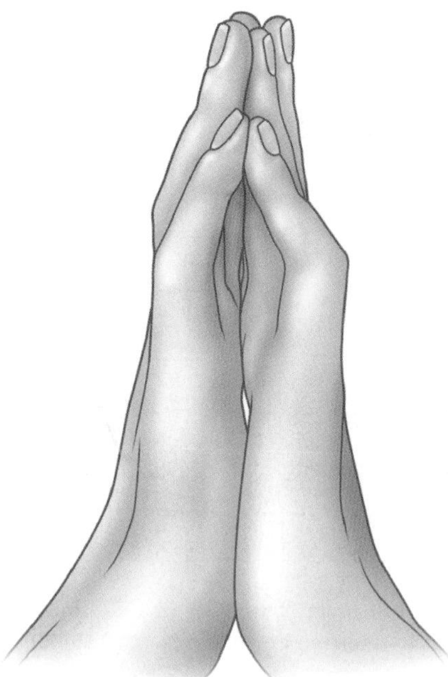

Figure 2.11. (Fig. 5.1 pg 132 From "Principles of airway management" by Finucane and Santora) Prayer sign—inability to oppose palms due to progressive stiffening of the joints caused by diabetes mellitus. It is estimated that about a third of long-term early onset diabetics develop stiff joint syndrome, and its presence is an extremely accurate predictor of difficult airway.

Systemic Conditions

Pregnancy

Pregnancy is associated with increased risk of difficult mask ventilation, difficult intubation, and rapid progression of hypoxemia[15]. Recent research shows that labor is associated with dynamic increases in Mallampati class, secondary to upper airway edema that settles over time after labor[16]. Rocke and colleagues[9] identified difficult intubation in 7.9 % of pregnant patients. Associated features for difficult intubation in pregnancy are pre/eclampsia, short neck, obesity, absent or excessively large maxillary incisors, and receding mandible.

Diabetes Mellitus

The association between diabetes and difficult airway relates to the glycosylation of joints and development of stiff joint syndrome[17]. The primary joints affected in patients with difficult laryngoscopy are the TMJ and the cervical spine, presenting limitation of mouth opening, mandibular subluxation, and head extension. The two tests described to identify stiff joint syndrome are the palm print test[18] and the prayer sign[19]. The former tests the ability to make full contact with a flat surface, and increasing risk of difficult airway is seen with decreasing surface contact. The prayer sign refers to the ability to place the palms together "in prayer," with diabetic stiff joint patients having progressive difficulty to achieve this (Figure 2.11). It is estimated that about a third of long-term early onset diabetics develop stiff joint syndrome[20], and its presence is an extremely accurate predictor of difficult airway[19].

Rheumatoid Arthritis

This is one of the more common autoimmune conditions with unique implications for airway management. Severe joint involvement of the TMJ, cervical spine, and extremities directly impacts access to the airway, visualization vector, and mandibular subluxation. The more important implication is cervical spine instability. Symptoms suggestive of nerve root or spinal cord compression, and limitation of neck movement should alert the practitioner to the risk of permanent neurological injury with direct laryngoscopy and intubation, although this is an extremely rarely reported outcome. Hoarseness, dysphonia, or stridor could suggest significant laryngeal distortion from joint involvement[21,22], and awake flexible bronchoscopic techniques or a surgical airway may be preferable in these cases.

Trauma

Trauma to the head and neck impacts the airway[23] typically due to direct injury with attendant airway distortion, bleeding, trismus, and airway edema. Stridor, inability to speak, laryngeal cartilage fracture, or neck emphysema suggests airway disruption and signals the emergent need for airway management by practitioners experienced in bronchoscopy and tracheotomy. Blind endotracheal intubation is likely to produce a catastrophic loss of airway with high risk of patient death in this clinical scenario. Injury precautions for the cervical spine are a mechanical impediment to achieving a satisfactory laryngoscopic visualization vector and may impair mouth opening. In the presence of known cervical spine injury, the force of laryngoscopy can worsen compression of the spinal cord and affect neurological outcome, by causing anterior bowing[8] and displacement of the mid-lower cervical vertebrae[24, 25].

Burns

Acute head and neck burns, exposure to explosions or fires in enclosed spaces, and airway burns are associated with difficult airway[26]. The mechanisms include airway edema secondary to thermal injury and tracheobronchial disruption from shock waves related to explosions. Difficult intubation is seen in patients with significant tongue edema and submental edema. Presence of hoarse voice, oral burns, singed nasal hairs, noncompliant submental tissues, and facial swelling should alert the practitioner to potentially difficult intubation, and emergent flexible bronchoscopic intubation should be performed where feasible[27]. Chronic anterior head and neck scarring from thermal and chemical burns produces extreme difficulty with the airway, through limitation in neck mobility and mouth opening. Chemical ingestion causes significant distortion of the upper airway, making identification of the glottic inlet impossible using conventional laryngoscopy in many patients, with false passages and grossly narrowed airway caliber[28].

Airway Tumors

Tumors developing from and close to the upper and lower airway present independent challenges to airway management[29]. Tumors within the airway lumen include oral cancers, laryngeal tumors, and bronchogenic carcinoma. Oral cancers can increase tongue volume or reduce pharyngeal and submental compliance, or affect mouth opening[30] (Figure 2.12). Laryngeal tumors predispose to sudden loss of airway and often present physical impediments to passage of endotracheal tubes[31]. Bronchogenic carcinoma produces significant airway narrowing and distortion. All these conditions are easily traumatized, causing bleeding into the airway.

Extrathoracic tumors that lie outside the lumen of the airway influence airway management in one of several ways[32–34]. Large goiters produce significant physical impediment to laryngoscopy and are associated with airway compression secondary to erosion of tracheal rings[35] (Figure 2.13). Anaplastic thyroid carcinoma has been known to erode the tracheal wall and cause airway collapse, distortion, or bleeding though this is very uncommon[36]. Thyroid masses are a physical impediment to successful surgical airway access. Life-threatening hemorrhage has followed thyroid injury during attempted tracheotomy.

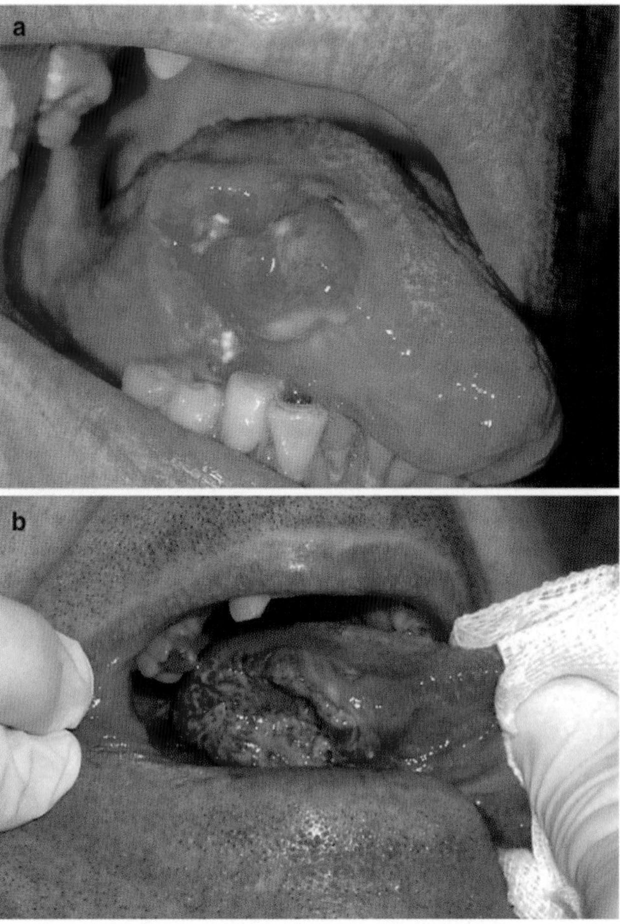

Figure 2.12. (Figs. 3.9.27 -a and b- pg 157; From "Diagnosis in Otorhinolaryngology" by Matin Onerci) Squamous cell carcinoma of the tongue causes swelling and induration, thereby reducing tongue and submental tissue compliance. Inability to compress the tongue into the submental space results in difficult laryngoscopy.

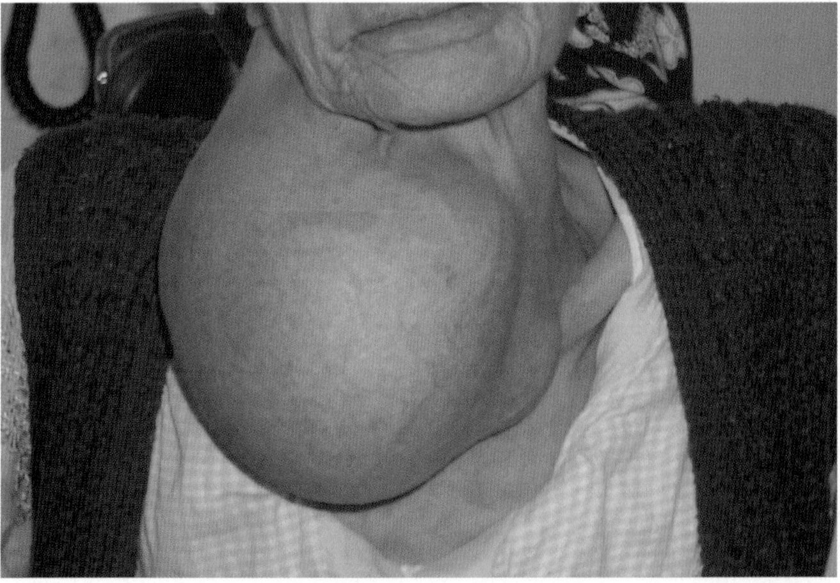

Figure 2.13. (Fig. 3.10.13- pg 167; From "Diagnosis in Otorhinolaryngology" by Matin Onerci) Anaplastic thyroid carcinoma. Long-standing goiters cause distortion of the trachea and tracheomalacia. Symptoms of airway obstruction in supine position should increase suspicion of tracheomalacia.

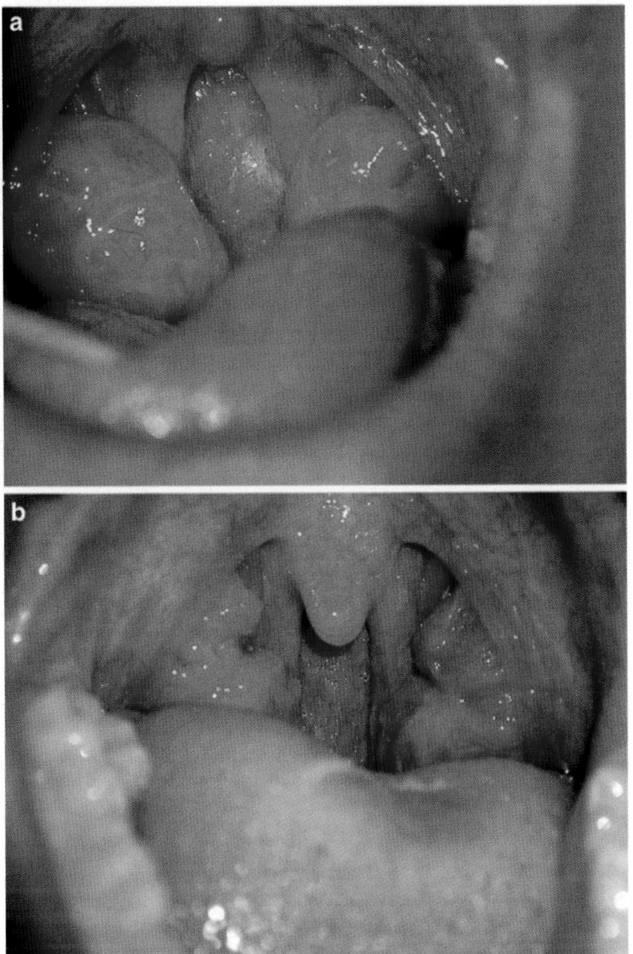

Figure 2.14. (3.1.6-a pg 124; From "Diagnosis in Otorhinolaryngology" by Matin Onerci) Chronic tonsillitis predisposes to tonsillar abscess formation. Such upper airway infections have the potential to result in rapid loss of airway under anesthesia.

Intrathoracic tumors related to the airway present several problems. Patients with these tumors can exhibit positional or dynamic airway obstruction. Superior vena cava syndrome can significantly impact the airway management[37]. Superior vena cava syndrome is associated with head and neck plethora, increased airway edema, and a risk of airway collapse. The loss of airway tone related to loss of consciousness in these patients is due to intrathoracic airway compression. Tracheal intubation may not be adequate to ventilate the patient due to the loss of airway patency distal to the endotracheal tube.

Upper Airway Infections

Infections related to the tonsils, teeth, epiglottis, and retropharyngeal tissues cause distortion of airway, reduced submental compliance, and increase risk of airway soiling due to accidental abscess rupture with instrumentation. Quincy or tonsillar abscesses are rare but significant causes of airway loss under sedation or anesthesia[38, 39] (Figure 2.14). Ludwig's angina refers to the multiplane infection of the submental tissues usually caused by molar root infection, resulting in brawny induration (Figure 2.15). Retropharyngeal abscess causes difficulty swallowing and typically presents with drooling, odynophagia, and significant airway narrowing secondary to posterior pharyngeal wall edema and abscess. All these conditions have significant risks of failed mask ventilation and difficult or

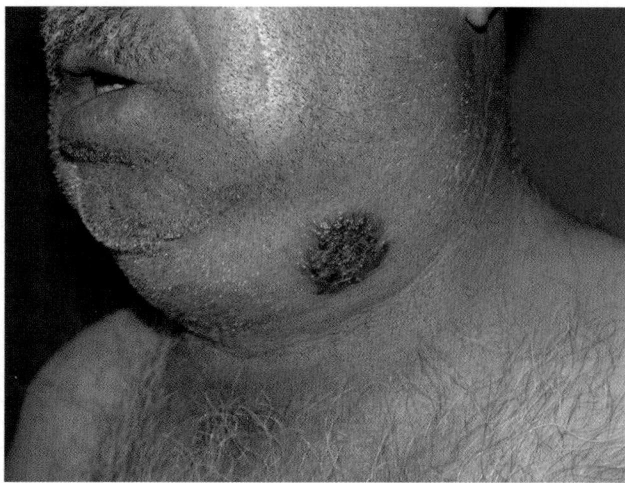

Figure 2.15. (3.10.12 - pg 166; From "Diagnosis in Otorhinolaryngology" by Matin Onerci) Deep neck space infection, commonly related to dental sepsis. The loss of submental tissue compliance coupled with increase in peri-airway soft tissue results in difficult airway. It is essential that a clear airway management plan and back-up plans are made in conjunction with ENT surgeons.

impossible intubation. Cautious flexible bronchoscopic or surgical airway access should be performed by experienced practitioners. While recognition of these conditions should prompt a high-index of suspicion that airway difficulties are highly probable, lingual tonsillar hyperplasia may be entirely occult and associated with difficult mask ventilation and laryngoscopic intubation[40].

Specific Airway Assessment

In this section we will look at some of the commonly used upper airway measurements and qualitative assessments.

Measures of Tongue-Pharyngeal Volume Disproportion

Modified Mallampati Test

The modified Mallampati classification[41] correlates tongue size to pharyngeal size. This test is performed with the patient in the sitting position, head in a neutral position, the mouth wide open, and the tongue protruding to its maximum. Patient should not be actively encouraged to phonate as it can result in contraction and elevation of the soft palate leading to a marked improvement in the Mallampati class. Classification is assigned according to the extent the base of tongue masks the visibility of pharyngeal structures (Figure 2.16):

Class I: Visualization of soft palate and uvula
Class II: Visualization of the soft palate and tonsillar pillars
Class III: Visualization of only the soft palate
Class IV: Visualization of only hard palate (this class is the additional modification by Samsoon to the original Mallampati classification[42])

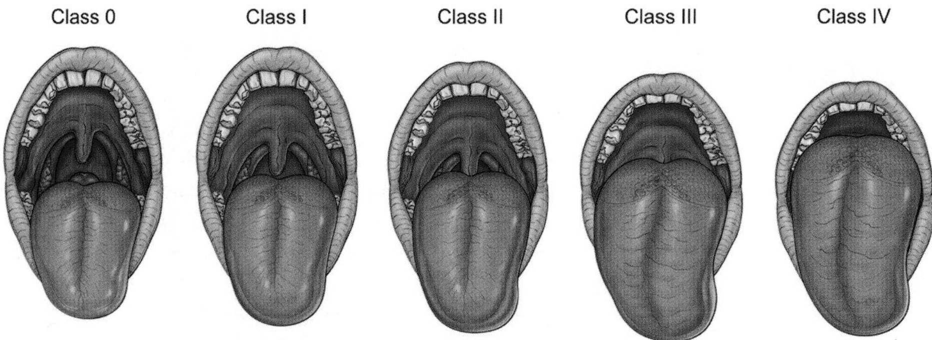

Figure 2.16. Modified Mallampati test. From Finucane, B.T., Tsui, B.C.H, and Santora, A.H., Principles of Airway Management, 4th ed., New York: Springer, 2010.

Extended Mallampati Score

The predictive value of the modified Mallampati class is improved when the patient's craniocervical junction is extended rather than neutral (Extended Mallampati Score) [43,44]. Compared to the modified Mallampati class and other tests, an extended Mallampati score class of 3 or 4 and a diagnosis of diabetes mellitus were the only statistically significant predictors of difficult laryngoscopy in the morbidly obese[43].

Measures of Laryngoscopic Visualization Vector

Neck Mobility

Head extension is measured or estimated with the patient sitting from the neutral head position. The examiner estimates the angle traversed by the occlusal surface of upper teeth with maximal head extension[5]. It is important to note that the movement of interest is at the head level, and shoulder movement should be discouraged as this will mask underlying limitation of head extension. Measurement can be by simple visual estimate or more accurately with a goniometer. Significant limitation defined as ≤20° movement from the neutral position or <80° of maximum extension from the fully flexed position.

Submental Space: Thyromental Distance

Thyromental distance is defined as the distance from the mentum to the thyroid notch with the patient's neck is fully extended. Reduced thyromental distance is <3 finger breadths or <6 cm in adults. Alternatively, the mentohyoid distance (mandibular length from mentum to hyoid with patient in full head extension) has been used to quantify the submental space with <4 cm suggesting reduced distance.

Mouth Opening

Reduced mouth opening is measured as less than 4 cm or two adult finger breadths between the incisors.

Mandibular Protrusion

This test is performed by asking the patient to protrude the lower jaw maximally forward to bite the upper lip[45]. The inability to achieve a more forward position of the lower incisors in relation to the upper incisors is a significant finding suggestive of significant maxillary overbite, recessed mandible, or poor subluxation at the TMJ.

Other Airway-Related Tests

Neck Circumference

Neck circumference >43 cm at the laryngeal cartilage level has been described for prediction of difficult intubation[46]. However, qualitatively assessed thick neck is sufficient to ascribe increased risk of airway closure during mask ventilation[10,11]. No difference has been described between muscular necks and excessive fat deposition in the neck region as both increase the weight on the upper airway predisposing to loss of patency in sleep and unconsciousness.

Beard

The presence of a beard increases the risk of difficult mask ventilation[10, 11]. In addition to the fact that this is a male phenomenon, the increased levels of testosterone predispose to upper airway collapse and OSA. Beards impede a quality seal of the face mask and may conceal a retrognathic mandible resulting in an unanticipated difficult intubation.

Clinical Prediction of the Difficult Airway

Clinical Prediction of Difficult Intubation

Difficult tracheal intubation is a relatively rare event with an incidence ranging from 1 to 3 % due to the varying definitions used[11, 47] though the inability to visualize the larynx by direct laryngoscopy may in fact be encountered in nearly 6 % of adults[48]. As a result, clinical prediction models for difficult intubation suffer from lack of positive predictive value. Most clinical prediction models described in the literature describe difficult laryngoscopy based on Cormack and Lehane[49] laryngoscopy views. This is technically different from difficult intubation, although grade III and IV views are associated with difficult intubation. In practice, difficulty in maneuvering the endotracheal tube in place is seen in some cases with grade II views. The presence of risk factors for difficult tracheal intubation and mask ventilation should alert the practitioner to the potential need for flexible endoscopic techniques to secure the airway or surgical airway access.

El-Ganzouri Multivariable Prediction of Difficult Laryngoscopy

El-Ganzouri and colleagues[50] identified seven independent predictors of difficult intubation namely reduced mouth opening, reduced thyromental distance, Mallampati class 3 (using the unmodified Mallampati scale), reduced neck mobility, inability to prognath, body weight >110 kg, and history of difficult tracheal intubation. The sensitivity was extremely low for individual test components. In other words, there were significantly greater numbers of false negatives compared to true positives. Thus each component had limited or no value individually for prediction of difficult airway. Combining two or more predictors in a simplified airway risk index reduced the false negative, rate significantly, and presence of four or more risk factors reduced the false positive rate to acceptable values. The small numbers of patients with difficult intubation and difficult mask ventilation potentially confound the robustness of the simplified airway risk index.

Rose and Cohen Clinical Predictors

The authors found that univariate risk factors for difficult tracheal intubation were male gender, age from 40 to 59 years, and obesity[51]. Clinical characteristics associated with difficult intubation by direct laryngoscopy were decreased mouth opening (relative risk, 10.3); shortened thyromental distance (relative risk, 9.7); poor visualization of the hypopharynx (relative risk, 4.5); and limited neck extension (relative risk, 3.2). Presence of any two of these characteristics (relative risk, 7.6), and more than two of these characteristics (relative risk, 9.4) increased the risk of difficult tracheal intubation. No summary measures of accuracy were described for the prediction of difficult intubation by direct laryngoscopy based on these risk factors.

Clinical Prediction of Difficult Mask Ventilation

Difficult Mask Ventilation

A range of definitions of difficult mask ventilation have been used in the literature, resulting in an incidence ranging from 1.5 to 5 %. Several studies have noted that obesity, presence of a beard, and advanced age are independent predictors of difficult mask ventilation. Although initial work by Langeron et al. identified edentulous dentition as an independent predictor of difficult mask ventilation, a more strict definition of difficult mask ventilation did not confirm the lack of teeth as a predictor. Of note, limited mandibular subluxation identified by an abnormal jaw protrusion test was identified as an important predictor of difficult mask ventilation in a study of more than 15,000 mask ventilation attempts.

Impossible Mask Ventilation

Impossible mask ventilation defined as the inability to exchange air during bag-mask ventilation attempts despite multiple providers, airway adjuvants, or neuromuscular blockade is a very rare event, with an estimated incidence of 0.15 %[11]. Neck radiation changes, male gender, sleep apnea, modified Mallampati class III or IV, and presence of a beard were identified as independent predictors of impossible mask ventilation. The caveats to this study include the presence of an active decision process to perform awake fiberoptic intubation in a significant number of patients, and as such the results represent the prediction of unanticipated impossible mask ventilation.

Difficult Mask Ventilation Combined with Difficult Intubation

The prediction of difficult mask ventilation or difficult direct laryngoscopy may be dismissed by some as an academic activity given the low positive predictive value of most indices. More importantly, predicting either airway outcome—mask ventilation or intubation—as a stand-alone entity does not reflect the primary goal of airway management, namely establishing a sustainable means of oxygenation and ventilation. Ostensibly, some patients that are difficult to intubate may be easily mask ventilated while those that are difficult to mask ventilate may be easily intubated. Clinical factors predictive of difficult mask ventilation combined with difficult intubation should be the foundation of an outcome-driven airway exam. The largest published series of difficult mask ventilation combined with difficult intubation events identified an incidence of 0.37 %. Limited jaw protrusion, obese neck anatomy, sleep apnea, snoring, and obesity were statistically significant predictors in a multivariate model.

Clinical Prediction of Need for Awake Surgical Airway

No studies have been performed to predict the need for or difficulty performing an awake surgical airway. Local practices affect rates of awake surgical airway, but by all published evidence, this is an extremely uncommon method of securing the airway in the absence of imminent airway obstruction. Gillespie and colleagues reviewed the indications and outcomes of emergent awake tracheotomy and cricothyroidotomy with failed mask ventilation or tracheal intubation[52]. The underlying medical conditions that resulted in the need for emergency airway management included cardiac or pulmonary arrest in 13 patients (37 %), head and neck cancer in 12 patients (34 %), and trauma in 10 patients (29 %). The following causes were identified: upper airway edema (40 %), difficult anatomy with inability to visualize the vocal cords (23 %), obstructing mass lesion of the oropharynx or larynx (20 %), or maxillofacial or neck trauma (17 %). In another study[53], the majority of patients presented with hoarseness, dyspnea, and stridor, underlining the importance of these findings in the emergent setting. Altman and colleagues[54] reviewed awake tracheotomies in another study and identified dyspnea in 50 %, dysphagia (75 %), odynophagia (22 %), hoarseness or voice change (56 %), and stridor (43 %) as the common presenting features in patients. In this study, 80 % of patients had aero-digestive cancer or neck tumors with direct compression of the airway.

Summary

Clinical screening for the difficult airway can be achieved by performing a series of simple tests that assess the tongue-pharyngeal volume disproportion, access to the airway, laryngoscopic visualization vector, and laryngeal anatomy. Attention to detail is critical to preventing false negative, and preempting a clinical situation resulting in hypoxemia should be the goal of airway management in the elective, urgent, and emergent scenarios. As a dictum in all cases, airway instrumentation should be preceded by primary and backup plans. The presence of two or more risk factors for difficult mask ventilation or difficult intubation should alert the practitioner to consider awake (endoscopic) intubation of the trachea. Finally, safe airway management especially in the compromised airway requires considerable expertise, and sufficient efforts to ensure that trained staff and equipment are available at all times is essential to preventing morbidity and mortality related to inability to secure the airway.

References

1. Caplan RA, Posner KL, Ward RJ, Cheney FW. Adverse respiratory events in anesthesia: a closed claims analysis. Anesthesiology. 1990;72:828–33.
2. Tsuiki SDDS, Isono SMD, Ishikawa TMD, Yamashiro YMD, Tatsumi KMD, Nishino TMD. Anatomical balance of the upper airway and obstructive sleep apnea. Anesthesiology. 2008;108:1009–15.
3. O'Grady K, Doyle DJ, Irish J, Gullane P. Biophysics of airflow within the airway: a review. J Otolaryngol. 1997;26:123–8.
4. Benumof JL. Obstructive sleep apnea in the adult obese patient: implications for airway management. Anesthesiol Clin North America. 2002;20:789–811.
5. Biebuyck JF, Benumof JL. Management of the difficult adult airway with special emphasis on awake tracheal intubation. Anesthesiology. 1991;75:1087–110.
6. Adnet F, Borron SW, Dumas JL, Lapostolle F, Cupa M, Lapandry C. Study of the "sniffing position" by magnetic resonance imaging. Anesthesiology. 2001;94:83–6.
7. Adnet F, Baillard C, Borron SW, Denantes C, Lefebvre L, Galinski M, et al. Randomized study comparing the "sniffing position" with simple head extension for laryngoscopic view in elective surgery patients. Anesthesiology. 2001;95:836–41.
8. Nichol HC, Zuck D. Difficult laryngoscopy—the "anterior" larynx and the atlanto-occipital gap. Br J Anaesth. 1983;55:141–4.
9. Rocke DA, Murray WB, Rout CC, Gouws E. Relative risk analysis of factors associated with difficult intubation in obstetric anesthesia. Anesthesiology. 1992;77:67–73.
10. Kheterpal S, Han R, Tremper KK, Shanks A, Tait AR, O'Reilly M, et al. Incidence and predictors of difficult and impossible mask ventilation. Anesthesiology. 2006;105:885–91.

11. Kheterpal S, Martin L, Shanks AM, Tremper KK. Prediction and outcomes of impossible mask ventilation: a review of 50,000 anesthetics. Anesthesiology. 2009;110:891–7.
12. Brown AC, Norton ML. Instrumentation and equipment for management of the difficult airway, atlas of the difficult airway. In: Norton ML, Brown AC, editors. St. Louis, MO: Mosby-Year Book; 1991.
13. Fahy L, Horton WA, Charters P. Factor analysis in patients with a history of failed tracheal intubation during pregnancy. Br J Anaesth. 1990;65:813–5.
14. Charters P. Analysis of mathematical model for osseous factors in difficult intubation. Can J Anaesth. 1994;41:594–602.
15. Barash PG, Cullen BF, Stoelting RK. Clinical anesthesia. 5th ed. Lippincott Williams & Wilkins: Philadelphia; 2006.
16. Kodali BS, Chandrasekhar S, Bulich LN, Topulos GP, Datta S. Airway changes during labor and delivery. Anesthesiology. 2008;108:357–62.
17. Salzarulo HH, Taylor LA. Diabetic "stiff joint syndrome" as a cause of difficult endotracheal intubation. Anesthesiology. 1986;64:366–8.
18. Nadal JL, Fernandez BG, Escobar IC, Black M, Rosenblatt WH. The palm print as a sensitive predictor of difficult laryngoscopy in diabetics. Acta Anaesthesiol Scand. 1998;42:199–203.
19. Reissell E, Orko R, Maunuksela EL, Lindgren L. Predictability of difficult laryngoscopy in patients with long-term diabetes mellitus. Anaesthesia. 1990;45:1024–7.
20. Buckingham B, Perejda AJ, Sandborg C, Kershnar AK, Uitto J. Skin, joint, and pulmonary changes in type I diabetes mellitus. Am J Dis Child. 1986;140:420–3.
21. Absalom AR, Watts R, Kong A. Airway obstruction caused by rheumatoid cricoarytenoid arthritis. Lancet. 1998;351:1099–100.
22. McGeehan DF, Crinnion JN, Strachan DR. Life-threatening stridor presenting in a patient with rheumatoid involvement of the larynx. Arch Emerg Med. 1989;6:274–6.
23. Langeron O, Birenbaum A, Amour J. Airway management in trauma. Minerva Anestesiol. 2009;75:307–11.
24. Robitaille A, Williams SR, Tremblay MH, Guilbert F, Theriault M, Drolet P. Cervical spine motion during tracheal intubation with manual in-line stabilization: direct laryngoscopy versus GlideScope videolaryngoscopy. Anesth Analg. 2008;106:935–41. Table of contents.
25. Turner CR, Block J, Shanks A, Morris M, Lodhia KR, Gujar SK. Motion of a cadaver model of cervical injury during endotracheal intubation with a Bullard laryngoscope or a Macintosh blade with and without in-line stabilization. J Trauma. 2009;67:61–6.
26. de Campo T, Aldrete JA. The anesthetic management of the severely burned patient. Intensive Care Med. 1981;7:55–62.
27. Norton ML, Kyff J: Key medical considerations in the difficult airway: sleep apnea, obesity, and burns, atlas of the difficult airway. In: Norton ML, Brown AC, editors. St. Louis, MO: Mosby-Year Book, Inc.; 1991.
28. Chen YW, Lai SH, Fang TJ, Li HY, Lee TJ. Pediatric dyspnea caused by supraglottic stenosis: a rare complication of alkali corrosive injury. Eur Arch Otorhinolaryngol. 2006;263:210–4.
29. Keon TP. Anesthesia for airway surgery. Int Anesthesiol Clin. 1985;23:87–116.
30. Shaha AR. Mandibulotomy and mandibulectomy in difficult tumors of the base of the tongue and oropharynx. Semin Surg Oncol. 1991;7:25–30.
31. Ferlito A, Rinaldo A, Marioni G. Laryngeal malignant neoplasms in children and adolescents. Int J Pediatr Otorhinolaryngol. 1999;49:1–14.
32. Shaw IC, Welchew EA, Harrison BJ, Michael S. Complete airway obstruction during awake fibreoptic intubation. Anaesthesia. 1997;52:582–5.
33. Voyagis GS, Kyriakos KP. The effect of goiter on endotracheal intubation. Anesth Analg. 1997;84:611–2.
34. Souza JW, Williams JT, Ayoub MM, Jerles ML, Dalton ML. Bilateral recurrent nerve paralysis associated with multinodular substernal goiter: a case report. Am Surg. 1999;65:456–9.
35. Shaha AR. Airway management in anaplastic thyroid carcinoma. Laryngoscope. 2008;118:1195–8.
36. Licker M, Schweizer A, Nicolet G, Hohn L, Spiliopoulos A. Anesthesia of a patient with an obstructing tracheal mass: a new way to manage the airway. Acta Anaesthesiol Scand. 1997;41:84–6.
37. Hammer GB. Anaesthetic management for the child with a mediastinal mass. Paediatr Anaesth. 2004;14:95–7.
38. Beriault M, Green J, Hui A. Innovative airway management for peritonsillar abscess. Can J Anaesth. 2006;53:92–5.

39. Fradis M, Goldsher M, David JB, Podoshin L. Life-threatening deep cervical abscess after infiltration of the tonsillar bed for tonsillectomy. Ear Nose Throat J. 1998;77:418–21.
40. Ovassapian A, Glassenberg R, Randel GI, Klock A, Mesnick PS, Klafta JM. The unexpected difficult airway and lingual tonsil hyperplasia: a case series and a review of the literature. Anesthesiology. 2002;97:124–32.
41. Samsoon GL, Young JR. Difficult tracheal intubation: a retrospective study. Anaesthesia. 1987;42:487–90.
42. Mallampati SR, Gatt SP, Gugino LD, Desai SP, Waraksa B, Freiberger D, et al. A clinical sign to predict difficult tracheal intubation: a prospective study. Can Anaesth Soc J. 1985;32:429–34.
43. Mashour GA, Kheterpal S, Vanaharam V, Shanks A, Wang LY, Sandberg WS, et al. The extended Mallampati score and a diagnosis of diabetes mellitus are predictors of difficult laryngoscopy in the morbidly obese. Anesth Analg. 2008;107:1919–23.
44. Mashour GA, Sandberg WS. Craniocervical extension improves the specificity and predictive value of the Mallampati airway evaluation. Anesth Analg. 2006;103:1256–9.
45. Khan ZH, Kashfi A, Ebrahimkhani E. A comparison of the upper lip bite test (a simple new technique) with modified mallampati classification in predicting difficulty in endotracheal intubation: a prospective blinded study. Anesth Analg. 2003;96:595–9.
46. Gonzalez H, Minville V, Delanoue K, Mazerolles M, Concina D, Fourcade O. The importance of increased neck circumference to intubation difficulties in obese patients. Anesth Analg. 2008;106:1132–6.
47. Yentis SM. Predicting trouble in airway management. Anesthesiology. 2006;105:871–2.
48. Shiga T, Wajima Z, Inoue T, Sakamoto A. Predicting difficult intubation in apparently normal patients: a meta-analysis of bedside screening test performance. Anesthesiology. 2005;103:429–37.
49. Cormack RS, Lehane J. Difficult tracheal intubation in obstetrics. Anaesthesia. 1984;39:1105–11.
50. el-Ganzouri AR, McCarthy RJ, Tuman KJ, Tanck EN, Ivankovich AD. Preoperative airway assessment: predictive value of a multivariate risk index. Anesth Analg. 1996;82:1197–204.
51. Rose DK, Cohen MM. The airway: problems and predictions in 18,500 patients. Can J Anaesth. 1994;41:372–83.
52. Gillespie MB, Eisele DW. Outcomes of emergency surgical airway procedures in a hospital-wide setting. Laryngoscope. 1999;109:1766–9.
53. Yuen HW, Loy AH, Johari S. Urgent awake tracheotomy for impending airway obstruction. Otolaryngol Head Neck Surg. 2007;136:838–42.
54. Altman KW, Waltonen JD, Kern RC. Urgent surgical airway intervention: a 3 year county hospital experience. Laryngoscope. 2005;115:2101–4.

3 The Role of Awake Intubation

P. Allan Klock Jr.

Introduction

In 1993 the American Society of Anesthesiologists (ASA) Task Force on Management of the Difficult Airway published its first set of guidelines for management of the difficult airway[1]. These guidelines brought consideration of awake intubation (intubation of the trachea under topical anesthesia with or without sedation) to the forefront of airway management. In the updated guidelines published in 2003, one of the first recommendations is that the

P.A. Klock Jr. (✉)
Department of Anesthesiology and Critical Care, University of Chicago Medical Center, Chicago, IL 60637, USA
e-mail: aklock@dacc.uchicago.edu

D.B. Glick et al. (eds.), *The Difficult Airway: An Atlas of Tools and Techniques for Clinical Management*, DOI 10.1007/978-0-387-92849-4_3, © Springer Science+Business Media New York 2013

1.Assess the likelihood and clinical impact of basic management problems:
   a.Difficult facemask ventilation
   b.Difficult ventilation with extraglottic airway
   c.Difficult tracheal intubation
   d.Difficulty with patient cooperation or consent
   e.Difficult tracheostomy
2.Actively pursue opportunities to deliver supplemental oxygen throughout the process of difficult airway management
3.Consider the merits and feasibility of basic management choices:

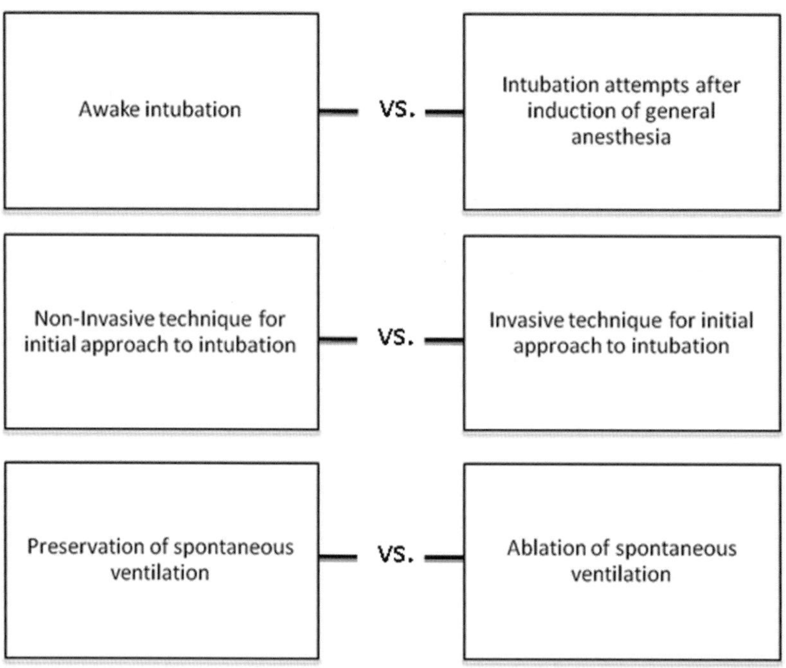

Figure 3.1. Modified ASA algorithm for management of the difficult airway. Modified from The American Society of Anesthesiologists Task Force on Difficult Airway Management. [2]

patient be evaluated to determine if the patient can safely be rendered unconscious and apneic prior to securing the airway or if spontaneous ventilation should be preserved [2]. The principles discussed herein generally apply to a wide variety of clinical settings apart from anesthesia, requiring management of a suspected or known difficult airway.

The 2003 guidelines recommend taking a history and performing a physical examination tailored to detect a possible difficult airway. After the patient has been evaluated, three airway management choices must be made: (1) awake intubation vs. intubation after the induction of general anesthesia, (2) use of invasive vs. noninvasive techniques to secure the airway, and (3) preservation of spontaneous ventilation vs. ablation of spontaneous ventilation (see Figure 3.1).

One of the most important decisions an airway manager must make before securing the airway is whether it is safe to induce apnea before intubating the trachea. Many anesthesiologists think that for certain patients awake intubation of the trachea is the safest and most conservative method for securing the airway. In a survey conducted of Canadian anesthesiologists asking how they would care for patients presenting with a challenging airway, the majority of the 833 respondents chose awake intubation for 5 of the 10 most challenging scenarios: a patient with cervical cord compression presenting for discectomy; a stridulous patient with a laryngeal tumor who requires a laryngectomy; a patient with a mediastinal mass who is stridulous when supine; a patient with a Mallampati class IV airway presenting for laparoscopic cholecystectomy; and a patient who cannot swallow due to a retropharyngeal abscess [3].

In many areas of medicine, no randomized controlled trials define the superiority of a current standard of care over earlier techniques. Studying the management of a difficult airway is challenging because many anesthesiologists believe that it would be unethical to randomly allocate patients to another treatment group. Although we may never have studies that demonstrate the superiority of awake intubation over intubation after induction of general anesthesia, it is clear in several settings the standard of care is to secure the airway before induction of general anesthesia.

Indications for Awake Intubation

A difficult airway can be defined as difficulty with (1) mask ventilation, (2) tracheal intubation, (3) securing a surgical airway, or (4) an uncooperative patient[4]. For the first three situations, awake intubation may be the best option (see Table 3.1).

In order to develop the appropriate management plan, it is helpful to know the probability of a difficult airway. A proper evaluation can help detect the presence of a difficult airway. The ASA standards for preanesthesia care require review of the available medical record, obtaining a pertinent medical history, and performing a focused physical examination. Prior anesthesia records are reviewed with careful attention to the airway techniques employed and their outcomes. Patient imaging studies should be reviewed with special attention paid to radiographs of the cervical spine and MRI and CT studies of the head, neck, and thorax. A patient who has a history consistent with a previous difficult mask ventilation or difficult intubation has a high likelihood of a difficult airway[5].

A difficult airway can be the result of many conditions. These are discussed in detail in Chap. 2.

Aside from an anticipated difficult airway, there are three other situations in which awake intubation may be desirable. First, if the patient has a tenuous neurologic status due to cervical spine pathology, it might be desirable to have the patient intubated prior to induction of general anesthesia. The patient can be intubated and positioned for surgery while awake or with minimal sedation, thereby protecting his own spinal integrity. The patient can then have a neurological assessment prior to induction of general anesthesia.

In addition to indications for awake intubation driven by patient anatomy or pathology, there are two physiologic indications for awake intubation. First, the patient who is hypotensive or in shock may not respond well to sedative or anesthetic induction agents. These agents may reduce sympathetic tone or have a deleterious effect on blood pressure due to negative inotropic or vasodilating properties. Often, a patient in extremis will tolerate laryngoscopy and intubation with minimal or no topical anesthesia and no sedation. The second physiologic indication for awake intubation is respiratory failure. The patient with minimal respiratory reserve may not tolerate even a brief period of apnea without suffering significant hypoxia. In this setting it may be most prudent to allow the patient to breathe spontaneously throughout the intubation procedure. Blockade of the nerves innervating the airway and/or topical anesthesia can be provided while the patient breathes with a well-sealed face mask with very brief interruptions to apply topical agents.

Table 3.1. Indications for awake intubation.

Previous history of difficult intubation
Anticipated difficult mask ventilation
Physical examination consistent with difficult intubation
Trauma to the face, neck, upper airway, cervical spine
High risk of aspiration
Cervical spine disease
Hypotension, shock
Respiratory failure

Contraindications to Awake Intubation

There are few absolute contraindications to awake intubation. If patient refusal or reluctance is encountered initially, with proper counseling and reassurance most patients will agree to awake intubation (see "psychological preparation" below). Uncooperative patients such as children and intoxicated adults may present special challenges. A documented allergy to all local anesthetics means a patient is not a candidate for awake intubation. Most patients who report an allergy to local anesthetics have had an intravascular injection of local anesthetic before a dental procedure. The signs and symptoms they report are usually consistent with systemic toxicity from local anesthetics or epinephrine. These patients may safely receive local anesthetics as part of preparation for awake intubation.

Advantages of Awake Tracheal Intubation

There are several advantages to awake intubation over asleep intubation. First, an awake patient maintains ventilation and oxygenation. There is truth to the aphorism, "It is hard to kill a spontaneously breathing patient." Because the patient is breathing and oxygenating, they will not desaturate as quickly, eliminating the time pressure associated with intubating an apneic patient. If the initial technique is unsuccessful, then alternative techniques can be attempted in a deliberate and methodical manner. In the unlikely event that none of the attempted intubation techniques works, elective surgery and anesthesia can be rescheduled without harming the patient. Unfortunately, this may not be the case when airway management is required for resuscitation purposes.

The second advantage of awake intubation is that the normal anatomic architecture of the upper airway is maintained. In an unconscious patient, the normal muscular tone of the tongue and upper airway structures relaxes[6].

This collapse can render ineffective the patient's efforts to inspire as seen in patients with obstructive sleep apnea. Airway collapse also can make efforts to assist spontaneous ventilation less effective and may make positive pressure ventilation with a face mask impossible leading to a cannot ventilate scenario.

When airway structures collapse, intubation of the trachea may become difficult, especially when a flexible bronchoscope is used to guide a tube into the trachea. Since unlike during direct or video laryngoscopy where a lifting force is applied to the anterior structures of the airway creating an open space, a flexible bronchoscope cannot create an open space and must navigate an open channel from the nose or mouth to the trachea.

The third advantage of awake intubation is that the risk for aspiration is reduced because the airway is secured while the patient is conscious. First, the lower esophageal sphincter and cricopharyngeal muscle tone are maintained. Second, if the patient does regurgitate, gastric contents that reach the mouth can be expelled. Finally, if the carina is not anesthetized with a topical local anesthetic, the patient will cough vigorously if gastric contents do enter the distal trachea. Upper airway reflexes are blunted by many anesthetic drugs, so it is important that the patient not be deeply sedated if maintenance of airway reflexes is desired[7–9].

Finally, the neurologic status of the patient can be monitored during the intubation and positioning process. Evaluating the neurologic status is especially important in patients with cervical spine pathology. Because tracheal intubation of an anesthetized patient often involves manipulation of the cervical spine, there is some degree of uncertainty about the integrity of the central and peripheral nervous system if the patient is anesthetized before the airway is secured. It is very reassuring to the patient and the care providers if the patient is intubated and positioned for surgery while awake. This is especially important for surgery that will be performed with the neck extended or with the patient in the lateral or prone position.

Keys to Successful Awake Intubation

There is an adage, "The key to successful awake fiberoptic intubation is good preparation, while the key to successful asleep fiberoptic intubation is good help." Good preparation starts by establishing a good rapport with the patient and obtaining excellent topical anesthesia.

Psychological Preparation

Probably one of the most underappreciated aspects of a successful awake intubation is the development of good rapport with the patient. Patients should be told that the awake intubation is in their best interest. A patient's mood will often mirror the mood of the anesthesiologist. If an anesthesiologist is calm and matter of fact, the patient will be calm. It is important for the anesthesiologist to listen to and address the patient's concerns. Patients are often worried about gagging and loss of control. They can be comforted by assurances that topical anesthesia will block the gag reflex. It is also helpful to tell patients that they will be appropriately sedated and can retain control by having the ability to pause the intubation process by holding up a hand. Patients are told that they will be given more local anesthetic or anxiolytics if they experience discomfort or anxiety during the procedure.

Dry the Airway

A patient's airway should be dry for two reasons. The first reason is that oral secretions hinder the ability of the anesthesiologist to view anatomic structures through fiberoptic devices. This is more of a concern for flexible bronchoscopes than other intubation devices because bronchoscopes traverse the most dependent portion of the airway where fluids tend to pool. The second reason for drying the mucous membranes is that a topically applied local anesthetic is much more effective when applied to dry mucous membranes. Oral secretions decrease the effectiveness of topical local anesthetics in several ways. First, saliva will dilute the local anesthetic. Second, the local anesthetic will need to diffuse through a layer of viscous saliva, reducing the concentration at the tissue surface and lengthening the onset time of the local anesthetic. Finally, if the mouth is wet, a larger portion of the topical local anesthetic may be swallowed increasing the risk for nausea and systemic toxicity[10].

Glycopyrrolate 0.2 mg i.v. is administered to reduce oral secretions. Glycopyrrolate causes less tachycardia than atropine and does not cross the blood–brain barrier, so the risk of delirium from the central anticholinergic effects of drugs like atropine and scopolamine is avoided. Intravenous glycopyrrolate has an onset time of 2–4 min and an antisialogogue effect lasting over 2 h[11].

If the mucous membranes are not dry when it is time to apply topical anesthesia, then manual drying techniques should be used. Gauze can be wrapped around a tongue depressor and then applied to the tongue to dry it. Alternatively, the patient can be given gauze to wrap around his or her finger for insertion into his or her mouth to dry the mucous membranes. Insertion of one's finger into the mouth of a patient who is not anesthetized can elicit a gag or bite reflex and is therefore not advised.

Supplemental Oxygen

Supplemental oxygen is applied to prevent hypoxemia if the patient hypoventilates as a result of sedation. A larger fraction of oxygen in the lungs will provide a margin of safety if the patient becomes hypopneic or apneic or if the airway becomes completely obstructed. Clearly, one should take every precaution to prevent apnea or airway obstruction, but if either should occur there will be more time before the patient desaturates if the patient has been breathing supplemental oxygen.

Anxiolysis and Sedation

Ideally the patient should be cooperative, calm, and not anxious. The patient should need little or no analgesia if local anesthesia is working well. Minimal or moderate sedation-analgesia as defined by the American Society of Anesthesiologists is the appropriate depth for most patients[12]. The patient should be responsive to verbal or light tactile stimulation, airway architecture will remain unchanged, and the airway will remain patent. The patient should have normal or near-normal ventilatory drive, and cardiovascular function is largely unaffected.

The cooperative patient will be able to control his airway if he vomits. He will also be able to inspire deeply when requested to do so. Deep inspiration has three desirable effects. First, if the patient's oxygen level is falling, one or two vital capacity maneuvers are usually enough to raise the oxygen saturation to an acceptable level. Second, active inspiration makes it easier for the endoscopist to identify the glottic opening. Third, the vocal cords abduct during deep inspiration easing the passage of the endotracheal tube into the trachea.

Several drugs may be used individually or in combination to produce the desired level of sedation. Midazolam is used frequently because it is an anxiolytic with a rapid onset of action, a relatively short duration of action, and minimal effect on respiratory or cardiovascular physiology. Midazolam's effects are reversed with flumazenil. The amnestic properties of midazolam are also beneficial, particularly if the patient has a condition that requires multiple anesthetics with awake intubation. Often fentanyl or remifentanil are used in conjunction with midazolam for two reasons. The opiates are a potent antitussive that reduces coughing associated with translaryngeal injection or instrumentation of the trachea with a bronchoscope, endotracheal tube, or other device. If nerve blocks are performed before the intubation, fentanyl reduces the discomfort associated with the injections. It is important to realize, however, that there is a synergistic interaction between benzodiazepines and opiates with respect to sedation/hypnosis and hypoventilation, hypoxemia, and apnea[13,14].

Dexmedetomidine also has several desirable properties for airway management. Patients sedated with dexmedetomidine are calm and cooperative. In a study that compared dexmedetomidine and midazolam, patient satisfaction was superior and hemodynamics were smoother in patients sedated with dexmedetomidine and a small amount of midazolam than with properly titrated doses of midazolam alone[15]. In patients who received dexmedetomidine, hypercarbic and hypoxic ventilatory drive were nearly normal. A beneficial effect of dexmedetomidine sedation is a very dry airway. The disadvantages of dexmedetomidine are its cost, slow onset, and the need for an infusion pump for most applications. In addition, there is no reversal agent for dexmedetomidine.

Anesthesia of the Airway

It is important to provide excellent anesthesia of the airway before attempting laryngoscopy or intubation. At a minimum, the posterior portion of the tongue, the hypopharynx, the larynx, and the proximal trachea must be anesthetized. If the plan is to intubate the trachea via the nose, then the nasopharynx also must be anesthetized.

For topical anesthesia, the right drug must be selected in the right concentration, and sufficient time must be allowed for it to work. Benzocaine produces anesthesia of the mucous membranes quickly, but is associated with methemoglobinemia and has been removed from the formulary of several hospitals[16]. Lidocaine is safe and effective for providing topical anesthesia of the airway. It is possible to provide adequate anesthesia with 2 % lidocaine, but the onset of action with this low concentration takes approximately 20 min. For this reason, 4 or 5 % lidocaine is preferred for topical anesthesia of the airway. With the higher concentrations, the airway is ready for instrumentation within 2 min[17].

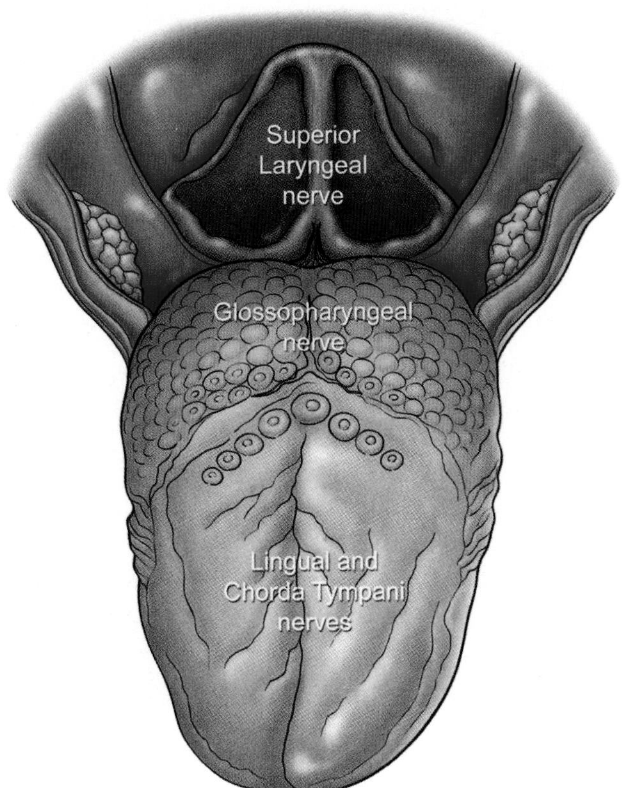

Figure 3.2. Sensory innervation of the tongue and upper airway (with kind permission from Springer Science+Business Media: Principles of airway management, 4th ed.; 2010. Finucane BT, Tsui BCH, Santora AH, Figure 1.6.).

Applied Airway Anatomy

The posterior third of the tongue, the tonsils, and the pharynx are innervated by the glossopharyngeal nerve (see Figure 3.2). This nerve passes through the palatoglossal arch, also known as the anterior tonsillar pillar. The nerve can be blocked with 1–2 mL of 1 % lidocaine injected into the anterior tonsillar pillar just cephalad to the tongue (see Figure 3.3).

Sensation of the larynx above the vocal cords is transmitted by the internal branch of the superior laryngeal nerve (see Figure 3.4). Anesthesia can be achieved with either topical application of local anesthetics or by blocking the nerve as it passes near the tip of the hyoid bone on each side (see Figure 3.5). The person performing the block palpates the hyoid bone with one hand to identify the tip of the bone. Lidocaine 1 % is injected at the tip of the hyoid bone. One milliliter is injected superficial to the hyothyroid ligament and another 1 mL is injected deep to the ligament. The procedure is then repeated on the opposite side.

Topical Anesthesia of the Tongue

The tongue can be well anesthetized with a topical local anesthetic. If the tongue is moist, it can be dried using a gauze pad wrapped around a tongue depressor, or the patient can be asked to blot his tongue dry with a gauze pad wrapped around his finger. Because the gag reflex is still intact at this point, allowing the patient to dry his own airway may be more comfortable for the patient. A dry tongue can be anesthetized with 5 % lidocaine ointment applied on a tongue depressor. It is important to note that 2 % lidocaine jelly

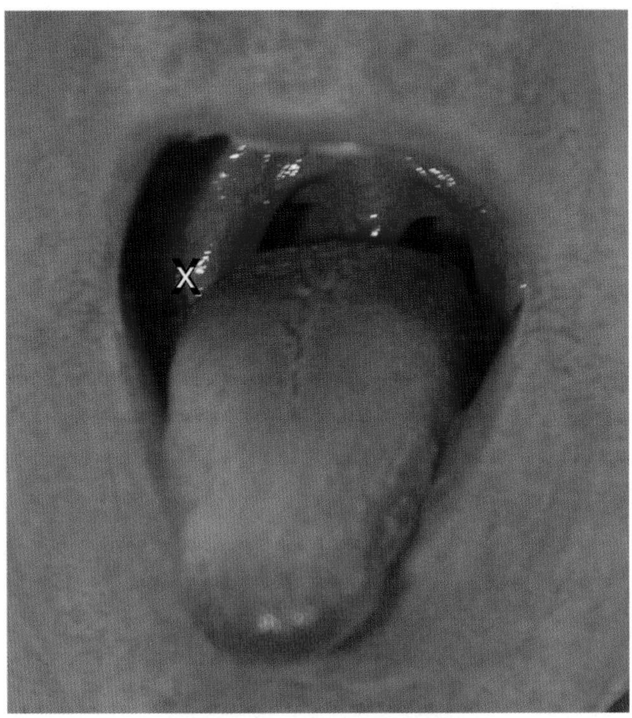

Figure 3.3. Injection site for glossopharyngeal nerve block. Local anesthetic is injected into the anterior tonsillar pillar 2 mm cephalad to the tongue at the spot indicated by the X.

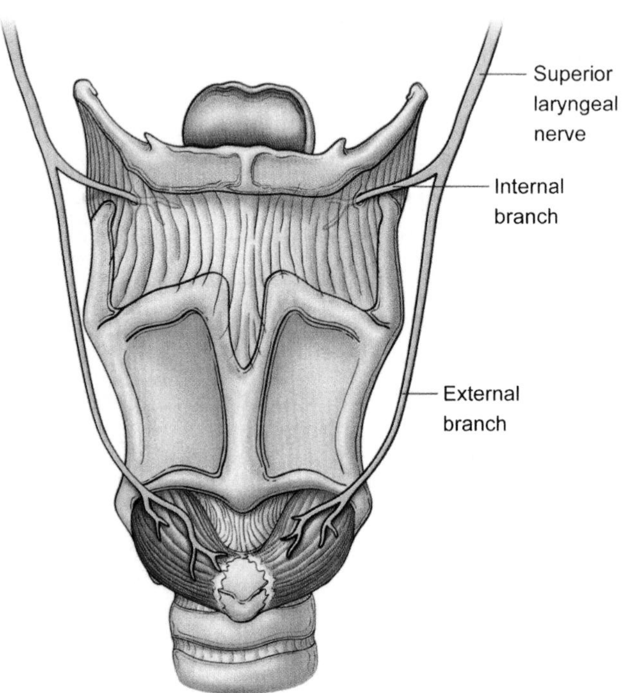

Figure 3.4. Innervation of the larynx. Sensory innervation of the larynx is provided by the internal branch of the superior laryngeal nerve (with kind permission from Springer Science+Business Media: Principles of airway management, 4th ed.; 2010. Finucane BT, Tsui BCH, Santora AH, Figure 1.19).

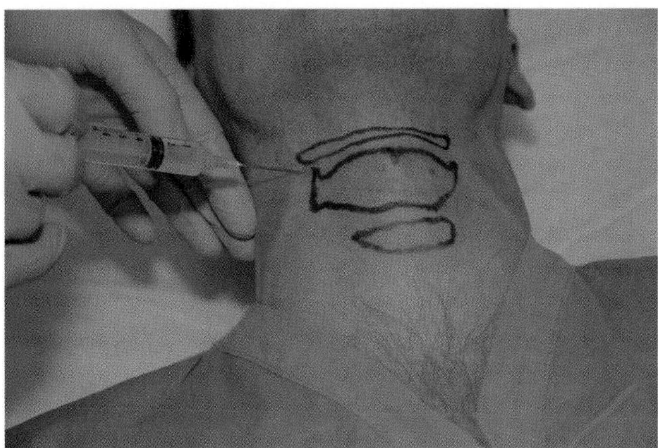

Figure 3.5. Blocking the superior laryngeal nerve. Local anesthetic is injected 2–3 mm caudad of the hyoid bone tip.

frequently does not produce adequate anesthesia of the tongue. To anesthetize the tongue, the operator starts in the middle of the tongue and gently applies the ointment with a painting side-to-side motion on the tongue (see Figure 3.6a, b). The tongue blade is slowly moved to the posterior aspect of the tongue (see Figure 3.6c). The goal is to deliver enough ointment to the posterior part of the tongue that some will melt and drip down into the hypopharynx, affecting the pyriform sinuses bilaterally and the vallecula.

After the lidocaine ointment has had 2–3 min to take effect, the application of topical anesthesia is completed by spraying the tongue, posterior pharynx, and larynx with 4 % lidocaine. An atomizer is used to deliver a directable spray. First the tongue and posterior pharynx are sprayed with approximately 1 mL (see Figure 3.7a). Then the atomizer is deflected to allow the spray to be directed to the pyriform sinus, applying approximately 0.5 mL on each side (see Figure 3.7b, c). Finally, the atomizer is placed in the posterior pharynx and directed in the midline toward the vocal cords. The patient is instructed to inspire deeply while 1 mL of lidocaine is injected quickly (see Figure 3.7d). This provides topical anesthesia of the epiglottis, vocal cords, distal larynx, and proximal trachea.

The trachea distal to the vocal cords is supplied by the recurrent laryngeal branch of the vagus nerve. While it is essential to thoroughly anesthetize this area, the recurrent laryngeal nerve is not amenable to direct neural blockade. To properly anesthetize the airway below the cords, topical anesthetic must be applied via one of two techniques; a translaryngeal injection or via a "spray as you go" technique[18].

To perform a translaryngeal block, the operator first identifies the cricothyroid ligament. The larynx is stabilized with the thumb and middle finger, while the ligament is palpated with the index finger. The other hand introduces a 20-gauge catheter or 22-gauge needle attached to a syringe containing 2–4 mL of 4 % lidocaine through the ligament into the airway. The plunger of the syringe is withdrawn, aspirating air into the lidocaine (see Figure 3.8). This "bubble contrast" technique is important to confirm that the needle is in the airway and not in tissue before injecting the local anesthetic. Once proper placement of the needle is confirmed, the patient is informed that he is likely to cough, and the local anesthetic is injected briskly into the airway. If a needle is used for the injection, it is removed immediately after the injection. If a catheter is used, it may be left in place or removed.

After an injection of local anesthetic through the cricothyroid ligament, the patient usually coughs, sometimes quite vigorously. Coughing spreads the local anesthetic proximally and distally in the airway, helping to anesthetize the larynx and trachea.

The "spray as you go" technique works well and is especially advantageous when it is undesirable to place a needle through the neck. In this technique the working channel of a fiberoptic bronchoscope is used to deliver local anesthetic to the larynx and trachea.

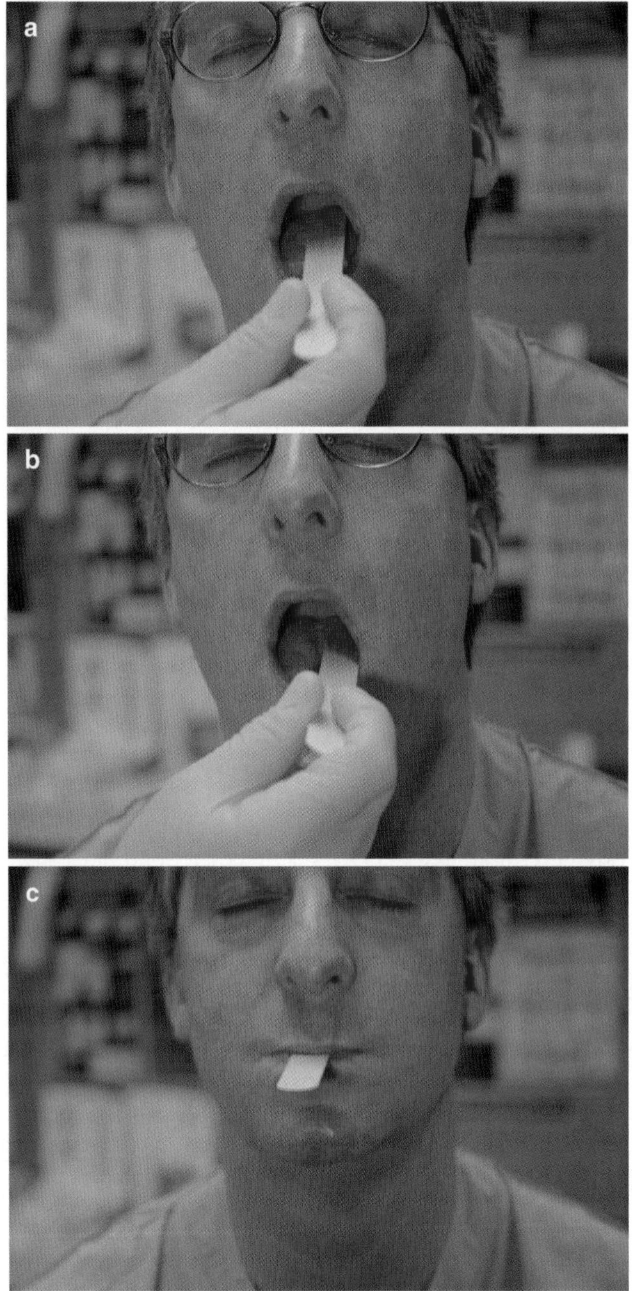

Figure 3.6. Application of Local anesthetic ointment. (**a**) Local anesthetic ointment is applied to the middle third of the tongue. The tongue blade is then moved side-to-side to anesthetize the entire tongue as seen in (**b**). The patient is then instructed to hold the local anesthetic-covered tongue blade over the posterior tongue in a manner similar to a lollipop (**c**),

For the technique to work, the velocity of the local anesthetic must be high enough to create a directable stream of fluid out of the end of the scope. Most adult bronchoscopes have a large (2.0–2.5 mm) working channel to allow for effective suctioning and passage of brushes and biopsy forceps. The large cross-sectional area of these channels produces a poor stream of fluid. This problem can be overcome by introducing an epidural catheter through the working channel. The small internal diameter of the catheter generates good flow characteristics (see Figure 3.9a). The epidural catheter is fed into the channel so that its tip is just inside the bronchoscope. At the same time, the scope is introduced in the airway and positioned to allow visualization of the larynx.

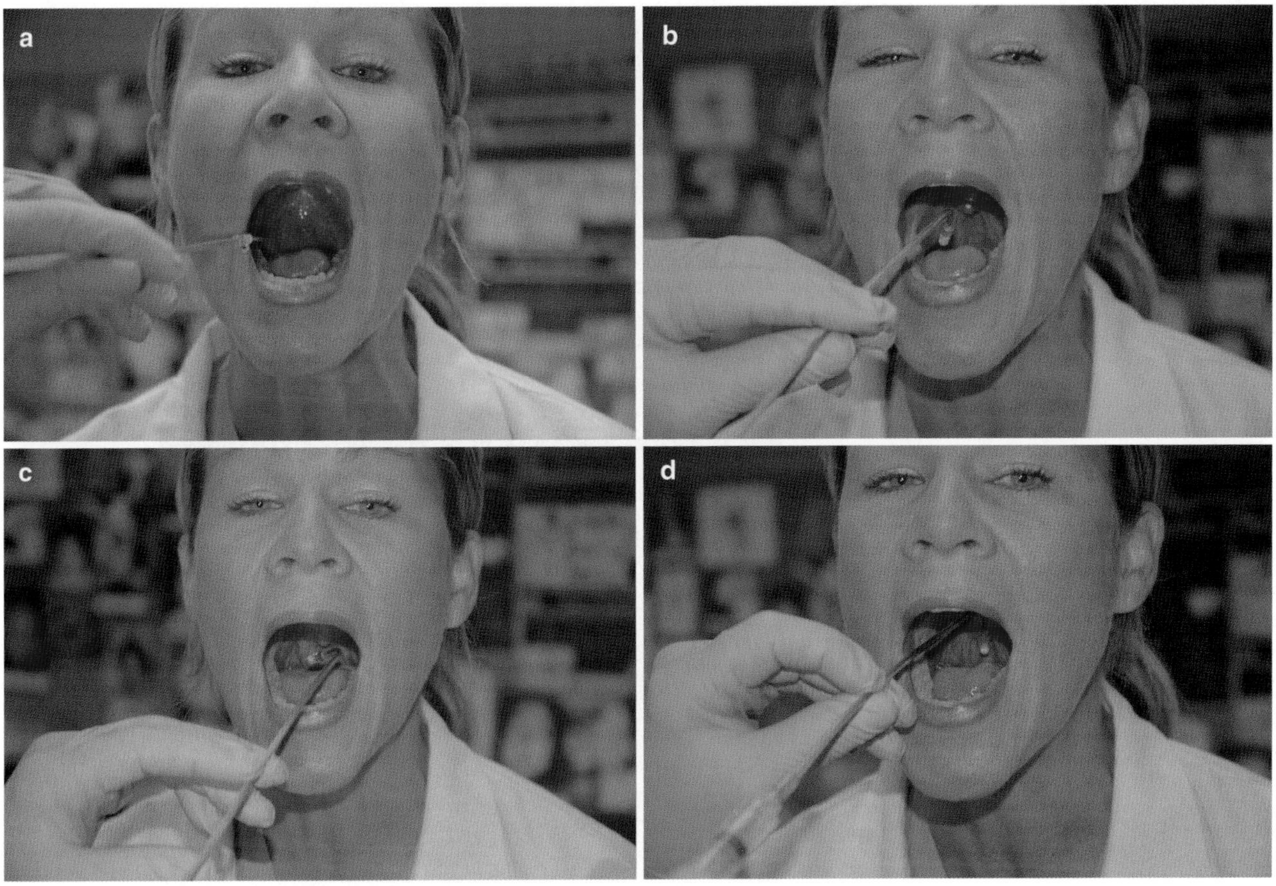

Figure 3.7. Translaryngeal injection. Local anesthetic is sprayed onto the oral and laryngeal mucosa. In (**a**) the tongue and posterior pharynx are anesthetized. The atomizer is then bent to allow the posterior tongue and larynx to be sprayed. (**b** and **c**) show the local anesthetic being directed laterally with the goal of anesthetizing the pirifom sinus and underlying internal branch of the superior laryngeal nerve on each side. Finally, the spray is directed in the midline and the patient is instructed to inspire deeply (**d**). This provides topical anesthesia of the vocal cords and proximal trachea.

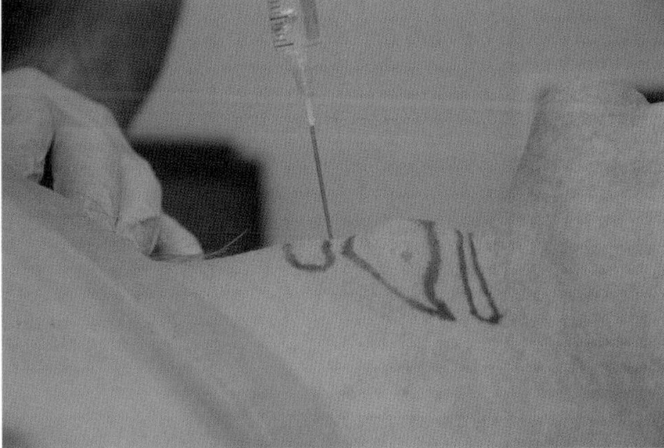

Figure 3.8. Translaryngeal injection. Local anesthetic is injected into the trachea via the cricothyroid ligament. It is important to confirm intra-tracheal needle position by aspirating air into the syringe prior to injecting local anesthetic.

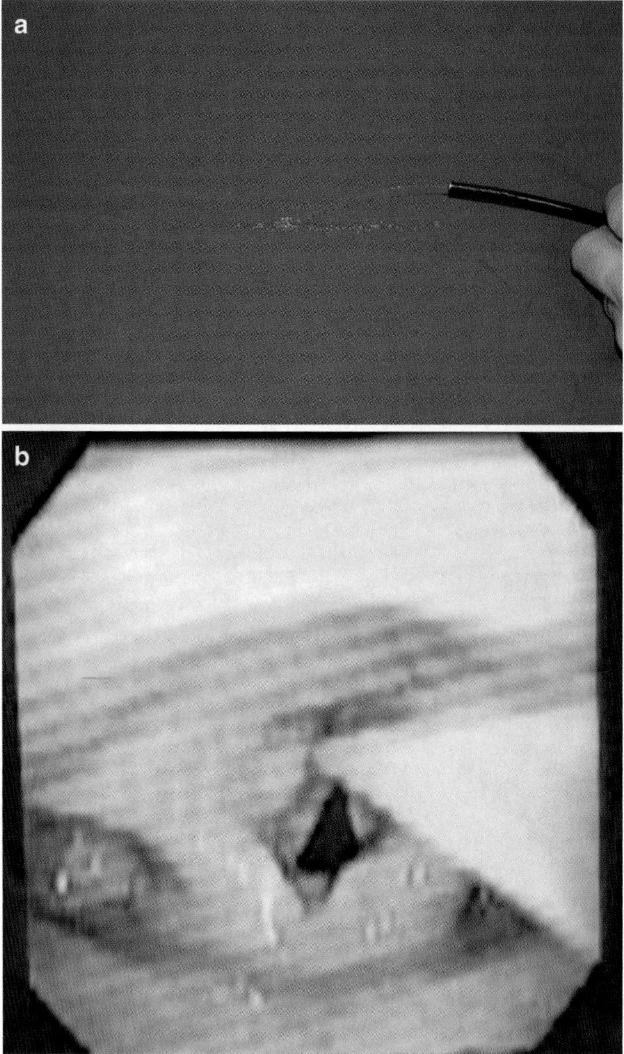

Figure 3.9. "Spray as you go" technique for providing topical anesthesia. (**a**) Fluid stream from an epidural catheter in the working channel of a fiberoptic bronchoscope. The small cross-sectional area of the epidural catheter makes it well-suited for producing a directable stream of local anesthetic. (**b**) Stream of local anesthetic applied to the anterior commisure of the vocal cords.

Once the larynx is in view, the catheter is advanced to extend 1–2 mm beyond the tip of the scope. The anterior commissure of the vocal cords is sprayed with 0.2–0.4 mL of lidocaine (see Figure 3.9b). If the cords remain open, the scope is aimed so that the next aliquot of lidocaine will hit the anterior wall of the trachea just distal to the vocal cords. It is important at this point to be patient. If the scope is advanced before the local anesthetic has a chance to work, the patient may cough or experience laryngospasm. After a period of 30–45 s, the scope is advanced into the trachea and the anterior surface of the proximal and mid trachea is sprayed.

If a bronchoscopic intubation is planned, the endotracheal tube can be advanced over the endoscope and into the trachea 45 s after the last application of local anesthetic. Passage of the endotracheal tube through the vocal cords is facilitated by asking the patient to inspire deeply before the tube is advanced. This maneuver will abduct the vocal cords allowing easier passage.

Intubating the Trachea

After proper intubating conditions have been created with airway anesthesia and appropriate sedation, the trachea can be intubated. In order from least to most stimulating, the common modes of tracheal intubation of the awake patient are: intubation over a flexible bronchoscope, video laryngoscopy, and direct laryngoscopy.

Flexible bronchoscopic intubation (FBI) allows the device to be gently steered through the open space in the airway with minimal contact and pressure on the base of the tongue and other airway structures. The one caveat to intubation with a flexible bronchoscope is that the scope must be passed through the vocal cords before the endotracheal tube is passed through the cords. If the trachea is not adequately anesthetized when the bronchoscope is passed through the cords, the patient may cough vigorously and/or develop laryngospasm.

Video laryngoscopes (VL) place more pressure on the base of the tongue than a flexible bronchoscope, thereby increasing the amount of stimulation, particularly pressure sensation on the base of the tongue. The shape of the blades used for video laryngoscopes vary considerably from one manufacturer to another, so the response to one device may be different than to another. Direct laryngoscopes (DL) need to create a straight line of sight from the upper incisors to the vocal cords exerting more pressure on the airway tissues than other techniques. VLs with the same shape as traditional DL blades (e.g., the Storz C-MAC) presumably produce similar amounts of pressure as the DL blades upon which they are based. VLs with highly curved blades (e.g., the Pentax AWS or the GlideScope) allow the operator to "see around the corner" of the airway and presumably produce less stimulation on the airway.

Other intubating techniques can be used with the awake patient. The Intubating LMA (LMA North America, San Diego) or C-Trach has been used for a hybrid "awake-asleep" intubation technique[19]. In this technique the oro-pharynx and hypopharynx are anesthetized with topical agents, while the larynx and trachea are not anesthetized. The C-Trach device is inserted and the video monitor applied. If the monitor shows a clear view of the vocal cords, general anesthesia is induced and the trachea is intubated through the device. This technique is especially good for patients when translaryngeal injection of lidocaine or tracheal anesthesia is undesirable.

Finally, surgical access to the trachea may be obtained in the awake patient with or without sedation. While surgical access to the airway is the technique of last resort in most difficult airway algorithms, there are times when it may be best to proceed with cricothyroidotomy or tracheostomy without anesthetizing or sedating the patient. Awake surgical techniques may be indicated in cases of massive airway hemorrhage, massive regurgitation, trauma to the face or neck, and cases of obstruction due to edema, infection, or foreign body. If the patient's airway is so tenuous that surgery is required prior to induction of general anesthesia, then extreme caution should be exercised with sedation. Often patients undergoing awake surgical airway access receive little or no sedatives or analgesia until the airway is secured. As always, the risk of supplemental oxygen must be recognized if the surgeon is to use electrocautery after the airway has been entered.

It is important for anesthesia providers to understand the role of awake airway management in the delivery of clinical anesthesia. Providers must be comfortable and competent in intubating the trachea prior to induction of general anesthesia. Establishing patient rapport to develop trust, providing appropriate antisialogogues and sedative agents to optimize conditions and cooperation, and applying appropriate techniques to anesthetize the airway are essential elements of successful awake intubation. As with all skills, these must be practiced regularly to maintain top proficiency. With proper technique and regular use, one should be able to perform an awake intubation in an efficient manner with little stress for the patient and provider.

References

1. The American Society of Anesthesiologists Task Force on Difficult Airway Management. Practice guidelines for management of the difficult airway. Anesthesiology. 1993;78(3): 597–602.
2. The American Society of Anesthesiologists Task Force on Difficult Airway Management. Practice guidelines for management of the difficult airway: an updated report by the American Society of anesthesiologists task force on management of the difficult airway. Anesthesiology. 2003;98(5):1269–77.
3. Jenkins K, Wong DT, Correa R. Management choices for the difficult airway by anesthesiologists in Canada. Can J Anaesth. 2002;49(8):850–6.
4. Klock PA, Benumof J. Definition and incidence of the difficult airway. In: Hagberg CA, editor. Benumof's difficult airway management. 2nd ed. Mosby Elsevier: Philadelphia; 2007. p. 215–20.
5. Lundstrøm LH, Møller AM, Rosenstock C, Astrup G, Gätke MR, Wetterslev J. A documented previous difficult tracheal intubation as a prognostic test for a subsequent difficult tracheal intubation in adults. Anaesthesia. 2009;64:1081–8.
6. Eastwood PR, Szollosi I, Platt PR, Hillman DR. Collapsibility of the upper airway during anesthesia with isoflurane. Anesthesiology. 2002;97:786–93.
7. Drummond GB. Influence of thiopentone on upper airway muscles. Br J Anaesth. 1989;63:12–21.
8. Murphy PJ, Langton JA, Barker P, Smith G. Effect of oral diazepam on the sensitivity of upper airway reflexes. Br J Anaesth. 1993;70:131.
9. Nishino T, Hiraga K, Sugimori K. Effects of i.v. lignocaine on airway reflexes elicited by irritation of the tracheal mucosa in humans anaesthetized with enflurane. Br J Anaesth. 1990;64:682–7.
10. Benumof JL, Feroe D. Swallowing topically administered 4 % lidocaine results in nausea and vomiting. Am J Anesthesiol. 1998;25(4):150–3.
11. Reed AP. Preparation of the patient for awake flexible fiberoptic bronchoscopy. Chest. 1992;101:244–53.
12. Practice Guidelines for Sedation and Analgesia by Non-Anesthesiologists. An updated report by the American Society of Anesthesiologists Task Force on Sedation and Analgesia by Non-Anesthesiologists. Anesthesiology. 2002; 96:1004–17.
13. Bailey PL, Pace NL, Ashburn MA, Moll JW, East KA, Stanley T. Frequent hypoxemia and apnea after sedation with midazolam and fentanyl. Anesthesiology. 1990;73(5):826–30.
14. Vinik HR, Bradley EL, Kissin I. Triple anesthetic combination: propofol-midazolam-alfentanil. Anesth Analg. 1994;78(2):354–8.
15. Bergese SD, Bender SP, McSweeney TD, Fernandez S, Dzwonczyk R, Sage K. A comparative study of dexmedetomidine with midazolam and midazolam alone for sedation during elective awake fiberoptic intubation. J Clin Anesth. 2010;22(1):35–40.
16. Nguyen ST, Cabrales RE, Bashour CA, Rosenberger TE, Michener JA, Yared JP, et al. Benzocaine-induced methemoglobinemia. Anesth Analg. 2000;90(2):369–71.
17. Takita K, Morimoto Y, Kemmotsu O. Tracheal lidocaine attenuates the cardiovascular response to endotracheal intubation. Can J Anesth. 2001;48(8):732–6.
18. Webb AR, Fernando SS, Dalton HR, Arrowsmith JE, Woodhead MA, Cummin AR. Local anaesthesia for fibreoptic bronchoscopy: transcricoid injection or the "spray as you go" technique? Thorax. 1990;45(6):474–7.
19. Ovassapian A. Awake-asleep sequential intubation using CTrach LMA. Anesthesiology. 2006;105:870.

4

Unanticipated Difficult Direct Laryngoscopy: Methods to Improve Its Success

Mark E. Nunnally and Michael R. Hernandez

M.E. Nunnally (✉)
Department of Anesthesiology and Critical Care, University of Chicago Medical Center,
Chicago, IL 60637, USA
e-mail: mnunnally@dacc.uchicago.edu

M.R. Hernandez
Anesthesia and Critical Care, University of Chicago Medical Center,
5841 S. Maryland Avenue MC 4028, Chicago, IL, 60637, USA
e-mail: mhernandez@dacc.uchicago.edu

D.B. Glick et al. (eds.), *The Difficult Airway: An Atlas of Tools and Techniques for Clinical Management*,
DOI 10.1007/978-0-387-92849-4_4,

Introduction

When faced with a difficult intubation, one might abandon direct laryngoscopy in favor of another intubation technique. As technology promises to render the improbable routine, it is difficult to generate interest in a traditional airway technique such as direct laryngoscopy, especially when it proves to be difficult. However, direct laryngoscopy has also benefitted from technological advances. Illumination has improved with brighter sources such as light emitting diodes (LED) or fiberoptic light transmission replacing the direct light of incandescent bulbs. Battery longevity in modern laryngoscope handles is improved, including rechargeable options. Magnetic resonance imaging compatible (non-ferromagnetic) blades and disposable laryngoscope blades and handles have been designed. Despite these advances, interest in direct laryngoscopy, especially when it becomes difficult, pales in comparison to the excitement surrounding the use of a multitude of newer video-driven airway devices. Innovation and technological advancement in airway management are inevitable and desirable, but the simplicity and sheer efficacy of direct laryngoscopy remain constant. New airway techniques must always be evaluated against a "gold standard," and for most airway devices, the gold standard is direct laryngoscopy. In the setting of difficult laryngoscopy, it is important to recognize that techniques and tools can facilitate difficult intubation and that a difficult airway need not be an absolute contraindication to the use of the technique.

Traditional techniques are often replaced by new ones, but direct laryngoscopy remains important to the practice of airway management. Direct laryngoscopy is cost-effective relative to newer techniques. Laryngoscopes are widely available and can be in many locations without an undue economic burden. They are relatively sturdy and do not depend upon fragile fiberoptic or video-based image capture or transmission. They are highly portable and suitable for use inside or out of the operating room. Although a video-based system lets the operator visualize structures without achieving a direct line of sight for intubation, freedom from direct vision comes at a cost. Operators see only what the camera can show them. Blood and secretions, which typically do not fully preclude direct laryngoscopy, have the potential to render a video-based technique impossible.

An interesting argument in the evolution of airway management is the notion that video laryngoscopes and similar devices should replace standard laryngoscopes as primary airway devices. Proponents of this notion argue that video laryngoscopes provide a better view and image than direct laryngoscopy with less manipulation of the blade and patient. Thus, it would seem prudent to start with the best tool for an optimal view. This argument assumes that the failure rate of a video laryngoscope or a similar device is known. The failure rate for intubation with direct laryngoscopy is low, but unless video laryngoscopes are widely adopted as first line airway devices, it is impossible to know how often they fail [1].

Interesting debates aside, direct laryngoscopy still holds a place in airway management and deserves consideration in any text about it. This chapter considers causes, techniques, equipment, and complications of direct laryngoscopy in the setting of difficult airway management.

Lingual Tonsil Hyperplasia

Unanticipated difficult direct laryngoscopy remains a challenge for the laryngoscopist. Multiple factors can contribute to an unanticipated difficult airway. Direct laryngoscopy relies on an unimpaired line of sight from the laryngoscopist to the patient's glottis. Structures that obscure the laryngoscopist's line of vision are an important source of unanticipated difficult direct laryngoscopy. Lingual tonsil hyperplasia (LTH) is one such example. LTH is not likely to be appreciated on exam preoperatively. There is evidence that LTH may be responsible for unanticipated difficult or failed intubation with direct laryngoscopy [2].

Copious Blood and Secretions

Unanticipated blood and secretions can partially or completely obstruct the laryngoscopist's view. Suctioning can help, but continued bleeding can still pose a challenge. Patients with histories of coagulation disorders or difficulty managing secretions can alert the laryngoscopist to potential difficulty. However, unanticipated difficulty can result from reflux of stomach contents, traumatic bleeding during laryngoscopy, or copious secretions. An antisialogogue, such as glycopyrrolate, may lessen secretions, but only if given in advance. Efforts to slow bleeding may be useful, particularly in the case of epistaxis. If it is not possible to clear the airway, laryngoscopists may orient themselves by looking for bubbles at the inlet to the airway of a spontaneously breathing patient.

Blades

In spite of their evident utility, near ubiquitous presence, and the value placed on expertise in their use, many essential details about laryngoscopic blades are underappreciated. Studies comparing blades frequently focus on blade shape, construction (disposable vs. reusable), and features (e.g., articulated parts). Additionally, prism, fiberoptic, and video-imaging modifications make indirect laryngoscopy possible with some of the devices. It is hard to compare the performance of different blades for difficult direct laryngoscopy because each clinical situation is unique and the circumstances vary. Using simulations to practice difficult intubation is not easy and may be inappropriate. Speed, success, and complications are relevant variables; however, reporting across studies is inconsistent. Most studies rely on mannequins, so often the ability to visualize glottic structures around a steep angle, the so-called "anterior airway," is compared. This comparison may or may not take into account patient variables, such as secretions, blood or masses, or the fidelity of the mannequin.

Shape

Apart from modifications and improvements, two basic blade designs dominate: straight blades, such as the Miller, and curved blades, such as the Macintosh. To improve direct laryngoscopy performance in difficult airways, attempts have been made to modify blade shape and angle, attach prisms, such as the Huffman prism (Figure 4.1), add mirrored surfaces, such as in the Siker blade (Figure 4.2), or add articulating tips, such as with the Corazelli, London, McCoy (CLM) blade (Figures 4.3 and 4.4). Among the numerous modifications to these designs, we will describe three: the Belscope; Corazelli, London, McCoy (CLM); and reduced-step designs.

A laryngoscope blade is both a retractor and an illuminator. A successful direct laryngoscopy surmounts conditions that hamper these actions. Figure 4.5 shows the parts of typical Macintosh and Miller designs. The enlarged flange and web of the Macintosh is designed

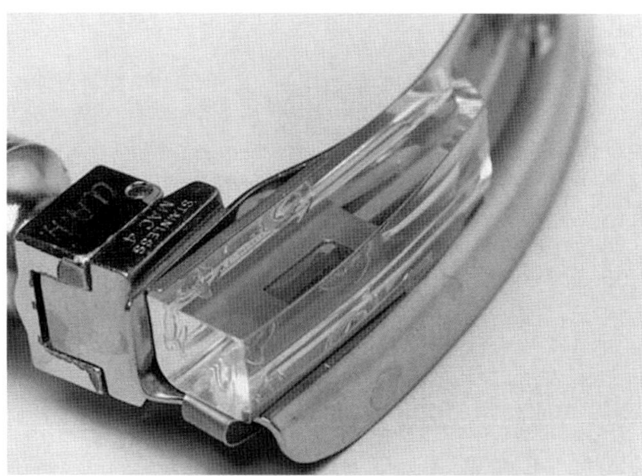

Figure 4.1. The Huffman prism projects images outside the line of sight, enabling visualization of anterior airway structures (with kind permission from Springer Science+Business Media: Principles of airway management. 4th ed. Springer: New York; 2011. Finucane BT, Tsui BCH, Santora A).

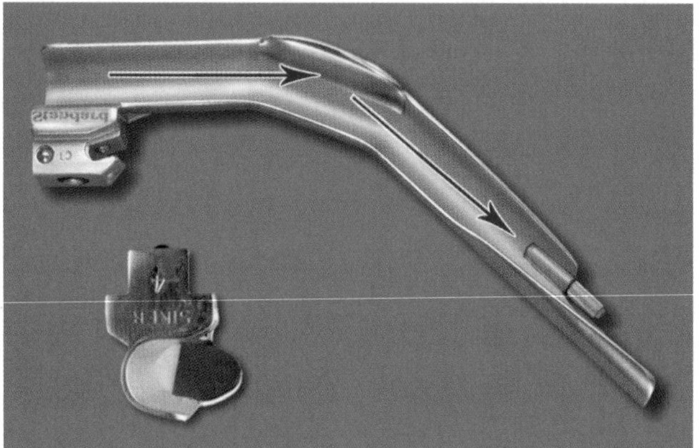

Figure 4.2. The Siker blade has a mirrored surface to reflect glottis structures anterior to the laryngoscopist's line of sight (figure provided by SunMed).

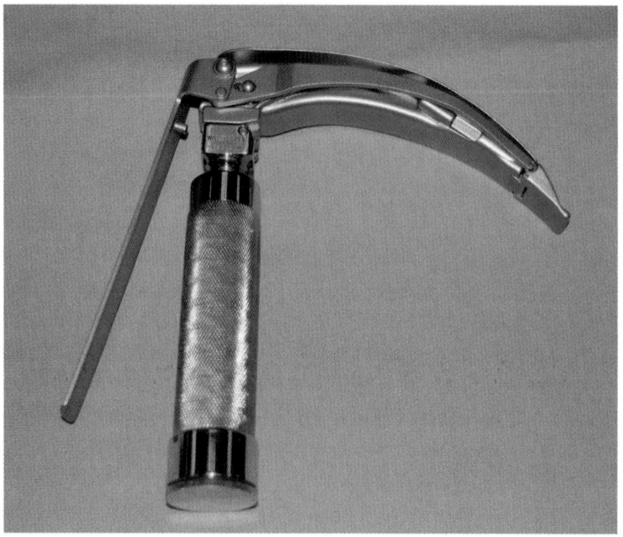

Figure 4.3. The Corazelli, London, McCoy (CLM) blade has an articulating tip to lift tissues directly, possibly minimizing trauma to soft tissues, the cervical spine, or teeth.

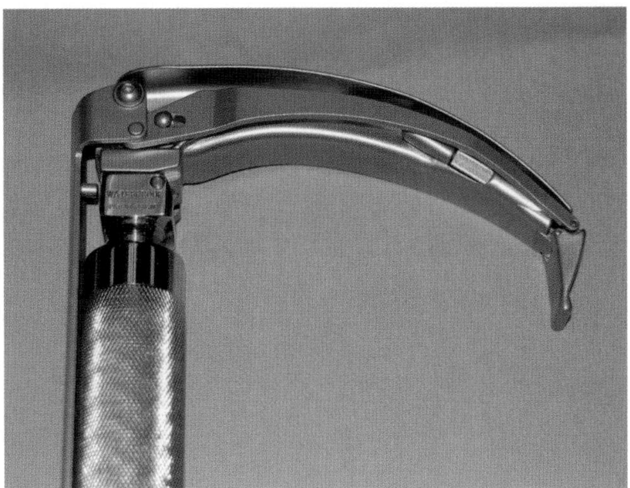

Figure 4.4. The Corazelli, London, McCoy (CLM) blade with the tip flexed.

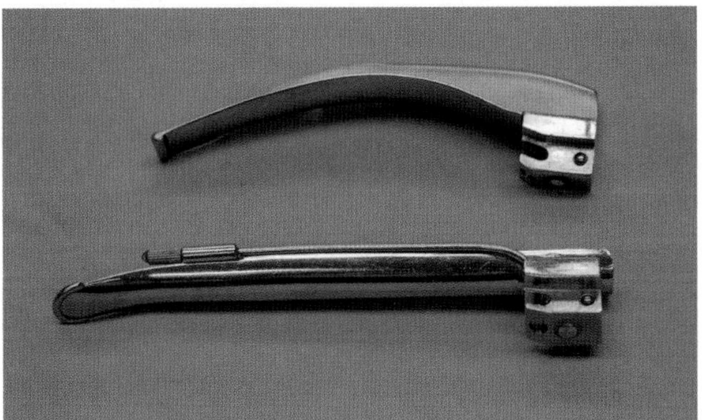

Figure 4.5. Macintosh (*top*) and Miller (*bottom*) blade designs. The web forms the *vertical* profile of the blade and is capped by the *horizontal* flange (the flanges of both blades are perpendicular to the viewer; the Macintosh flange extends into the table, the Miller flange is not visible, but forms the *top* of the partial tube created by the blade). The proximal face of both blades, on the right of the photo, is called the heel.

to retract the tongue from the right side of the mouth and oropharynx. For this reason, some studies find speed and ease of intubation are better with the Macintosh than with the Miller, but the Miller's shape and profile provide a better view of laryngeal structures [3]. The Macintosh design favors indirect epiglottic retraction, whereas the Miller blade is intended to elevate the epiglottis directly, potentially more helpful if an epiglottis is enlarged, stiff, or irregularly shaped. Although the Macintosh and Miller designs are by far the most popular laryngoscope blades [4], these designs are not consistent. Variability in both blade designs has been blamed for poor performance during difficult intubations [5,6].

The Belscope blade is a double-angle blade modification (Figure 4.6). Designed to retract the epiglottis directly, its shape improves the glottic view and minimizes dental contact better than a straight design, at least under some study conditions [7]. The blade can be fitted with a prism for viewing anterior structures. Although literature has reviewed the Belscope blade favorably [8], the device requires considerable experience to master [9].

The CLM design modification (Figures 4.3 and 4.4) features an articulating tip connected to a lever on the laryngoscope handle. It is available in Miller and Macintosh designs. By flexing the tip, the operator can sometimes expose the glottic view with less force to soft tissues, the cervical spine, and teeth [10,11]. However, in some patients the laryngoscopic view is not satisfactory with the CLM [12,13].

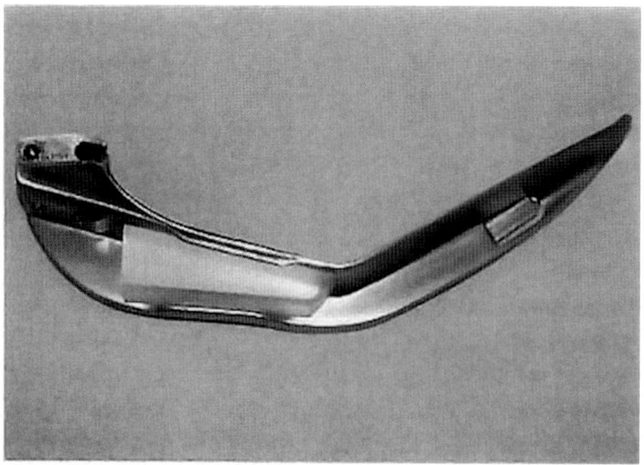

Figure 4.6. Belscope blade with double angle modification, fitted with a prism. This shape is meant to improve the glottis view and minimize dental contact. The tip of the blade is designed to retract the epiglottis directly (from Gajraj NM, Chason DP, Shearer VE, Cervical spine movement during orotracheal intubation: comparison of the Belscope and Macintosh blades. Anaesthesia 1994;49(9):772–4).

Other modifications reduce the height of the step or flange to optimize the glottic view and reduce the risk of dental trauma. These modifications are associated with less force on the teeth [14–17], but may not be as useful with the Miller design [18].

Construction

Reducing infections and cost and keeping light performance consistent have motivated the development of plastic, disposable blades. Some studies have found few problems with plastic blades, [19] others report blade breakage [20, 21], and less intubation success with plastic than with metal blades [22–24].

Lights

The airway is dark and illumination is important for successful laryngoscopy. Thus, good lighting is vital for a difficult intubation. Brightness and other characteristics of lighting influence the operator's view during direct laryngoscopy. Light performance is highly variable between and within blade types: [25] light can be too dim or too bright [26, 27], and subjective assessment of optimal lighting varies substantially [28, 29]. The area of illumination and the spectral characteristics of the light produced are important factors [30]. Xenon and halogen bulbs, used in light-in-handle designs, have higher green and blue light spectra. These, in theory, should provide better contrast illumination than vacuum bulbs in bulb-in-blade designs, which feature more red and yellow spectra [31]. Because no study has examined lighting during actual difficult laryngoscopy, most evidence is speculative.

It seems logical that optimal lighting during a difficult direct laryngoscopy is different from optimal lighting under routine laryngoscopy, and certainly different from lighting for laryngoscopy in mannequins. Vocal folds, lighter than surrounding tissues, should illuminate brighter than other peri-glottic tissues and require less light output for illumination, but when these cannot be adequately visualized, more illumination might be necessary. Adjustable, or at least brighter, light sources might improve the laryngoscopic view during a difficult direct laryngoscopy. This concept remains largely unexplored.

Several factors regarding lighting during a difficult direct laryngoscopy deserve consideration. Although most studies of lighting are performed on mannequins, human tissue has reflectivity properties that can change during difficult direct laryngoscopy. Secretions and blood make good lighting necessary in practice. If the pharynx is full of bloody or thick secretions, better lighting might help the laryngoscopist visualize the dark shape of the glottic opening. A wider field of illumination can reveal peripheral structures even though luminance is sacrificed.

Most blades are battery-powered; their light sources are either bulbs in the blade itself or light in the handle that is transmitted to the tip. With the light in the handle, high heat bulbs pose no risk of burning the patient, are easy to clean, improve the integrity of the bulb-power contacts, and diminish the risks associated with bulb parts falling into the airway. In theory, handle-lit blades offer brighter illumination, but this theory is subject to several practical constraints. First, any given blade will perform differently based on the charge and size of the batteries. Second, bulbs and light optics degrade with time, and blade light performance decreases with use. Fiberoptic laryngoscope blades with external light sources [32] may be particularly useful when intubating through secretions or blood. Single-use blades may offer a reliable lighting profile [26], but present their own risks, as described above. Taking all considerations into account, improving the brightness of a light source could be useful during difficult direct laryngoscopy.

Several manufacturers have begun to use LEDs as the light source. This prolongs the duty cycle with greater illumination, less battery consumption, and heat production as well as a wider range of color choices. Potentially this will result in better tissue illumination and contrast.

Adjuncts to Direct Laryngoscopy

Because laryngoscopy retracts and aligns airway tissues, it can facilitate the use of other airway devices. When a tube cannot be inserted into the trachea under direct laryngoscopy, the skilled laryngoscopist chooses other tools. These include introducers, fiberscopes, or hybrids of the two. Without a direct view of the glottis, these devices facilitate intubation "around the corner" of view-occluding tissues. Adjuncts may be particularly useful if poor visualization is anticipated, or for techniques that require cricoid pressure, which can be associated with a worsened glottic view [33, 34].

Stylets and Introducers

In this context, *stylet* refers to a malleable rod for shaping an endotracheal tube to ease its insertion. *Introducers*, on the other hand, are rigid or semi-rigid rods that are inserted semi-blindly into the trachea before an endotracheal tube is passed over them. Many use the terms "bougie" or "gum elastic bougie" to refer to these devices, inexact terms derived from the history of the devices [35]. Introducers come in a variety of shapes, sizes, and consistencies, but share three common traits of design: an endotracheal tube can be passed over them, their tips are angulated, and they can be bent to some degree. One example of an introducer is the Eschmann introducer, a 15 French rigid polyfiber rod with a blunt tip angulated at 30°. Variations of the introducer have different degrees of malleability at the tip, single-use or multiple-use design, and a hollow working channel.

Some landmarks should be identified before an angled introducer tip is passed into an unseen glottic opening. Classic landmarks include the epiglottis (especially if it is down-folded or large) and the posterior glottic structures described by the Cormack and Lehane grade III or IIb views, respectively. The operator has a sensation of "clicks" as the blunt tip slides across anterior tracheal rings and a "stop" encountered at depths ranging from 30 to 40 cm in average-sized adults [36] as the tip becomes lodged in small bronchi [37].

In investigations, the sensitivity for clicks ranges from 55 to 98%, and the specificity from 80 to 100%. For stops, the sensitivity range is 33–100%, and the specificity ranges from 67 to 100% [38, 39]. Visualization of landmarks increases success. If no recognizable glottic or supraglottic structures are seen, the risk of esophageal intubation is clinically significant. After the introducer is passed, the endotracheal tube can be slid over it into the trachea. As with flexible bronchoscope use, tube passage may be difficult, especially if the tip of the endotracheal tube is lodged on glottic structures. Counterclockwise rotation of the endotracheal tube may help remedy this problem [34]. Placing an introducer correctly is a skill like laryngoscopy, and the intubating clinician should verify final tube placement. Modifications to the introducer technique include capnographic sampling [40] or application of an aspirating device through a working channel to confirm tracheal placement [41]. Use in conjunction with a mirror [42] is also described. Cooling the introducer can decrease tip deformability [43].

Success with introducer use in conjunction with laryngoscopy is high. As a primary intubation strategy, large studies suggest a success rate of 99% or higher [44]. As rescue in the case of a poor laryngoscopic view, success rates range from 75 to 94% [35]. Introducers have been advocated as part of a comprehensive airway management strategy. When used as a backup technique when rigid laryngoscopy had failed, success with the introducer was 91% though first-pass success was achieved in only half the cases; they have also been advocated in intubation plans for patients with a receding chin [45, 46].

It has been argued that success rates with single-use introducers are lower than multiple-use devices [47, 48]. Conversely, cracks and deformities on multiple-use introducers limit the number of times they can be re-used [49, 50]. Inline cervical stabilization may decrease success with the technique [51]. Although the tip is blunt, there is a risk of soft tissue trauma when an introducer is passed. Holding the shaft closer to the tip may increase the force applied and the subsequent risk of complications [52].

Hybrid fiberoptic optical stylets have a variety of designs. Examples of such devices are the Bonfils (Karl Storz), Clarus Video System, Shikani SOS (Clarus Medical), Levitan FPS (Clarus Medical), and the SensaScope (Acutronic). These are discussed in detail in Chap. 9. They are useful adjuncts to direct laryngoscopy, enabling the operator to see around tissues and maneuver the endotracheal tube under visual control. Figure 4.7 demonstrates the use of a fiberoptic stylet in the setting of difficult direct laryngoscopy.

Laryngoscope Optical Modifications

The Truview EVO_2™ combines a 15 mm optical viewport with a direct laryngoscope to facilitate the laryngeal exposure. This can be connected to a digital camera. This is a low cost portable device that combines some aspects of a videolaryngoscope with a rigid laryngoscope. Intubation with the Truview EVO™ blade led to a better laryngoscopic view, less application of force to the soft tissues of the neck, but increased time to intubation in comparison with the Macintosh blade in adult patients. This device is discussed in greater detail in Chap. 5 [53].

Technique of Direct Laryngoscopy

Patient positioning is a key component of successful direct laryngoscopy. Patient physiology and comorbidities, however, influence the laryngoscopist's choice of patient position and affect the success of direct laryngoscopy. In the setting of difficulty, position modifications can facilitate an improved glottic view.

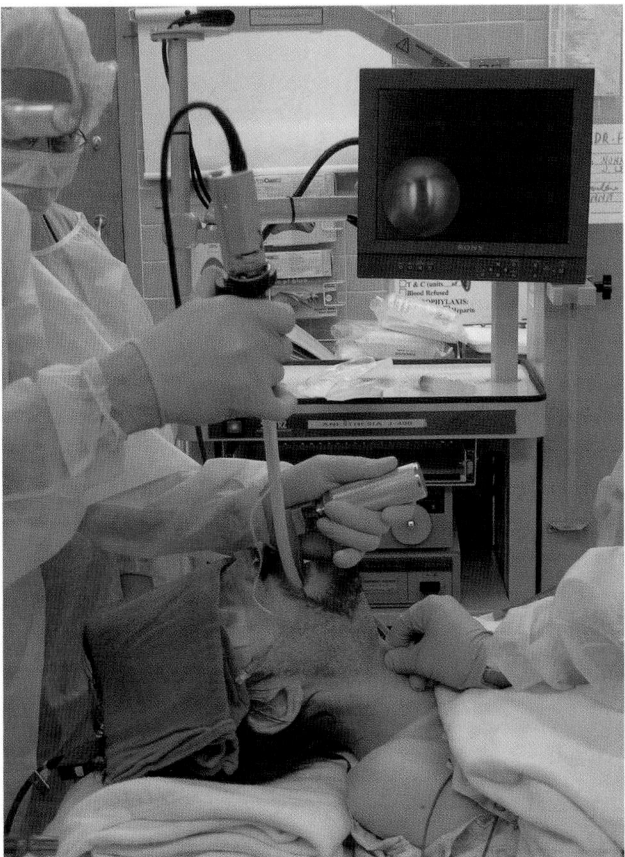

Figure 4.7. Fiberoptic stylet used with direct laryngoscopy for a difficult airway. The stylet can be fitted to a camera, as is shown here. Without a good traditional laryngoscopic view, the laryngoscopist can visualize the glottis opening and pass the tube under visual control.

Sniffing Position

The sniffing position is generally advocated for patient positioning during direct laryngoscopy. Evidence supporting the sniffing position as the best for direct laryngoscopy is lacking. It involves a combination of occipito-atlanto-axial extension and neck flexion, theoretically aligning the visual axis from oropharynx to glottis. It seems unlikely that a true sniffing position is achieved in the majority of the patients undergoing direct laryngoscopy. Although this line of sight is often not achieved [54], a difficult intubation is a rare phenomenon [2]. Some argue that the sniffing position does not represent the ideal condition for direct laryngoscopy.

Head Extension

As one component of the sniffing position, head extension may be sufficient and no worse for direct laryngoscopy in nonobese patients [55]. In fact, simple head extension is the only patient positioning needed for many patients.

Neck Flexion

Another component of the sniffing position is neck flexion. Several studies have suggested that the laryngeal view may be improved with head elevation and resultant neck flexion [56, 57]. Neck flexion at the cervicothoracic vertebrae was associated with a better laryngeal

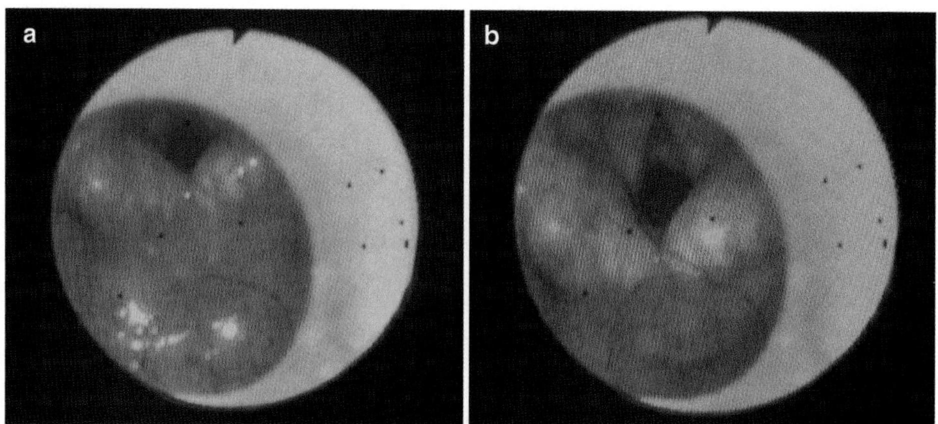

Figure 4.8. Visualization of the glottis opening before (**a**) and after (**b**) neck flexion using a Macintosh blade fitted with a camera. Flexion allows visualization of all of the glottis structures.

view during direct laryngoscopy. Head elevation with resultant cervicothoracic neck flexion may provide the laryngoscopist with a better view than the traditional sniffing position, especially in obese patients [58]. Figure 4.8 shows the glottic view before (4.8a) and after (4.8b) neck flexion.

Obesity and the Sniffing Position

The sniffing position makes assumptions about typical anatomy that may not hold for obese patients. Placing a pillow under a supine patient's head may be sufficient to achieve head extension and neck flexion in a patient of normal body habitus, but not in the obese patient. Additional mass and tissue in the chest and abdomen interfere with direct laryngoscopy in the supine position. It is difficult to manipulate an obese patient's neck, clearance for the laryngoscope handle is minimal, and neck flexion is difficult in a supine obese patient. Obese patients are more likely to benefit from elevation of shoulders and head with a ramp-like support (Figure 4.9). The ramp is created with multiple blankets arranged to elevate the head and upper thorax. This position displaces the chest for better external neck manipulation and clearance for the handle of the laryngoscope. The ramped position may be superior to the sniffing position for direct laryngoscopy in obese patients [58]. A preformed ramp (the Troop pillow) is also available to facilitate positioning of obese patients for intubation (Figure 4.10).

Building a ramp of blankets before direct laryngoscopy of an obese patient may improve the laryngoscopic view and intubation but lead to problems afterwards. A blanket ramp remaining during a surgical procedure might interfere with surgical exposure or predispose to positioning injuries. Brachial plexus injuries may result when the chest is elevated and arms hyper-extended. Therefore, it is prudent to remove the additional blankets and padding after an airway is secured. Removal can be a sizeable and physically demanding task. Most modern operating room tables feature motorized patient positioning. In one study, a combination of flexion of an obese patient at the torso/thigh section and then elevation of the back of the bed was equivalent to a classic ramp built of blankets [59]. Such a technique shifts the physical burden of patient positioning from hospital staff to the motorized bed.

Laryngeal Manipulation

Posterior displacement of the cricoid cartilage, the Sellick maneuver, is designed to prevent reflux of gastrointestinal contents during induction of anesthesia and direct laryngoscopy [60]. Regurgitation issues aside, cricoid manipulation may improve or worsen the view

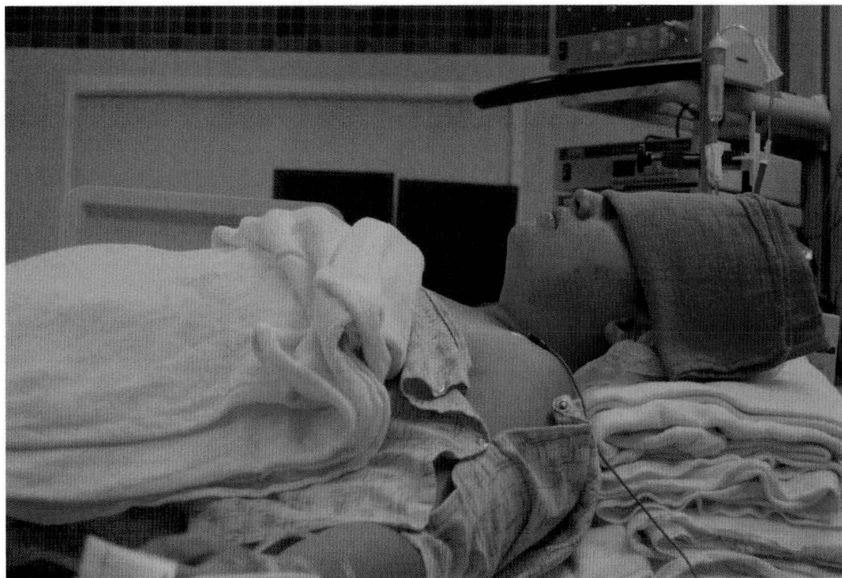

Figure 4.9. Ramp support of an obese patient. Blankets under the shoulders position the head and thorax to optimize laryngoscopic visualization. Notice the sternal notch and external auditory meatus are aligned in a *horizontal* plane.

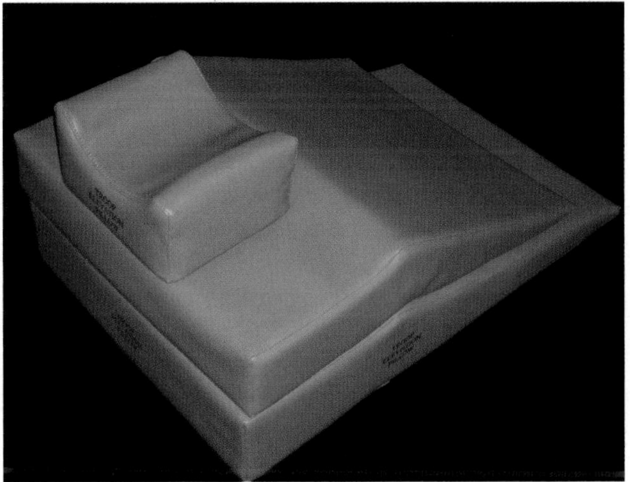

Figure 4.10. Troop pillow. The pillow is designed to facilitate positioning of obese patients for optimal larygoscopy (CR Enterprises, LLC, Frisco, Texas).

during direct laryngoscopy. Arytenoids or vocal cords once initially too anterior for direct vision can be displaced posteriorly into view. On the other hand, cricoid pressure applied with too much force can worsen the view. The force necessary during the Sellick maneuver is sufficient to compress the esophagus, but also airway structures, hampering identification of anatomical landmarks. It may also tilt the laryngeal axis making it more anterior. It is important to recognize this possibility, because many laryngoscopies planned with cricoid pressure are rapid sequence intubations with limited time before oxygen desaturation.

It is important to distinguish between "cricoid pressure" and "optimal external laryngeal manipulation." Failure to do so leads to confusion on the purpose of these respective maneuvers and may result in neither achieving its intended goal. Laryngeal manipulation is one technique for improving the laryngoscopist's view of airway structures during laryngoscopy. The manipulation can be performed by the laryngoscopist with the free hand. Alternatively, an assistant manipulates the larynx under the direction of the laryngoscopist. In another external laryngeal manipulation, bimanual laryngoscopy, the operator manipulates the larynx externally, while assessing the impact on the view during the laryngoscopy. An assistant then holds the best position while the operator passes the endotracheal tube. Laryngeal manipulation is a trial and error process, although some maneuvers are associated with an improved view. The "BURP" (*B*ackward *U*pward *R*ightward *P*ressure) maneuver has been described as a helpful technique [61]. In the BURP maneuver, posterior pressure is applied with superior and lateral pressure. Application of the BURP maneuver improved laryngoscopic visualization in some studies [62]. In another the BURP maneuver and cricoid pressure worsened laryngoscopic views during direct laryngoscopy, whereas bimanual laryngoscopy improved laryngeal view [63].

Cervical Spine Injury

The risks of direct laryngoscopy maneuvers are minimal in a patient with normal anatomy. The risk/benefit analysis is less clear in patients with potential or diagnosed cervical spine injuries. The rate of secondary neurologic injury and its causes in cervical spine-injured patients is not known. No mechanism for secondary neurologic injury due to airway management has been clearly defined. Decreasing cervical spine motion during laryngoscopy of injured patients, although intuitive, has not been demonstrated to prevent secondary neurologic injury, but can make direct laryngoscopy more difficult. Collective experience worldwide with multiple techniques in the airway management of cervical spine injuries has not shown an appreciable number of secondary neurologic injuries attributable to airway management. Nonetheless, most practitioners attempt to minimize spine motion during laryngoscopy in these patients.

Numerous studies have sought to clarify the anatomical ramifications of typical airway management maneuvers. Some studies have used cadavers; others have assessed anatomic changes in living patients. In fact, there is evidence that simply performing a "jaw thrust," or cricoid pressure on a patient causes more cervical spine motion than direct laryngoscopy [64, 65]. It is not easy to assess the anatomic changes to a cervical spine during direct laryngoscopy. The force exerted and how it varies among operators using similar techniques are potential confounders in any study. All injuries of the cervical spine are not alike, and the nature and location of the pathology have an impact on a potential injury during direct laryngoscopy. Therefore, the "safest" technique for intubation in patients with cervical spine injuries is unknown. Despite this uncertainty, available data suggest a low rate of secondary neurologic injury.

The impact of different laryngoscope blade types on cervical anatomy, although studied, is also not certain. One study suggests that the Miller blade results in less axial distraction of the cervical spine during direct laryngoscopy than the Macintosh blade [66]. Another study failed to find a difference between the effects of the two [67]. The clinical implications of any potential differences of laryngoscope blades for patients with cervical spine injuries are difficult to determine. No study has been designed in a clinically representative population, and therefore data are only suggestive. More than the laryngoscope blade, the experience of the laryngoscopist and the anatomic factors influencing the laryngoscopic view are more important considerations.

Efforts to minimize potential motion of the cervical spine during a typical direct laryngoscopy include axial traction, manual inline stabilization, or both. An orotracheal intubation by direct laryngoscopy will cause craniocervical extension between the C1 and C2 vertebrae [68]. Both axial traction and manual inline stabilization seek to oppose this potential craniocervical extension. Axial traction is classically applied in a cephalad direction by an assistant with enough force to stabilize the cervical spine. The necessary amount of force is ambiguous and completely dependent on the assistant. Furthermore, traction likely has differing effects on the injured cervical spine depending on the mechanism and location of injury. There is evidence that it has potential for causing a secondary neurologic injury. Axial traction caused both subluxation and increased distraction in a series of cadavers with lethal trauma and cervical spine injury [69]. As a result, axial traction is no longer recommended as an adjunct to direct laryngoscopy in a cervical spine injury patient.

Manual inline stabilization is another technique designed to minimize the risk of secondary neurologic injury during direct laryngoscopy of the patient with a cervical spine injury. Manual inline stabilization is typically performed by an assistant either at the head or the side of the bed, exerting a downward force on the patient's mastoid processes. This maneuver ensures that the patient's head is not lifted during direct laryngoscopy. Although studies of manual inline stabilization have been limited by the availability of a suitable study population and variability in technique and injury, it appears that inline stabilization lessens spine movement. Manual inline stabilization resulted in less spine movement during direct laryngoscopy than did no stabilization, or stabilization with a rigid neck collar [67]. Correlation with reduced secondary neurologic injury is lacking.

A lack of proven benefit of manual inline stabilization has led some to question its utility as a routine measure during airway management of a patient with a potential cervical spine injury. Although it is technically easy to perform, the technique may cause additional morbidity during airway management. It is associated with a need for greater lifting force [70] and has the potential to worsen the view during direct laryngoscopy [71]. A difficult intubation because of a sub-optimal laryngeal view with manual inline stabilization increases the chances of oxygen desaturation, hypoxemia, and a lost airway in a patient who may have a neurologic injury. If manual inline stabilization interferes with intubation via direct laryngoscopy, consideration should be given to alternative techniques that do not require direct vision or as much manipulation in order to minimize neck movement. These may demand special skill or equipment and take more time than direct laryngoscopy. If urgency, personnel, or equipment considerations indicate direct laryngoscopy, allowing some neck movement for improved laryngeal view may be justified. Given a choice between less movement of the cervical spine and the ability to successfully secure the airway, the latter choice is more prudent.

Cervical spine injury patients will often be placed in a rigid neck collar to restrict neck movement. Such collars present numerous challenges during direct laryngoscopy, and indeed, may be used as an experimental means of creating a more challenging intubation [72]. They can restrict the patient's mouth opening, complicating the introduction of a laryngoscope blade and worsening the laryngeal view. The rigid collar also becomes a possible laryngoscope fulcrum potentiating a secondary neurologic injury [66].

Techniques for Difficult Laryngoscopy

The typical technique for direct laryngoscopy involves a midline approach with the laryngoscope blade. Alternative techniques such as the paraglossal and retromolar approach have been suggested as useful for difficult direct laryngoscopies. The paraglossal approach places the laryngoscope blade off midline beside the tongue. As the blade is advanced, the tip is angled medially, and anterior force is applied. This technique may have benefit when a midline approach might not displace the tongue and soft palate tissue sufficiently to expose the glottis. An additional modification to the paraglossal approach is retromolar laryngoscopy, in which the patient's head is turned to the left while the laryngoscope blade is maintained over the patient's molars. An endotracheal tube may be more difficult to pass with the retromolar approach, and an assistant may be needed to retract the side of the patient's mouth [73].

The paraglossal and retromolar approaches are traditionally described with a straight laryngoscope blade introduced from the right side. A left-sided approach for the paraglossal and retromolar techniques with a curved blade has also been described. The left-sided method has been advocated as superior to a right-sided approach when a curved blade is used, but this opinion is not universally shared [74]. Despite this assertion, others have found that successfully placing an endotracheal tube with the left paraglossal or retromolar approach is difficult [75]. The decision to use one approach over the others ultimately becomes one of personal preference and comfort for the laryngoscopist.

Complications

In the setting of difficult direct laryngoscopy, the risk of complications increases. In a large series of surgical patients, dental injuries increased with an odds ratio of 11 [76]. Emergency intubation has been associated with increased risk of tracheal rupture [77]. Arytenoid cartilage dislocation [78] and hypopharyngeal perforation [79] are also associated with intubation; it is likely that the same factors increase the risks of these injuries as well. Pharyngeal or tracheal injuries with introducer stylets are possible [80], as is pulmonary hemorrhage [81], and likely pneumothorax, although available literature is scant [82]. The ultimate complication of difficult direct laryngoscopy is loss of the airway, making both the mastery of other techniques and decision skills in abandoning unsuccessful laryngoscopy critical.

Conclusion

Laryngoscopy remains a mainstay of airway management, in spite of an increasing number of alternative airway management tools. Difficult direct laryngoscopy is not a contraindication to continuing with the technique *per se*, though caution must be exercised to avoid repetition of unproductive efforts and the application of increasing force in an effort to achieve better laryngeal exposure. Such an approach may increase the risk of converting a cannot intubate situation into a cannot ventilate one. Knowledge of factors influencing and methods of improving laryngoscopic success is important for expertise in airway management. Unexpected difficulties can arise from airway masses (especially lingual tonsils), blood or secretions, positioning considerations, cricoid pressure, or cervical spine precautions. Blade selection, bright or adjustable lighting, adjuncts, careful positioning, and alternative laryngoscopic approaches are all methods to increase the success of the most common intubating technique in use today.

References

1. Burkle CM, Walsh MT, Harrison BA, et al. Airway management after failure to intubate by direct laryngoscopy: outcomes in a large teaching hospital. Can J Anaesth. 2005;52:634–40.
2. Ovassapian A, Glassenberg R, Randel GI, et al. The unexpected difficult airway and lingual tonsil hyperplasia: a case series and a review of the literature. Anesthesiology. 2002;97:124–32.
3. Arino JJ, Velasco JM, Gasco C, Lopez-Timoneda F. Straight blades improve visualization of the larynx while curved blades increase ease of intubation: a comparison of the Macintosh, Miller, McCoy, Belscope and Lee-Fiberview blades. Can J Anaesth. 2003;50:501–6.
4. Maleck WH, Koetter KP, Lenz M, et al. A randomized comparison of three laryngoscopes with the Macintosh. Resuscitation. 1999;42:241–5.
5. Asai T, Matsumoto S, Fujise K, et al. Comparison of two Macintosh laryngoscope blades in 300 patients. Br J Anaesth. 2003;90:457–60.
6. Raw D, Skinner A. Miller laryngoscope blades (correspondence). Anaesthesia. 1999;54:500.
7. Bellhouse CP. An angulated laryngoscope for routine and difficult tracheal intubation. Anesthesiology. 1988;69:126–99.
8. Watanabe S, Suga A, Asakura N, et al. Determination of the distance between the laryngoscope blade and the upper incisors during direct laryngoscopy: comparison of a curved, and angulated straight, and two straight blades. Anesth Analg. 1994;79:638–41.

9. Hodges UM, O'Flaherty D, Adams AP. Tracheal intubation in a manikin: comparison of the Belscope with the Macintosh laryngoscope. Br J Anaesth. 1993;71:905–7.
10. McCoy EP, Mirakhur RK, Rafferty C, et al. A comparison of the forces exerted during laryngoscopy. The Macintosh versus the McCoy blade. Anaesthesia. 1996;51:912–5.
11. Haridas RP. The McCoy levering laryngoscope blade. Anaesthesia. 1996;51:91.
12. Cook TM, Tuckey JP. A comparison between the Macintosh and the McCoy laryngoscope blades. Anaesthesia. 1996;51:977–80.
13. Iohom G, Franklin R, Casey W, et al. The McCoy straight blade does not improve laryngoscopy and intubation in normal infants. Can J Anaesth. 2004;51:155–9.
14. Bucx MJL, Snijders CJ, van der Vegt MH, et al. Reshaping the Macintosh blade using biomechanical modeling. Anaesthesia. 1997;52:662–7.
15. Gerlach K, Wenzel V, von Knobelsdorff G, et al. A new universal laryngoscope blade: a preliminary comparison with Macintosh laryngoscope blades. Resuscitation. 2003;57:63–7.
16. Lee J, Choi JH, Lee YK, et al. The Callander laryngoscope blade modification is associated with a decreased risk of dental contact. Can J Anaesth. 2004;51:181–4.
17. Mireskandari S-M, Asjaruzadeh N, Darabi M-E, et al. The Callendar modification of the Macintosh laryngoscope blade reduces the risk of tooth-blade contact in children. Pediatr Anaesth. 2008;18:1035–9.
18. Kimberger O, Fischer L, Plank C, et al. Lower flange modification improves performance of the Macintosh, but not the Miller laryngoscope blade. Can J Anaesth. 2006;53:595–601.
19. Galinski M, Adner F, Tran D, et al. Disposable laryngoscope blades do not interfere with ease of intubation in scheduled general anaesthesia patients. Eur J Anaesth. 2003;20:731–5.
20. Itoman EM, Kajioka EH, Loren G, et al. Dental fracture risk of metal vs plastic laryngoscope blades in dental models. Am J Emerg Med. 2005;23:186–9.
21. Jefferson P, Perkins V, Edwards VA, et al. Problems with disposal laryngoscope blade (correspondence). Anaesthesia. 2003;58:385–6.
22. Armour J, Mermion F, Birenbaum A, et al. Comparison of plastic single-use and metal reusable laryngoscope blades for orotracheal intubation during rapid sequence induction of anesthesia. Anesthesiology. 2006;104:60–4.
23. Twigg SJ, McCormick B, Cook TM. Randomized evaluation of the performance of single-use laryngoscopes in simulated easy and difficult intubation. Br J Anaesth. 2003;90:8–13.
24. Jabre P, Leroux B, Brohon S, et al. A comparison of plastic single-use with metallic reusable laryngoscope blades for out-of-hospital tracheal intubation. Ann Emerg Med. 2007;50:258–63.
25. Levitan RM, Kelly JJ, Kinkle WC, et al. Light intensity of curved laryngoscope blades in Philadelphia emergency departments. Ann Emerg Med. 2007;50:253–7.
26. Howes BJ. The reliability of laryngoscope lights. Anaesthesia. 2006;61:488–91.
27. Malan CA, Wilkes AR, Hall JE, et al. An evaluation of the filtration performance of paediatric breathing system filters at low flows. Anaesthesia. 2007;62:644.
28. Scholz A, Faqrnum N, Wilkes AR, et al. Minimum and optimum light output of Macintosh size 3 laryngoscopy blades: a manikin study. Anaesthesia. 2007;62:163–8.
29. Malan CA, Scholz A, Wilkes AR, et al. Minimum and optimum light requirements for laryngoscopy in paediatric anaesthesia: a manikin study. Anaesthesia. 2008;63:65–70.
30. Tousignant G, Tessler MJ. Light intensity and area of illumination provided by various laryngoscope blades. Can J Anaesth. 1994;41:865–9.
31. Crosby E, Cleland M. An assessment of the luminance and light field characteristics of used direct laryngoscopes. Can J Anaesth. 1999;46:792–6.
32. Arthurs GJ. Fibre-optically lit laryngoscope. Anaesthesia. 1999;54:873–4.
33. Noguchi T, Koga K, Shkiga Y, et al. The gum elastic bougie eases tracheal intubation while applying cricoid pressure compared to a stylet. Can J Anaesth. 2003;50:712–7.
34. McNelis U, Syndercombe A, Harper J, et al. The effect of cricoid pressure on intubation facilitated by the gum elastic bougie. Anaesthesia. 2007;62:456–9.
35. Henderson JJ. Development of the 'gum-elastic bougie'. Anaesthesia. 2003;58:103–4.
36. Jabre P, Combes X, Leroux B, et al. Use of gum elastic bougie for prehospital difficult intubation. Am J Emerg Med. 2005;23:552–5.
37. Kidd JF, Dyson A, Latto P. Successful difficult intubation. Anaesthesia. 1988;43:437–8.
38. Bair AE, Laurin EG, Schmitt BJ. An assessment of a tracheal tube introducer as an endotracheal tube placement confirmation device. Am J Emerg Med. 2005;23:754–8.
39. Shah KH, Kwong BM, Hazan A, et al. Success of the gum elastic bougie as a rescue airway in the emergency department. J Emerg Med. 2011;40(1):1–6.
40. Green DW. Gum elastic bougie and simulated difficult intubation. Anaesthesia. 2003;58:391–2.

41. Kadry T, Harvey M, Wallace M, et al. Frova intubating catheter position can be determined with aspirating oesophageal detection device. Emerg Med Australas. 2007;19:203–6.
42. Weisenberg M, Warters D, Medalion B. Endotracheal intubation with a gum-elastic bougie in unanticipated difficult direct laryngoscopy: comparison of a blind technique versus indirect laryngoscopy with a laryngeal mirror. Anesth Analg. 2002;95:1091–3.
43. Mingo O, Suaris P, Charman S, et al. The effect of temperature on bougies: a photographic and manikin study. Anaesthesia. 2008;63:1135–8.
44. Latto IP, Stacey M, Mecklenburgh J, et al. Survey of the use of the gum elastic bougie in clinical practice. Anaesthesia. 2002;57:379–84.
45. Combes X, LeRoux B, Dumerat M, et al. Unanticipated difficult airway in anesthetized patients: prospective validation of a management algorithm. Anesthesiology. 2004;100:1146–50.
46. Semjen F, Bordes M, Cros A-M. Intubation of infant with Pierre Robin syndrome: the use of the paraglossal approach combined with a gum-elastic bougie in six consecutive cases. Anaesthesia. 2008;63:147–50.
47. Annamaneni R, Hodzovic I, Wilkes AR, Latto IP. A comparison of simulated difficult intubation with multiple-use and single-use bougies in a manikin. Anaesthesia. 2003;53:45–9.
48. Marfin AG, Pandit JJ, Hames KC, et al. Use of the bougie in simulated difficult intubation. II. Comparison of single-use bougie with multiple-use bougie. Anaesthesia. 2003;58:852–5.
49. Latto P. Fracture of the outer varnish layer of a gum elastic bougie. Anaesthesia. 1999;54:497–8.
50. Kumar DS, Jones G. Is your bougie helping or hindering you? Anaesthesia. 2001;56:1121.
51. Kim DK, Kim H-K, Lee KM, et al. Poor performance of the pediatric airway exchange catheter in adults with cervical spine immobilization. Can J Anaesth. 2008;55:748–53.
52. Hodzovic I, Wilkes AR, Latto IP. Bougie-assisted difficult airway management in a manikin—the effect of position held on placement and force exerted by the tip. Anaesthesia. 2004;59:38–43.
53. Barak M, Philipchuck P, Abecassis P, Katz Y. A comparison of the Truview blade with the Macintosh blade in adult patients. Anesthesia. 2007;62:827–31.
54. Shiga T, Wajima Z, Inoue T, Sakamoto A. Predicting difficult intubation in apparently normal patients: a meta-analysis of bedside screening test performance. Anesthesiology. 2005;103:429–37.
55. Adnet F, Baillard C, Boron SW, et al. Randomized study comparing the "sniffing position" with simple head extension for laryngoscopic view in elective surgery patients. Anesthesiology. 2001;95:836–41.
56. Levitan RM, Mechem CC, Ochroch EA, Shofer FS, Hollander JE. Head-elevated laryngoscopy position: improving laryngeal exposure during laryngoscopy by increasing head elevation. Ann Emerg Med. 2003;41:322–30.
57. Schmitt HJ, Mang H. Head and neck elevation beyond the sniffing position improves laryngeal view in cases of difficulty direct laryngoscopy. J Clin Anesth. 2002;4:335–8.
58. Collins JS, Lemmens HJ, Brodsky JB, et al. Laryngoscopy and morbid obesity: a comparison of the "sniff" and "ramped" positions. Obes Surg. 2004;14:1171–5.
59. Rao SL, Kunselman AR, Schuler HG, DesHarnais S. Laryngoscopy and tracheal intubation in the head-elevated position in obese patients: a randomized, controlled, equivalence trial. Anesth Analg. 2008;107:1912–8.
60. Sellick BA. Cricoid pressure to control regurgitation of stomach contents during induction of anaesthesia. Lancet. 1961;2:404–6.
61. Knill RL. Difficult laryngoscopy made easy with a BURP. Can J Anaesth. 1993;40:279–82.
62. Takahata O, Kubota M, Mamiya K, et al. The efficacy of the "BURP" maneuver during a difficult laryngoscopy. Anesth Analg. 1997;84:419–21.
63. Levitan RM, Kinkle WC, Levin WJ, Everett WW. Laryngeal view during laryngoscopy: a randomized trial comparing cricoid pressure, backward-upward-rightward pressure, and bimanual laryngoscopy. Ann Emerg Med. 2006;47:548–55.
64. Donaldson 3rd WF, Heil BV, Donaldson VP, et al. The effect of airway maneuvers on the unstable C1-C2 segment. A cadaver study. Spine. 1997;22:1215–8.
65. Donaldson 3rd WF, Towers JD, Doctor A, et al. A methodology to evaluate motion of the unstable spine during intubation techniques. Spine. 1993;18:2020–3.
66. Gerling MC, Davis DP, Hamilton RS, et al. Effects of cervical spine immobilization technique and laryngoscope blade selection on an unstable cervical spine in a cadaver model of intubation. Ann Emerg Med. 2000;36:293–300.

67. Majernick TG, Bieniek R, Houston JB, Hughes HG. Cervical spine movement during orotracheal intubation. Ann Emerg Med. 1986;15:417–20.
68. Legrand S, Hindman BJ, Franklin D, et al. Craniocervical motion during direct laryngoscopy and orotracheal intubation with the Macintosh and Miller blades. Anesthesiology. 2007;107:884–91.
69. Bivins HG, Ford S, Bezmalinovic Z, Price HM, Williams JL. The effect of axial traction during orotracheal intubation of the trauma victim with an unstable cervical spine. Ann Emerg Med. 1988;17:25–9.
70. Santoni BGPD, Hindman BJMD, Puttlitz CMPD, Weeks JBMPT, Johnson NBS, Maktabi MAMD, et al. Manual in-line stabilization increases pressures applied by the laryngoscope blade during direct laryngoscopy and orotracheal intubation. Anesthesiology. 2009;110:24–31.
71. Heath KJ. The effect on laryngoscopy of different cervical spine immobilisation techniques. Anaesthesia. 1994;49:843–5.
72. Agro F, Barzoi G, Montecchia F. Tracheal intubation using a Macintosh laryngoscope or a GlideScoope® in 15 patients with cervical spine immobilization. Br J Anaesth. 2003;90:705.
73. Henderson JJ. The use of paraglossal straight blade laryngoscopy in difficult tracheal intubation. Anaesthesia. 1997;52:552–60.
74. Yamamoto K, Tsubokawa T, Ohmura S, Itoh H, Kobayashi T. Left-molar approach improves the laryngeal view in patients with difficult laryncoscopy. Anesthesiology. 2000;92:70–4.
75. Cuvas O, Basar H, Gursoy N, Culhaoglu S, Demir A. Left-molar approach for direct laryngoscopy: is it easy? J Anesth. 2009;23:36–40.
76. Warner ME, Benenfeld SM, Warner MA, et al. Perianesthetic dental injuries: frequency, outcomes, and risk factors. Anesthesiology. 1999;90:1302–5.
77. Miñambres E, Burón J, Ballesteros MA, et al. Tracheal rupture after endotracheal intubation: a literature systematic review. Eur J Cardiothorac Surg. 2009;35:1056–62.
78. Rubin AD, Hawkshaw MJ, Moyer CA, et al. Arytenoid cartilage dislocation: a 20 year-experience. J Voice. 2005;19:687–701.
79. Hawkins DB, Seltzer DC, Barnett TE, et al. Endotracheal tube perforation of the hypopharynx. West J Med. 1974;120:282–6.
80. Arndt GA, Cambray AJ, Tomasson J. Intubation bougie dissection of tracheal mucosa and intratracheal airway obstruction. Anesth Analg. 2008;7:603–4.
81. Hosking E, Morris EA, Johnson CJ. Assessing the difficult airway. Anaesthesia. 2003;58:811.
82. Hodzovic I, Latto IP, Henderson JJ. Bougie trauma—what trauma? Anaesthesia. 2003; 58:192–3.

5

The Role of Rigid Fiberoptic Laryngoscopes

Richard M. Cooper

Introduction

Direct laryngoscopy (DL) has seen no substantive advances since its introduction by Janeway[1] or modifications by Miller[2] and Macintosh[3]. The difficulty in seeing around the corner beyond the tip of the laryngoscope blade has been a persistent challenge in a limited, but often unpredicted group of patients. The new possibilities offered by fiberoptics and embedded miniature video cameras may enable us to overcome many of the limitations of the direct line-of-sight.

R.M. Cooper (✉)
Department of Anesthesia, University of Toronto, Toronto General Hospital, Toronto, Canada

Department of Anesthesia and Pain Management, Ontario, Canada, M5G 2C4
e-mail: richard.cooper@uhn.ca

D.B. Glick et al. (eds.), *The Difficult Airway: An Atlas of Tools and Techniques for Clinical Management*, DOI 10.1007/978-0-387-92849-4_5, © Springer Science+Business Media New York 2013

Limitations of Direct (Line-of-Sight) Laryngoscopy

The sniffing position was intended to align the axes of the mouth, pharynx, and trachea[4] but this contention has recently been challenged[5–7]. Adnet and colleagues have suggested that neither the sniffing position nor simple extension actually achieves this objective[8,9]. Yet generally direct (line-of-sight) laryngoscopy does provide a partial or complete view of the larynx. How do we achieve this? We do so by exerting force on the soft and skeletal tissues, distracting and compressing the tongue, displacing the mandible anteriorly, elevating the epiglottis, and occasionally applying external force to the anterior neck.

A number of studies involving non-obstetrical, adult patients reveal the extent of the problem. We unexpectedly fail to achieve a view of the larynx in 6–10% of laryngoscopies [10–12]. An Intubation Difficulty Score was developed, incorporating seven parameters including laryngeal exposure, the number of attempts, and a requirement for ancillary equipment. A score of >5, signifying a moderate or major difficulty, was unexpectedly encountered in 6.3% and 16% of intubations performed inside and outside the OR respectively[13,14]. External laryngeal manipulation (ELM) was required in 23% of cases to bring the larynx into view; more than three laryngoscopies were performed in 3% of intubations. The lowest IDS was seen in a surprisingly low 55% of attempted intubations and minor intubation difficulties were very common (37% of 1,170). Overall, moderate, or major difficulties were seen in 8% of adult laryngoscopies. Rose and Cohen found that difficulties with direct laryngoscopy were most commonly dealt with by repeated attempts. These were significantly associated with hypoxia, trauma, and unanticipated ICU admission[15]. Adnet found that a higher IDS was associated with longer laryngoscopy times and greater perceived difficulty by the operator[13]. More than two attempts at laryngoscopy are associated with additional risk of serious complications, including hypoxemia, bradycardia, regurgitation, and aspiration[16]. When laryngoscopy is difficult, we often use more force and make repeated efforts.

Rigid Fiberoptic Laryngoscopes

In 1968 a flexible fiberoptic endoscope was first used in the airway. It could navigate tortuous pathways, obviating the need for the anatomical axial alignment or the soft tissue compression or distraction required by direct laryngoscopy. But it was not intended primarily for intubation and required a different set of skills. Several rigid fiberoptic devices specifically for intubation appeared. These still required a new skill set, and although they lacked the versatility of the flexible scope, they provided protection for the fragile fiberoptic elements and a view of the vocal folds throughout the intubation. These included devices such as the UpsherScope (UL), the Bullard (BL), and the WuScope (WS). These all have optical eyepieces but when coupled with video cameras, they became the progenitors of video laryngoscopes. These are task-specific devices—laryngoscopy and intubation. None can be passed through a tracheotomy or nasal passage; neither can they be used to position a bronchial blocker or endobronchial tube nor perform pulmonary toilet. The BL was introduced in 1988; the UL and WS arrived shortly after. While some have strong advocates, they are few[17–19]. These tools require an investment of time to become competent. Increasingly, they are challenged by newer, easier to use and more familiar devices. In fact, the UpsherScope (Mercury Medical, Clearwater FL) and the WuScope (Achi Corporation, Freemont CA) have recently been withdrawn from the market and will be mentioned only briefly.

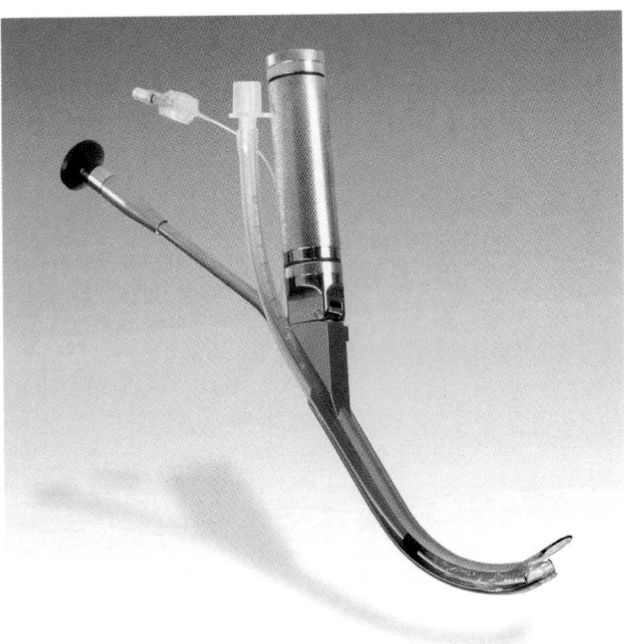

Figure 5.1. The UpsherScope Ultra, now discontinued, is shown with a battery handle attachment. An endotracheal tube is positioned in the tube slot. A video camera can be attached to the eyepiece.

UpsherScope[20–23]

The UL or its successor the UpsherScope Ultra™ represent the simplest design of this class, consisting of a fully immersible J-shaped stainless steel blade protecting its fiberoptic bundle, an optical eye-piece, and a "tube guide" for an endotracheal tube (ETT) up to size 8.5 mm ID (Figure 5.1). Secretions, fogging, difficulty elevating the epiglottis, and directing the ETT through the vocal cords were often encountered[21,22] and a coudé-tipped introducer was generally required to facilitate ETT placement[21]. It offered little or no advantage over DL in either easy or challenging airways.

WuScope™[20,24–26]

The WS was manufactured by Achi Corporation (Freemont, CA). It consists of a customized flexible nasopharyngoscope inserted within two semicircular rigid blades. An ETT is introduced into a tube slot (Figure 5.2). A video camera can be attached to the eyepiece to allow the image to be displayed on a monitor (Figure 5.3).

An anti-sialogogue and anti-fogging spray are recommended. The cuff of an ETT is completely deflated, lubricated, and preloaded into the tube slot of the WS (Figure 5.2). A coudé-tipped suction catheter, Eschmann or Frova introducer, is inserted into the ETT (Figure 5.4). Oxygen insufflation at 1–2 LPM via a nipple (Figure 5.5) may reduce fogging. The WS is introduced into the midline and rotated around the base of the tongue, preferentially positioned in the vallecula. The suction catheter or intubation guide is advanced into the trachea and the ETT is then advanced under visual control. Then the ETT is secured, the suction catheter removed, the bi-valved blade is disassembled, and rotated out of the mouth (Figure 5.6).

The WS has been advocated for routine use as well as settings typically challenging for DL[24]. Ideal intubating conditions were achieved in 17/24 (71%) and 38/45 (84%) of patients with and without features predictive of a difficult (direct) laryngoscopy[27]. A Cormack-Lehane (C/L) grade I view was obtained in 97% of patients. Problems included

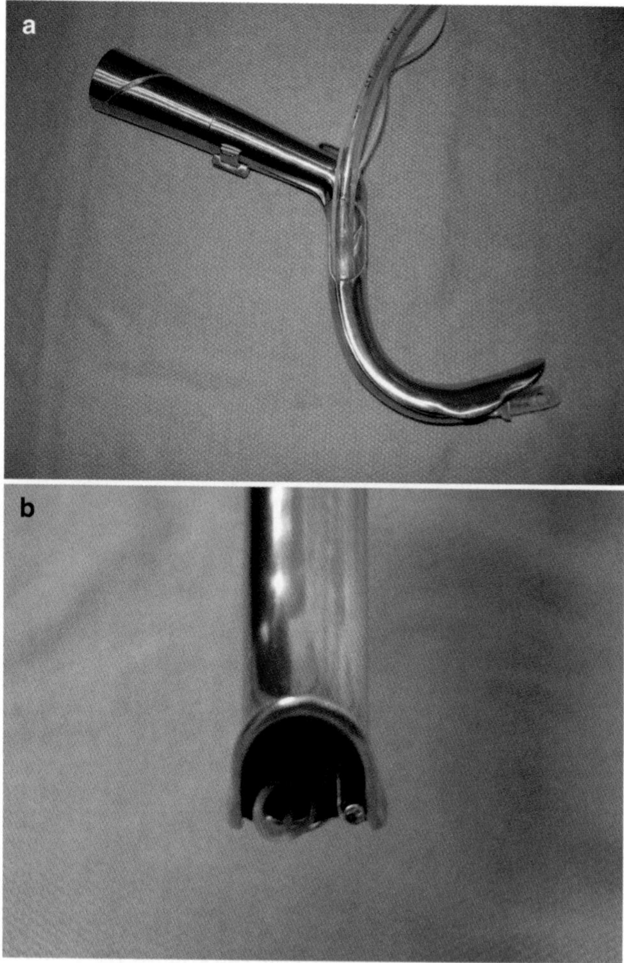

Figure 5.2. (**a**) Two components of the WuScope, now discontinued, are assembled with an endotracheal tube positioned in the tube slot. A lock/release is seen on the lower aspect at the mid-portion of a tapering barrel. Release of this lock allows the two components to be disassembled for removal of the endotracheal tube. (**b**) This close-up of the distal aspect of the WuScope with an endotracheal tube in the tube slot and a proprietary flexible bronchoscope in a dedicated channel on the right. Not shown in this figure is the flexible bronchoscopic attachment. See Figure 5.3.

a damaged cuff (1), secretions or blood obscuring the view (8), and fogging (4). Manual in-line axial stabilization still resulted in an IDS of zero (ideal) in 79% using the WS compared with 18% using DL[28].

Lingual tonsil hyperplasia (LTH) may present as an unanticipated failed laryngoscopy and not infrequently, ventilation too may be very difficult[29–34]. The WS was used successfully in two patients, one unsuspected and the other with known LTH[35]. The WS has also been used to perform ETT tube exchanges in patients with difficult airways[36,37].

Bullard

The BL is manufactured by Gyrus ACMI (Norwalk, OH). Available in three sizes, its distinguishing feature is a blade thickness of only 6 mm. This houses the image and light bundles as well as a 3.7-mm working channel. Oxygen can be insufflated through the working channel to reduce fogging. This channel can also be used for topical anesthesia.

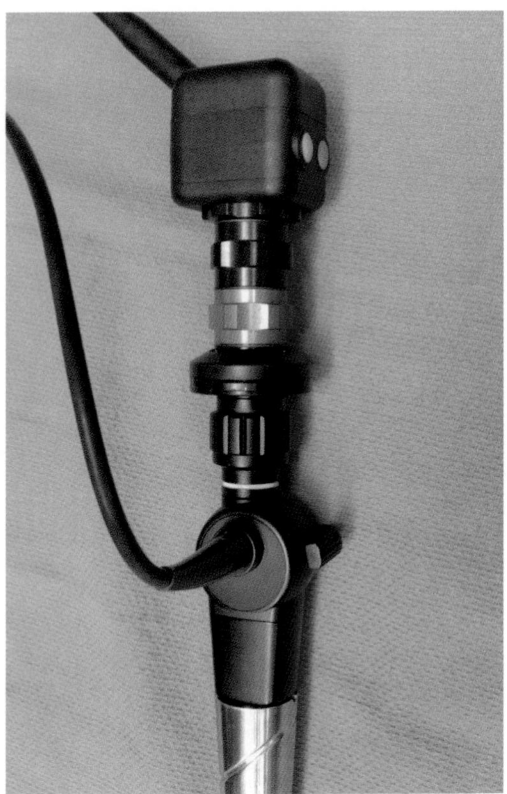

Figure 5.3. An operating room video camera is attached to the eyepiece of the WuScope to allow viewing on a video monitor.

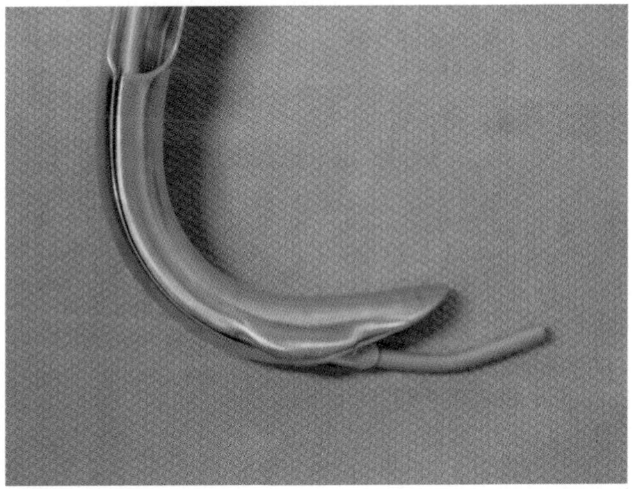

Figure 5.4. A Frova (or coudé-tipped catheter) has been passed through an endotracheal tube positioned in the tube slot of the WuScope.

The ETT can be introduced with a malleable stylet or with either the Bullard "intubating stylet" or "multifunctional stylet." The "intubating stylet" mounts on the body and should reside in a groove on the under-surface of the blade (Figure 5.7). When loading the ETT, the stylet is passed through the Murphy Eye. The authors recommend retracting and

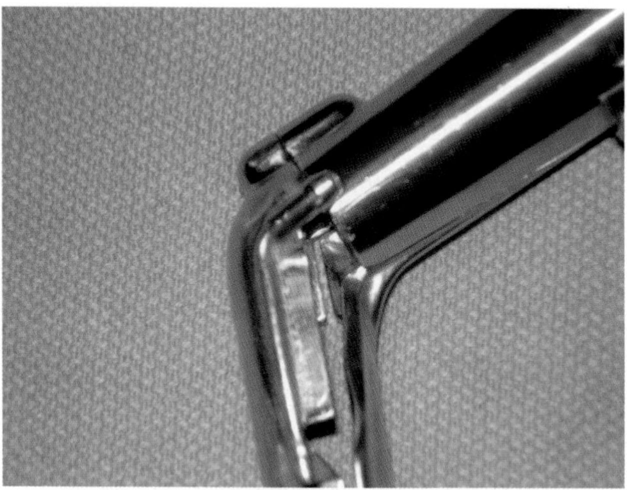

Figure 5.5. An oxygen nipple can be connected to O_2 tubing allowing low-flow insufflation during laryngoscopy. This may help clear secretions, reduce fogging, and oxygen desaturation.

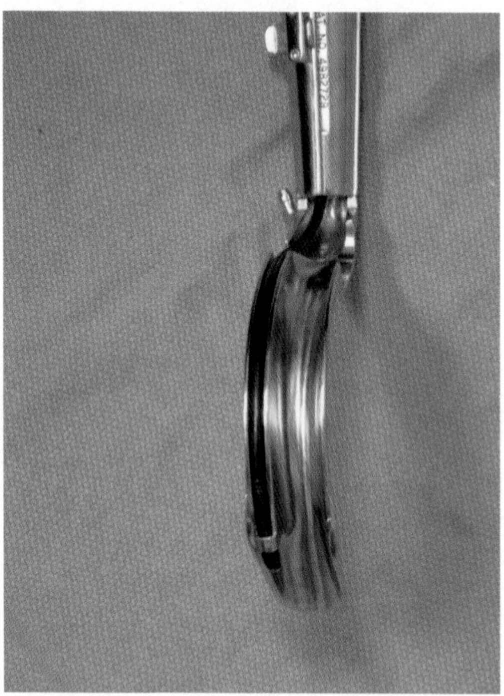

Figure 5.6. This shows a disarticulated WuScope with the proprietary flexible endoscope in its channel. After positioning the endoscope, the upper component would be attached and locked into place, the endotracheal tube would be introduced into the central channel, and oxygen tubing could be attached to the nipple seen on the left.

rotating the ETT 180° so that the leading edge of the bevel points to the left (Figure 5.8). Control of the stylet and ETT during laryngoscopy is essential. The hollow "straight-tipped multifunctional stylet" is sufficiently long to accommodate a double lumen tube. An ETT is introduced over the multifunctional stylet and the intubation guide is inserted through the stylet (Figure 5.9). A plastic blade extender can be attached to the distal end of the laryngoscope blade (Figure 5.10) when the distance to the epiglottis is greater than normal[38].

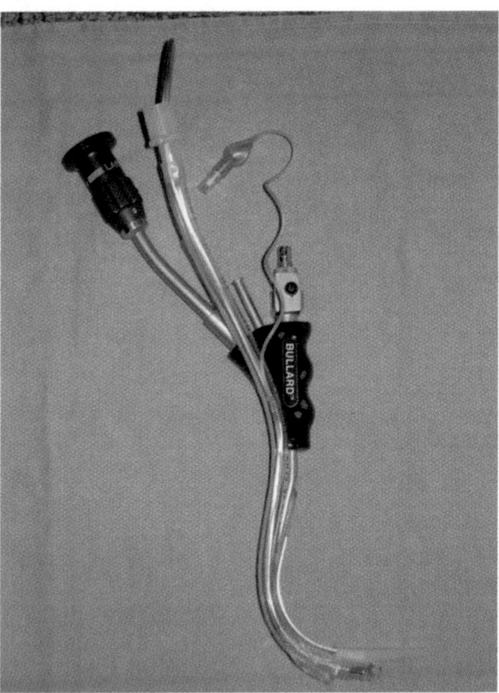

Figure 5.7. A Bullard laryngoscope is shown with a dedicated proprietary stylet and endotracheal tube attached and properly positioned beneath the laryngoscope blade. A light source is not shown. A laryngoscope battery handle can be used; however if a video camera is attached to the eyepiece, an external light source is preferred. This would be attached to the vertical fiberoptic post. A working channel can be used to insufflate oxygen or instill local anesthesia. For direct viewing through the eyepiece, a diopter adjuster allows the operator to focus the image.

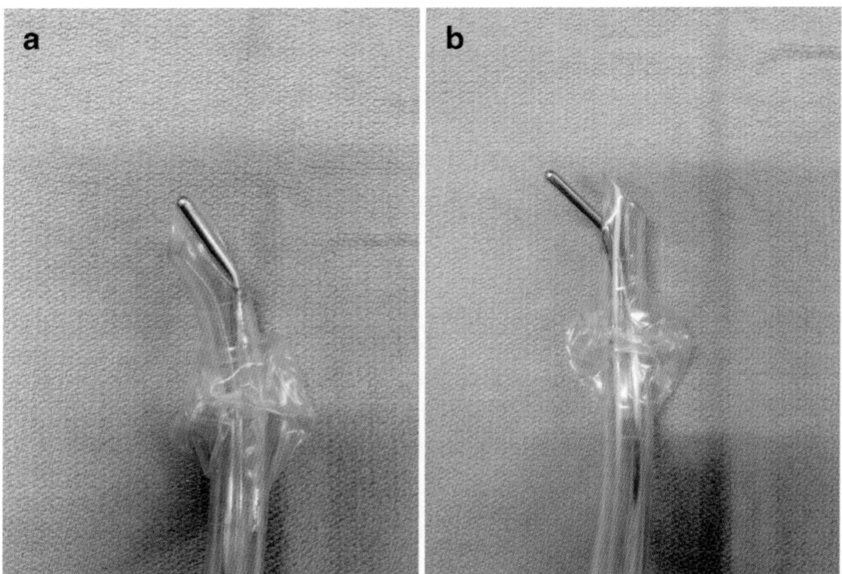

Figure 5.8. (**a**) The endotracheal tube is mounted on the proprietary stylet and passed through the Murphy eye. (**b**) The author prefers to rotate the endotracheal tube 180° redirecting the bevel so that it is less likely to impinge on the right vocal cord or arytenoid. It is essential that Bullard laryngoscope is held such that the stylet and ETT remain in intimate contact and the stylet is always seen through the viewer (see Figure 5.11)

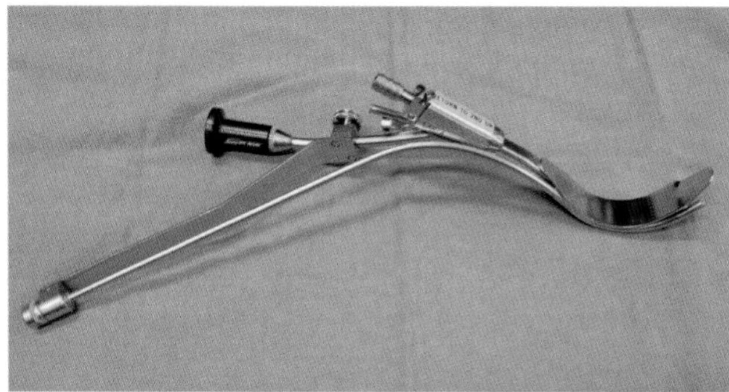

Figure 5.9. The Bullard multifunctional stylet is tubular and lacks the distal angulation. It is longer and was intended for compatibility with double lumen tubes; however this will be dependent upon the ID of the bronchial lumen. Like the proprietary stylet in Figure 5.8, it sits on the right side of the under-surface of the laryngoscope blade so as to keep the stylet/ETT in close contact

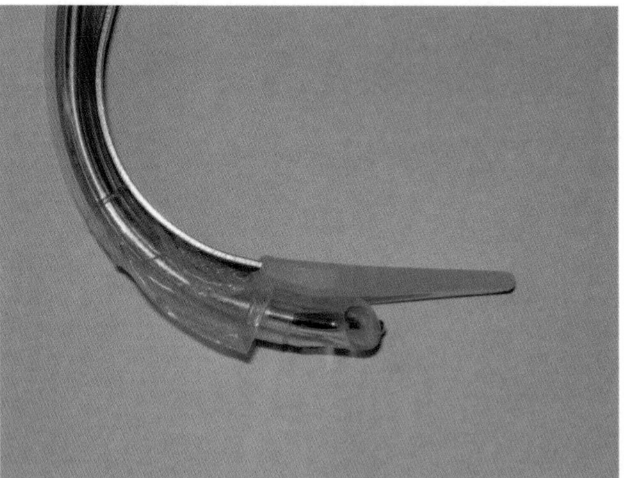

Figure 5.10. A single-use plastic blade extender can be added to the Bullard laryngoscope. It must be properly secured during use and removed prior to sterilization of the scope. In this photo, the ETT has been loaded onto the stylet and is held close to the undersurface of the blade

An anti-sialogogue and an anti-fogging solution should be used. The eyepiece should be focused and if a video camera is used, a white balance and further focusing should also be performed. For awake intubations, lidocaine ointment or EMLA cream can be applied with the blade and an epidural catheter can be introduced through the working channel and attached to a syringe containing local anesthesia to apply topical anesthesia via the working channel.

With the patient's head in a neutral position, the BL is introduced in the midline. The blade is rotated around the base of the tongue until the epiglottis is seen. A tongue pull or jaw thrust elevates the epiglottis, which is picked up by the blade. The glottic image should be centered such that the dedicated stylet points toward the left vocal fold

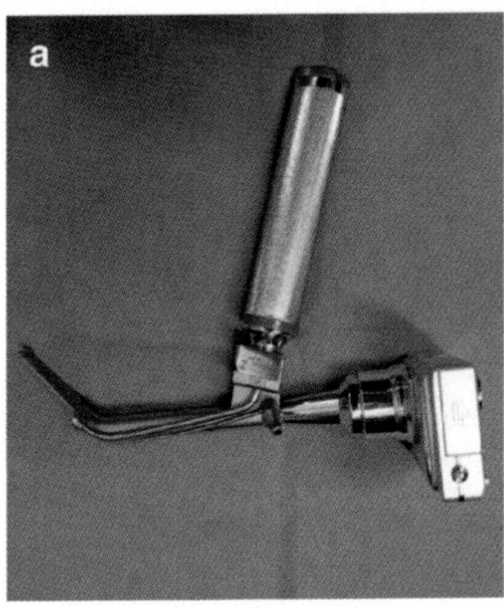
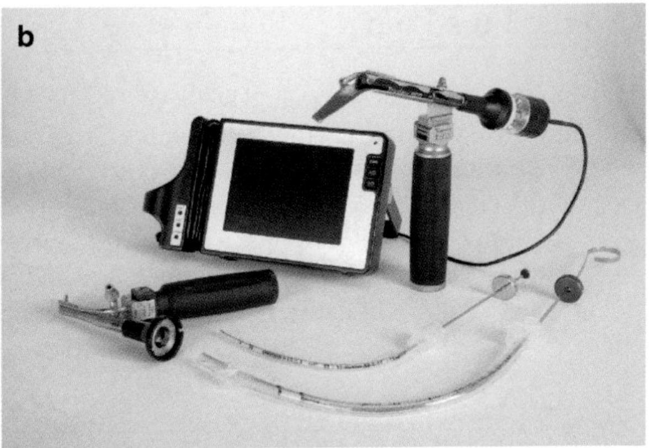

Figure 5.11. (**a**) The Truphatek Truview EVO2 is shown with a mounted (optional) camera, capable of recording still (jpeg) or video (mpeg) images. There is an oxygen nipple which may delay the development of hypoxia and reduce fogging. (**b**) In the lower left, the pediatric size Truphatek PCD laryngoscope is seen with an oxygen nipple and a magnetic eyepiece that couples with a video camera. The coupled assembly is seen in adult size on the right. The camera is attached to a proprietary battery-powered monitor. Also shown are pediatric and adult size stylets with adjustable tube stops (to prevent the stylet from protruding beyond the endotracheal tube) (photograph provided courtesy of Truphatek International and is reprinted with their consent).

(or the multifunctional stylet points to the tracheal lumen). It is very important to optimally align the ETT with the glottic chink since only minor adjustments are possible once the ETT is advanced off the stylet. The tip of the multifunctional stylet, on the other hand, is pointed toward the center of the laryngeal orifice so that the ETT, when advanced, avoids contact with the right arytenoid[39,40].

The BL has been used in a wide variety of clinical settings, including routine airway management[41] as well as simulated[42] and anticipated difficult DLs[43] and unanticipated failures of DL[10,44]. These include awake[31,45] and asleep intubations, oral and nasal intubations in children and adults, intubations in the morbidly obese[46], and in pregnant patients[46], or in patients with cervical spine instability or limitation[47–49], when double lumen tube insertion is required[50], and in patients with LTH[31].

Truview EVO2™

The Truview (TV) EVO2™ (or Viewmax) is manufactured by Truphatek (Netanya, Israel) and distributed in the USA by Teleflex Medical (Research Triangle Park, NC). It is available with a dedicated digital camera that attaches to the optical viewport, providing a low cost, highly portable system with an LCD display capable of still or video image capture (Figure 5.11a). The two blades corresponding roughly to a 2.5 and 3.5 Macintosh have an anterior deflection of ~45°.

In a manikin study simulating normal and difficult airways[51] and in patients[52,53], the TV EVO2 provided better laryngeal views and required less force but did not reduce intubation time or difficulty compared with Macintosh DL. Advanced paramedics observed no advantage over the Macintosh DL in manikins with a simulated difficult airway[54].

A new Truview PCD was released in 2010 but there is very limited experience with this device; this is available in four blade sizes with a magnetically coupled video camera head and a proprietary LCD monitor. There are as yet no published reports of its clinical performance.

Conclusion

The rigid fiberoptic devices were developed specifically for laryngoscopy. While they lack the versatility of flexible fiberoptic endoscopes, they are more robust and provide a supraglottic vantage point, allowing the insertion and advancement of the ETT to be viewed. Despite the effectiveness of some of these devices, they failed to achieve widespread use and have been largely eclipsed by the newer video laryngoscopes that incorporate cameras and dedicated monitors. The UpsherScope/Ultra and WuScope were recently withdrawn from the market. The Bullard still has a place alongside devices such as the flexible bronchoscope and video laryngoscopes due to its very low profile.

References

1. Janeway HH. Intra-tracheal anesthesia from the standpoint of the nose, throat and oral surgeon with a description of a new instrument for catheterizing the trachea. Laryngoscope. 1913;23(11):1082.
2. Miller RA. A new laryngoscope. Anesthesiology. 1941;2(3):317–20.
3. Macintosh RR. New inventions. A new laryngoscope. Lancet. 1943;1(6):205.
4. Bannister FB, Macbeth RB. Direct laryngoscopy and tracheal intubation. Lancet. 1944;1:651–4.
5. Adnet F, Borron SW, Lapostolle F, Lapandry C. The three axis alignment theory and the "sniffing position": perpetuation of an anatomic myth? Anesthesiology. 1999;91(6):1964–5.
6. Hochman II, Zeitels SM, Heaton JT. Analysis of the forces and position required for direct laryngoscopic exposure of the anterior vocal folds. Ann Otol Rhinol Laryngol. 1999;108(8):715–24.
7. Levitan RM, Mechem CC, Ochroch EA, Shofer FS, Hollander JE. Head-elevated laryngoscopy position: improving laryngeal exposure during laryngoscopy by increasing head elevation. Ann Emerg Med. 2003;41(3):322–30.
8. Adnet F, Borron SW, Dumas JL, Lapostolle F, Cupa M, Lapandry C. Study of the "sniffing position" by magnetic resonance imaging. Anesthesiology. 2001;94(1):83–6.
9. Adnet F, Baillard C, Borron SW, et al. Randomized study comparing the "sniffing position" with simple head extension for laryngoscopic view in elective surgery patients. Anesthesiology. 2001;95(4):836–41.
10. Crosby ET, Cooper RM, Douglas MJ, et al. The unanticipated difficult airway with recommendations for management. Can J Anaesth. 1998;45(8):757–76.
11. Rose DK, Cohen MM. The incidence of airway problems depends on the definition used. Can J Anaesth. 1996;43(1):30–4.
12. Shiga T, Wajima Z, Inoue T, Sakamoto A. Predicting difficult intubation in apparently normal patients: a meta-analysis of bedside screening test performance. Anesthesiology. 2005;103(2):429–37.
13. Adnet F, Borron SW, Racine SX, et al. The intubation difficulty scale (IDS): proposal and evaluation of a new score characterizing the complexity of endotracheal intubation. Anesthesiology. 1997;87(6):1290–7.
14. Adnet F, Racine SX, Borron SW, et al. A survey of tracheal intubation difficulty in the operating room: a prospective observational study. Acta Anaesthesiol Scand. 2001;45(3):327–32.
15. Rose DK, Cohen MM. The airway: problems and predictions in 18,500 patients. Can J Anaesth. 1994;41(5 Pt 1):372–83.
16. Mort TC. Emergency tracheal intubation: complications associated with repeated laryngoscopic attempts. Anesth Analg. 2004;99(2):607–13.
17. Rosenblatt WH, Wagner PJ, Ovassapian A, Kain ZN. Practice patterns in managing the difficult airway by anesthesiologists in the United States. Anesth Analg. 1998;87(1):153–7.
18. Jenkins K, Wong DT, Correa R. Management choices for the difficult airway by anesthesiologists in Canada. Can J Anesth. 2002;49(8):850–6.
19. Ezri T, Szmuk P, Warters RD, Katz J, Hagberg CA. Difficult airway management practice patterns among anesthesiologists practicing in the United States: have we made any progress? J Clin Anesth. 2003;15(6):418–22.

20. Cooper RM, Law JA, Hung O, Murphy MF, Law JA. Rigid and semi-rigid fiberoptic and video-laryngoscopy and intubation. Management of the difficult and failed airway. New York: McGraw Hill Medical; 2007.
21. Yeo V, Chung DC, Hin LY. A bougie improves the utility of the Upsherscope. J Clin Anesth. 1999;11(6):471–6.
22. Pearce AC, Shaw S, Macklin S. Evaluation of the Upsherscope. A new rigid fibrescope. Anaesthesia. 1996;51(6):561–4.
23. Fridrich P, Frass M, Krenn CG, Weinstabl C, Benumof JL, Krafft P. The UpsherScope in routine and difficult airway management: a randomized, controlled clinical trial. Anesth Analg. 1997;85(6):1377–81.
24. Wu TL, Chou HC. A new laryngoscope: the combination intubating device. Anesthesiology. 1994;81(4):1085–7.
25. Law JA, Hagberg CA. The evolution of upper airway retraction: new and old laryngoscope blades. Benumof's airway management principles and practice, vol. 2. Philadelphia PA: Mosby Elsevier; 2007. p. 532–75.
26. Sprung J, Weingarten T, Dilger J. The use of WuScope fiberoptic laryngoscopy for tracheal intubation in complex clinical situations. Anesthesiology. 2003;98(1):263–5.
27. Smith CE, Sidhu TS, Lever J, Pinchak AB. The complexity of tracheal intubation using rigid fiberoptic laryngoscopy (WuScope). Anesth Analg. 1999;89(1):236–9.
28. Smith CE, Pinchak AB, Sidhu TS, Radesic BP, Pinchak AC, Hagen JF. Evaluation of tracheal intubation difficulty in patients with cervical spine immobilization: fiberoptic (WuScope) versus conventional laryngoscopy. Anesthesiology. 1999;91(5):1253–9.
29. Davies S, Ananthanarayan C, Castro C. Asymptomatic lingual tonsillar hypertrophy and difficult airway management: a report of three cases. Can J Anaesth. 2001;48(10):1020–4.
30. Ovassapian A, Glassenberg R, Randel GI, Mesnick PS, Klafta JM. Difficult airways because of lingual tonsil hyperplasia. Anesthesiology. 2001;95:A1214.
31. Crosby E, Skene D. More on lingual tonsillar hypertrophy. Can J Anesth. 2002;49(7):758.
32. Ovassapian A, Glassenberg R, Randel GI, Klock A, Mesnick PS, Klafta JM. The unexpected difficult airway and lingual tonsil hyperplasia: a case series and a review of the literature. Anesthesiology. 2002;97(1):124–32.
33. Al Shamaa M, Jefferson P, Ball DR. Lingual tonsil hypertrophy: airway management. Anaesthesia. 2003;58(11):1134–5.
34. Tokumine J, Sugahara K, Ura M, Takara I, Oshiro M, Owa T. Lingual tonsil hypertrophy with difficult airway and uncontrollable bleeding. Anaesthesia. 2003;58(4):390–1.
35. Andrews SR, Mabey MF. Tubular fiberoptic laryngoscope (WuScope) and lingual tonsil airway obstruction. Anesthesiology. 2000;93(3):904–5.
36. Andrews SR, Norcross SD, Mabey MF, Siegel JB. The WuScope technique for endotracheal tube exchange. Anesthesiology. 1999;90(3):929–30.
37. Sprung J, Wright LC, Dilger J. Use of WuScope for exchange of endotracheal tube in a patient with difficult airway. Laryngoscope. 2003;113(6):1082–4.
38. Crosby ET, Cleland MJ. Bullard laryngoscope: keeping its act together. Anesth Analg. 1999;89(1):266.
39. Katsnelson T, Farcon E, Schwalbe SS, Badola R. The Bullard laryngoscope and the right arytenoid. Can J Anaesth. 1994;41(6):552–3.
40. Katsnelson T, Farcon E, Cosio M, Schwalbe SS. The Bullard laryngoscope and size of the endotracheal tube. Anesthesiology. 1994;81(1):261–2.
41. Cooper SD, Benumof JL, Ozaki GT. Evaluation of the Bullard laryngoscope using the new intubating stylet: comparison with conventional laryngoscopy. Anesth Analg. 1994;79(5):965–70.
42. MacQuarrie K, Hung OR, Law JA. Tracheal intubation using Bullard laryngoscope for patients with a simulated difficult airway. Can J Anaesth. 1999;46(8):760–5.
43. Gorback MS. Management of the challenging airway with the Bullard laryngoscope. J Clin Anesth. 1991;3(6):473–7.
44. Connelly NR, Ghandour K, Robbins L, Dunn S, Gibson C. Management of unexpected difficult airway at a teaching institution over a 7-year period. J Clin Anesth. 2006;18(3):198–204.
45. Cohn AI, Zornow MH. Awake endotracheal intubation in patients with cervical spine disease: a comparison of the Bullard laryngoscope and the fiberoptic bronchoscope. Anesth Analg. 1995;81(6):1283–6.
46. Cohn AI, Hart RT, McGraw SR, Blass NH. The Bullard laryngoscope for emergency airway management in a morbidly obese parturient. Anesth Analg. 1995;81(4):872–3.

47. Wahlen BM, Gercek E. Three-dimensional cervical spine movement during intubation using the Macintosh and Bullard laryngoscopes, the bonfils fibrescope and the intubating laryngeal mask airway. Eur J Anaesthesiol. 2004;21(11):907–13.
48. Shulman GB, Connelly NR. A comparison of the Bullard laryngoscope versus the flexible fiberoptic bronchoscope during intubation in patients afforded inline stabilization. J Clin Anesth. 2001;13(3):182–5.
49. Abrams KJ, Desai N, Katsnelson T. Bullard laryngoscopy for trauma airway management in suspected cervical spine injuries. Anesth Analg. 1992;74(4):623.
50. Shulman GB, Connelly NR. Double lumen tube placement with the Bullard laryngoscope. Can J Anaesth. 1999;46(3):232–4.
51. Miceli L, Cecconi M, Tripi G, Zauli M, Della Rocca G. Evaluation of new laryngoscope blade for tracheal intubation, Truview EVO2: a manikin study. Eur J Anaesthesiol. 2008;25(6): 446–9.
52. Barak M, Philipchuck P, Abecassis P, Katz Y. A comparison of the TruviewR blade with the Macintosh blade in adult patients. Anaesthesia. 2007;62(8):827–31.
53. Li JB, Xiong YC, Wang XL, et al. An evaluation of the TruView EVO2 laryngoscope. Anaesthesia. 2007;62(9):940–3.
54. Malik MA, Maharaj CH, Harte BH, Laffey JG. Comparison of Macintosh, Truview EVO2(R), Glidescope(R), and Airwayscope(R) laryngoscope use in patients with cervical spine immobilization. Br J Anaesth. 2008;101(5):723–30.

6 Role of Rigid Video Laryngoscopy

Richard M. Cooper and Corina Lee

Introduction

The previous two chapters (Chaps. 4 and 5) discussed the limitations of line-of-sight (direct) laryngoscopy. Many of these shortcomings could be circumvented by rigid fiberoptic laryngoscopes, however, unless coupled to an external video camera, only the

R.M. Cooper (✉)
Department of Anesthesia and Pain Management, University of Toronto,
Toronto General Hospital, Toronto, ON, Canada M5G 2C4
e-mail: richard.cooper@uhn.ca

C. Lee
Department of Anesthesia and Pain Management,
200 Elizabeth Street, Toronto, ON, Canada, M5G 2C4

D.B. Glick et al. (eds.), *The Difficult Airway: An Atlas of Tools and Techniques for Clinical Management*,
DOI 10.1007/978-0-387-92849-4_6, © Springer Science+Business Media New York 2013

laryngoscopist could see, the image was small and the field of view was limited. If a camera head was attached, a more powerful external light source and monitor were required. This rather complex setup has been greatly simplified by embedding miniature video cameras into modified laryngoscope blades, illuminated by intense but low heat-emitting LEDs (light emitting diodes) and small, dedicated, high-resolution LCD monitors. These integrated video laryngoscopes (VLs) can be battery powered and portable. Some are resistant to fogging and able to capture time-annotated images of the laryngoscopy and intubation. This chapter will describe several such devices. They will be classified as channeled devices (e.g. Airtraq and AirwayScope) or non-channeled (McGrath, GlideScope, and Storz Direct Coupled Interface [DCI]/V-MAC and C-MAC). With channeled VLs, the scope and ETT are manipulated as a single unit; the ETT is directed by adjusting the orientation of the scope. With non-channeled VLs, the scope and ETT are independently maneuvered, generally using a stylet. This is a rapidly developing field characterized by technological leapfrogging. Existing indirect VLs will be modified, new devices will appear and some may disappear. Every effort has been made to be accurate up to the time of preparation.

Channeled Scopes

Airtraq

The Airtraq® Optical Laryngoscope (Prodol Meditec S.A., Vizcaya, Spain) was developed by Pedro Acha Gandarias. It is a *single-use*, portable, anatomically shaped, battery-powered device with two adjacent channels. One channel transmits the image through prisms and fog-resistant lenses to an optical viewer. The other channel acts as a conduit to guide the endotracheal (ETT) tube. Illumination is provided for up to 90 min by a low temperature LED located at the distal part of the blade. The Airtraq is available in a total of seven sizes or configurations—4 for oral ETT intubation, 2 for nasal intubation, and 1 for double lumen tube (DLT) insertion (see Figure 6.1a). Please see Table 6.1 for the sizes and required mouth openings[1–4]. The operator may view the image through the eyepiece, on a generic video display or on a proprietary monitor linked wirelessly to a transmitter attached to the laryngoscope (see Figure 6.1b, c).

The Airtraq is inserted into the mouth along the midline of the tongue. Insertion may be facilitated by placing the patient in the neutral position and opening the mouth with a crossed scissor technique. Digital pressure applied behind the lower incisors may create an internal jaw thrust[5] (Figure 6.2). The Airtraq is then gently passed around the dorsum of the tongue toward the larynx. The tip of the device is inserted into the vallecula and the epiglottis is indirectly elevated. Alternatively, the Airtraq may be passed posterior to the epiglottis allowing direct elevation. Once the vocal cords are exposed, the ETT is advanced slowly until the cuff is passed the cords. The ETT is then disengaged from the channel, and held in place with the right hand, while the Airtraq is removed (Figure 6.3).

Initial studies have shown that compared with Macintosh DL, the Airtraq provides comparable or superior intubating conditions in patients with a normal airway[6]. It also has advantages over the Macintosh in the management of the difficult airway as shown in both manikin[7–9] and human studies[10]. In a trial comparing Airtraq and Macintosh laryngoscopy, 40 patients with more than three features suggestive of a difficult laryngoscopy were randomly assigned to one or the other technique performed by experienced anesthesiologists. All 20 patients were successfully intubated using the Airtraq, 19 on the first attempt and all with Cormack–Lehane grade 1 views. By contrast 4 patients who could not be intubated by DL were successfully intubated with the Airtraq on the first attempt. The Airtraq was associated with lower intubation difficulty scores[11], improved glottic exposure, shorter time to tracheal intubation, less oxygen desaturation and minor airway trauma, and less stimulation of heart rate and blood pressure than Macintosh DL[10]. Another study compared the Airtraq and Macintosh DL in morbidly obese patients[12]

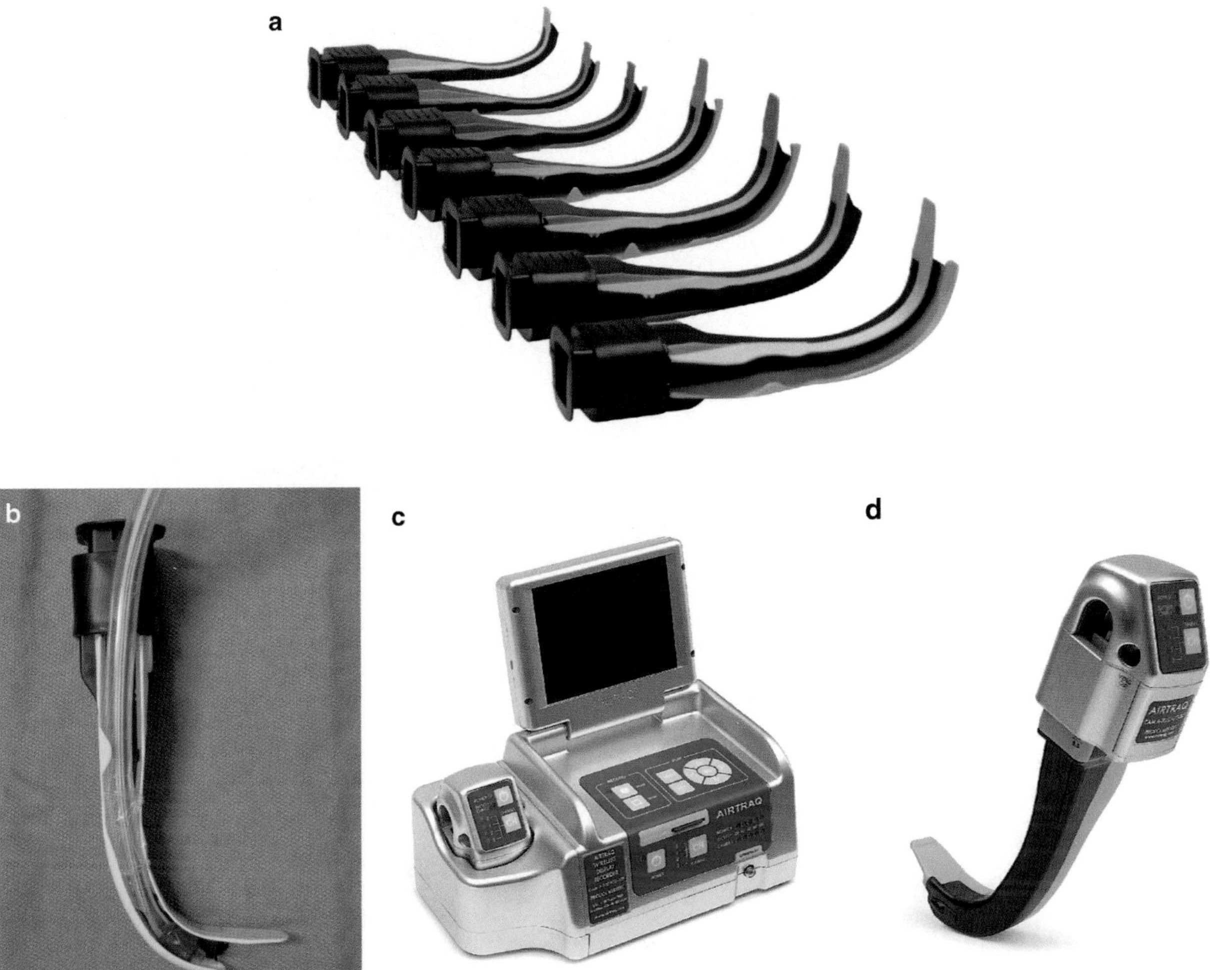

Figure 6.1. (**a**) At present, there are seven configurations of the Airtraq OL as described in the text. These are distinguished by their colors. The *yellow* laryngoscope has a wider tube slot for DLTs. The *orange* and *light gray* laryngoscopes lack posterior components to their "tube slots." These devices are strictly for visualizing and are intended for nasotracheal intubation. The photograph was provided by Prodol and is reprinted with their consent. (**b**) This shows the Airtraq OL DLT model with the tube in situ. (**c, d**) When the rubber cover seen in (**a**) is removed, a proprietary camera can be attached. This can be connected with a generic monitor or a dedicated wireless monitor (**c**). (**a**), (**c**), and (**d**) appear with the permission of Prodol Meditec S.A.

Table 6.1. Airtraq® sizes.

Description	Size	ETT sizes	Mouth opening	Color
Adult oral	3	7.0–8.5 mm ID	18 mm	Blue
Adult oral	2	6.0–7.5 mm ID	16 mm	Green
Pediatric oral	1	4.0–5.5	12.5	Purple
Infant oral	0	2.5–3.5	12.5	Gray
Adult nasal		N/A	18 mm	Orange
Infant nasal		N/A	12.5	White
Double lumen		35–41 Fr	19	Yellow

These are single-use products, and the batteries housed in the main body should be removed and discarded separately

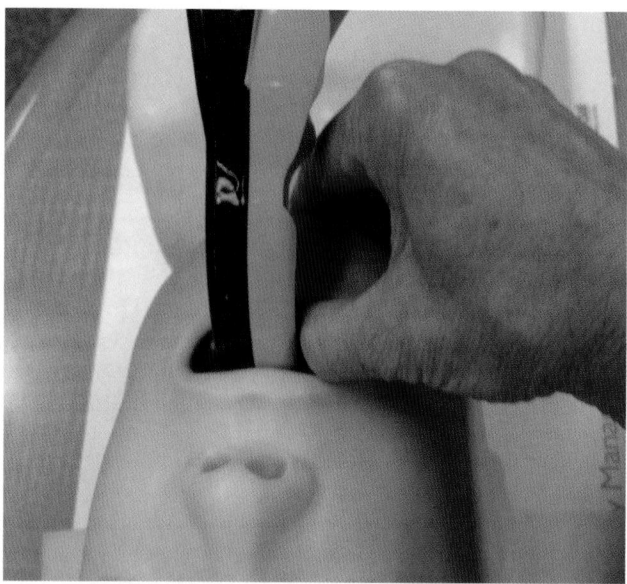

Figure 6.2. This demonstrates an internal jaw thrust. The same maneuver is helpful with the Bullard (Figure 5.11), lightwand, and flexible bronchoscopic intubation. This is accomplished with the thumb and index finger pulling the mandible anteriorly, raising the epiglottis, and creating more space in the hypopharynx.

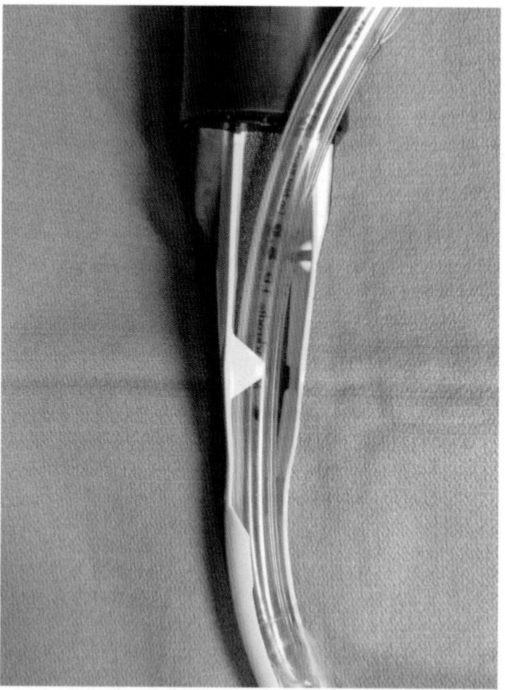

Figure 6.3. The endotracheal tube is retained within the tube slot by a small plastic tab. The endotracheal tube can be released by deflecting it around the tab and slightly rotating the endotracheal tube and laryngoscopes in opposite directions making sure that the tube is not withdrawn.

showing reductions in intubation time and oxygen desaturation using the Airtraq. In a simulated difficult airway study using a (Laerdal SimMan®) manikin, in a comparison of the GlideScope, McGrath, Airtraq, and Macintosh, the indirect laryngoscopes consistently outperformed the Macintosh DL and the Airtraq consistently resulted in the most rapid intubation[13].

When direct laryngoscopy has failed despite optimal positioning and use of a gum elastic bougie, the Airtraq has been used successfully as a "rescue device." A case series of 7 patients with Cormack–Lehane grade 4 views by Macintosh DL and failed intubation were converted to Cormack–Lehane grade 1 views and successfully intubated with the Airtraq[12]. Compared with Macintosh DL, hemodynamic stimulation was also reduced using the Airtraq® [6,10,14].

Despite having a guide channel for ETT insertion, obtaining a full view of the glottis with the Airtraq does not always guarantee successful intubation at the first attempt[15], with occasional failures despite repositioning. Dhonneur et al.[16] conducted a retrospective review of video recordings of the internal view obtained using the Airtraq in 109 laryngoscopies performed on 50 patients in whom more than one attempt was required. They found that successful intubation was most often associated with positioning the glottic opening in the vertical center, slightly below its horizontal midline (Figure 6.4)[1,16]. In-line stabilization to reduce cervical spine movement also helps to center the position of the glottic opening on the screen[4,16].

Insertion of the device into the pharynx of obese patients can be challenging due to narrowing between the oral and pharyngeal space and the rigid structure of the Airtraq[14,16]. Dhonneur et al. have described an alternative insertion method[17]. Lean and morbidly obese patients were randomized to the conventional technique or a "reverse maneuver," wherein the device is inserted 180° opposite to that conventional method and rotated into position once in the pharynx, much like a Guedel airway (Figure 6.5). The reverse method was associated with a higher first-pass success rate in morbidly obese patients and reduced the time to exposure of the glottis by half. In the morbidly obese group, but not in the lean group, total intubation time was reduced. In this study, among obese patients, the conventional method required the application of significant pressure on the distal part of the blade to place the Airtraq into the pharyngeal space and resulted in more incidents of minor trauma compared with reverse insertion. Regardless of insertion technique, the Airtraq has been associated with significantly less trauma compared to the Macintosh in cases of difficult tracheal intubation[10]. Dhonneur et al.[18] and Holst et al.[19] and their respective coworkers have identified soft tissue injuries that might go unnoticed when using the Airtraq device. In the former publication, these were more common in obese patients. In the latter study, also involving the Airtraq, a 2-cm nasopharyngeal laceration gave rise to a large clot retrieved from the oropharynx prior to extubation. They referred to this as the "coroner's clot" since it can give rise to complete airway obstruction following extubation, and they advocate caution when introducing a bulky device providing a relatively limited field of view into the airway.

Like the other indirect laryngoscopes, the ability to "see around the corner" suggests that less cervical spine movement may be required to visualize and intubate the glottis. This was confirmed fluoroscopically[20,21]. While cervical spine immobilization has been used experimentally as a model for difficult laryngoscopy[22], it may actually improve the glottic view offered by the Airtraq[18,23], at least in patients with otherwise normal airway anatomy.

The Airtraq has a rapid learning curve among novice users for both normal and difficult airways, with increased first-pass success and shorter time to tracheal intubation compared with Macintosh DL[6,7,24–26].

Studies assessing skill acquisition need to be evaluated critically. Was the study population relevant for the skill being considered? Was the training realistic? Was the skill evaluated on patients or manikins? Do these simulators accurately reflect the task being evaluated? Do some manikins favor specific devices? Skill retention is rarely evaluated but similar questions should be raised.

Maharaj et al. demonstrated that the intubation skills of minimally trained medical students, without interval exposure to laryngoscopy, diminish at 6 months when evaluated using an intubation manikin. Skill retention was also greater for the Airtraq compared with the Macintosh and the performance differences widened as the task became more complex[27]. Missaghi et al. suggest that, following formal education with the Airtraq with

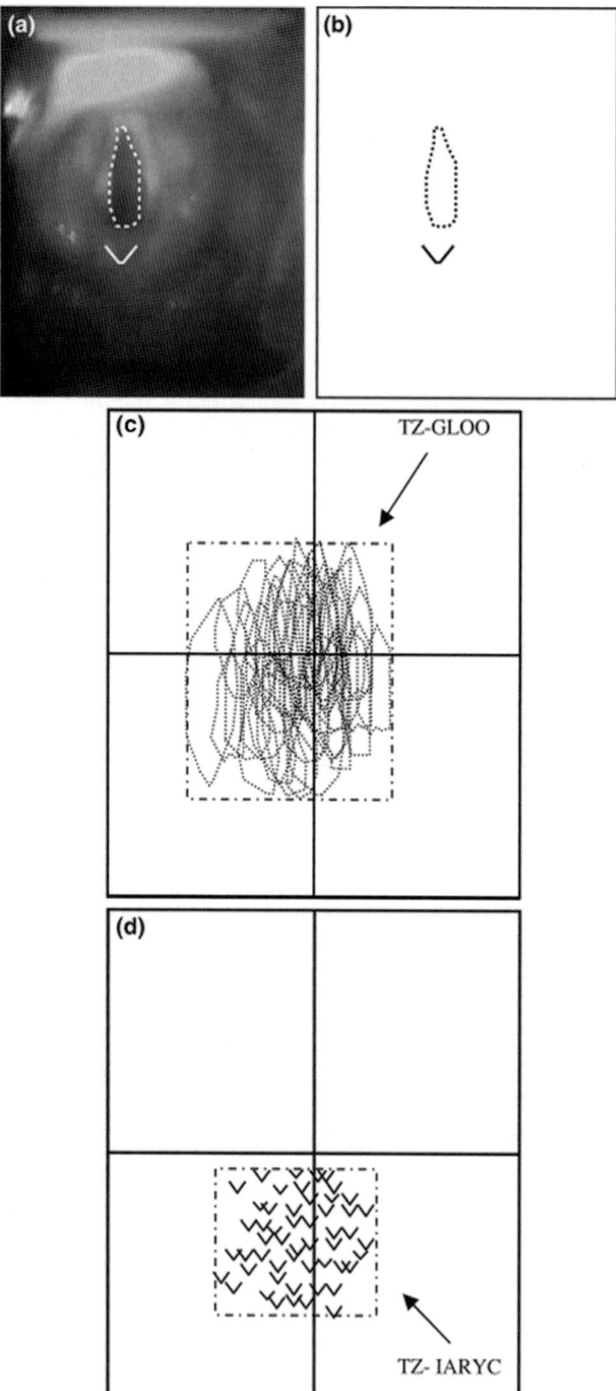

Figure 6.4. (**a**) This shows the image of the larynx with the laryngeal aperture and inter-arytenoid cleft identified. The former is identified by a cylindrical hatched line; the latter is shown as a V. (**b**) If the visual field seen through the Airtraq is divided into quadrants, the panel marked. (**c**) Represents the position of the laryngeal aperture associated with successful intubations. The panel marked (**d**) represents the position of the interarytenoid cleft associated with successful intubations. Their study involving 109 intubation attempts indicated that success was most often achieved if the inter-arytenoid cleft was positioned medially and below the center of the visual field (from Dhonneur et al.[16] and reprinted with permission of the publisher).

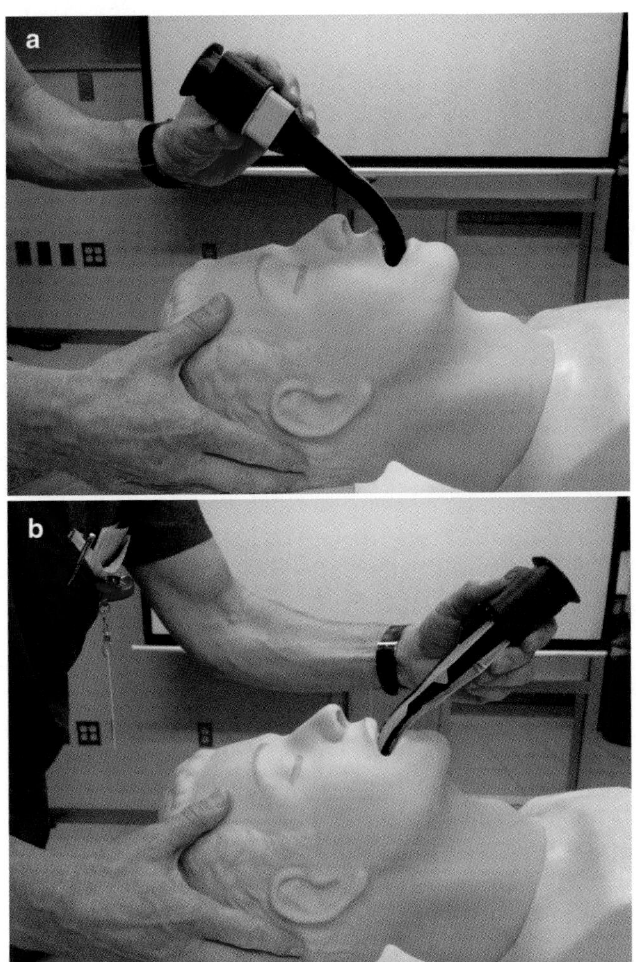

Figure 6.5. In patients with large chests or breasts and decreased cervical extension, insertion of the Airtraq may be difficult. In such a situation, it is worth attempting to insert the device like a Guedel airway (**a**), carefully introducing it into the oropharynx and rotating it 180° after passage beyond the tongue base (**b**). Care must be taken to avoid soft tissue injuries.

a manikin, novice users achieve acceptable clinical performance and competence within ten supervised uses[4]. Education in using the Airtraq may also be aided by the use of a video camera, which clips onto the viewfinder of the Airtraq. This can then be connected to an external monitor or to the Airtraq Wireless Monitor for viewing and recording.

Alongside routine and difficult airway use, the Airtraq may be useful in other scenarios. There are two reports of the Airtraq being used to successfully intubate awake patients with difficult airways[28,29], and being better tolerated than direct laryngoscopy. A modified version of the Airtraq in which the tube-guide is removed, leaving only the flange on the right of the blade, is available for nasotracheal intubation[16,29], and a version is also available for DLT insertion, accommodating endobronchial tubes up to size 41F (Figure 6.1)[16,30]. The Airtraq can also be used to facilitate visualized tracheal tube exchange of a difficult airway. Using an airway exchange catheter (see Chap. 16), the existing ETT is withdrawn over an exchange catheter, and its replacement is advanced over the catheter using the Airtraq to monitor the exchange[31].

In summary, the Airtraq Optical Laryngoscope has several advantages: it is lightweight, disposable, portable and requires minimal setup time, making it useful in emergency situations, especially in remote locations. It provides excellent laryngeal exposure, albeit with a low-quality image. It is useful in difficult airways, morbidly obese patients, when manual in-line stabilization (MILS) is required, as a rescue device when direct

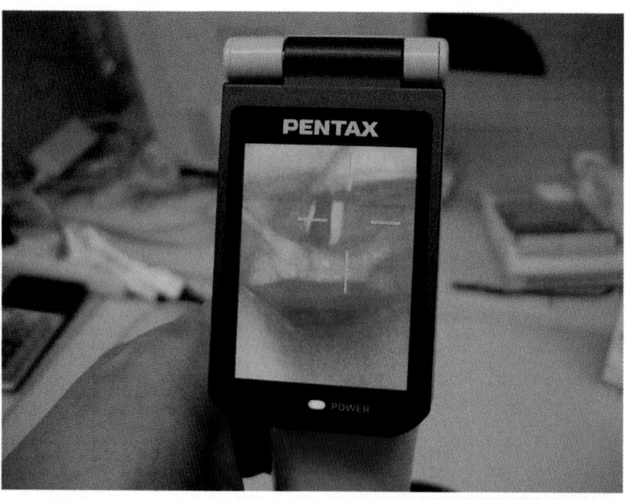

Figure 6.6. The crosshairs in the Pentax Airway Scope monitor are shown. This photograph was provided by Ambu and is reprinted with their permission.

laryngoscopy has failed, and may reduce hemodynamic stimulation. Skill acquisition is fast regardless of level of experience, and images can be easily recorded. The main disadvantages are cost/use, an adverse environmental impact, poor quality image, difficulty inserting the device into the pharynx, and difficulty obtaining the optimal viewing position of the glottis for successful intubation.

Pentax AWS100

The Airway Scope 100 consists of a portable, water-resistant, flexible charge-coupled device (CCD), powered by 2-AA alkaline batteries, illuminated by a dual-type white LED that conveys a high-resolution image to a 2.4 in. LCD, located on the handle of the device. The small screen swivels in a single plane, allowing it to be adjusted to an appropriate viewing angle. Crosshairs are superimposed upon the display, showing the approximate trajectory of the ETT after advancement (Figure 6.6). The "PBlade" is a rigid polycarbonate, disposable ETT conduit that accommodates the flexible scope (on the left) and an endotracheal tube (on the right) (Figure 6.7). The camera is recessed approximately 3 cm from the tip of the blade. A midline 12F channel can be used for suction, oxygen insufflation, or the instillation of topical anesthesia. There is no antifogging feature. A composite video signal port allows for easy image transport to an analogue recorder or external video display. At present, there is only one size PBlade, which accepts ETTs with an OD of 8.5–11.0 mm (generally corresponding to ID 6.5–8.0 mm). The external dimensions of the PBlade are as follows: length 131 mm; width 49 mm; depth 96 mm; and height 18 mm.

This device was initially developed as a collaboration between neurosurgeons, anesthesiologists, and Pentax Corporation[32], so cervical stabilization was a high priority. The head can remain in a neutral position for laryngoscopy. Like other indirect laryngoscopes—with the exception of the Storz DCI/V-Mac and C-MAC—the AWS is introduced in the midline and advanced beyond the base of the tongue. Unlike the Airtraq, the AWS must be advanced between the epiglottis and the posterior pharyngeal wall, directly elevating the epiglottis. Although the blade design looks very similar to the Airtraq, the trajectory of the ETT is different and demands a different technique[33].

Studies involving manikins have been performed with naïve[34] and experienced operators[35], simulating normal[36] and abnormal airways[37]. Although such studies provide controlled conditions, it is uncertain whether extrapolation to clinical conditions is valid.

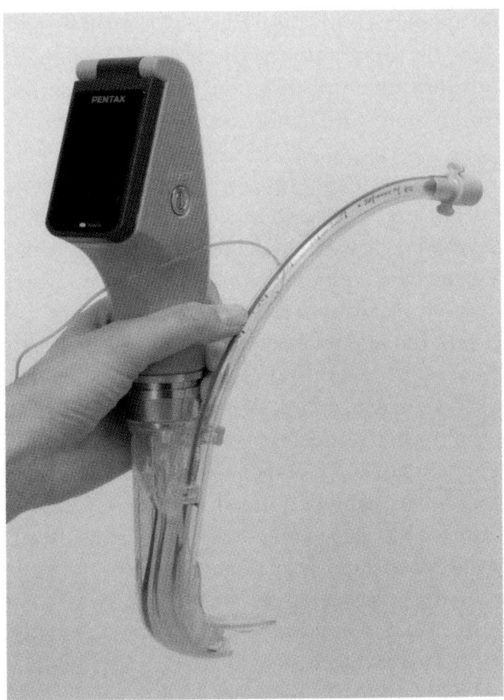

Figure 6.7. An endotracheal has been loaded into a lubricated tube slot and retracted to a position behind the camera until the laryngoscope is optimally positioned. The monitor can be adjusted to a convenient viewing angle. This photograph was provided by Ambu and is reprinted with their permission.

In an early study, the AWS was used by 74 operators in 405 patients, including 13 in whom Macintosh DL had yielded a C/L III or IV view[38]. Intubation was attempted after and before induction of anesthesia in 390 and 15 patients, respectively. Laryngeal exposure was achieved in every case and intubation was successful on the first attempt in 95% (383/405) of cases. The 14 operators who had used the AWS more than ten times achieved intubation within 24.7 ± 4.6 s. Suzuki et al. performed two laryngoscopies on each of 320 elective, adult surgical patients with adequate mouth opening. Using Macintosh DL and the AWS, they compared the modified Cormack and Lehane glottic views[39], the percent of glottic opening (POGO score)[40], the intubation difficulty score[11], time to tracheal intubation, and the number of required attempts[41]. All 46 patients with modified C/L scores ≥3 by DL were grade 1 (45) or grade 2a (1) with the AWS. AWS laryngoscopy yielded C/L 1 scores in 317/320 patients. The POGO scores and IDS were also significantly improved using the AWS but there was no significant difference in the time to tracheal intubation. In 308 cases, the first attempt using the AWS was successful. In 14 cases, the ETT became impinged upon laryngeal structures, but this was easily corrected by adjusting the scope and redirecting the ETT. Only 4 patients presented particular challenges. These included one patient in halo fixation, one patient with mouth opening limited to 1.9 cm following oropharyngeal irradiation, one patient with contractures resulting from a burn and laryngeal trauma following DL while the last patient had temporomandibular arthritis.

The AWS has also been used as a rescue device when DL failed[42] and in a multicentered study involving 270 patients in whom DL had been difficult and 23 patients prior to induction of anesthesia with features predictive of difficulty for mask ventilation *and* (DL) intubation[43]. In the multicentered study they permitted two DLs and up to two AWS attempts, allowing use of an Eschmann Introducer (gum elastic bougie) if the larynx could be seen but the ETT could not be advanced into the larynx. The AWS improved a DL C/L ≥3 view to grade ≤2 in 255 of the 256 patients. Tracheal intubation was accomplished in 268 of the 270 patients who had routine inductions, 255 on the first attempt. This is a "rescue rate" of 99.3% (268/270). The two failures occurred in patients in whom it was not possible to elevate the epiglottis with the PBlade (1) or the epiglottis could not be seen (1). Intubation was accomplished, prior to the induction of anesthesia, in 22 of the 23 patients in whom both difficult intubation and bag mask ventilation were anticipated. One failure occurred in a patient with a post-carotid endarterectomy hematoma producing airway obstruction.

The cervical spine movement was compared in 20 adults, performing both Macintosh DL and AWS laryngoscopy on each[44]. All had apparently normal cervical spines and airway anatomy; their heads were positioned neutrally and their necks were not stabilized. A single radiograph was taken when optimal laryngeal exposure was achieved. They observed significantly less movement at all measured segments with the AWS, however, a single radiograph may not reveal the maximal cervical excursion. Enomoto et al. applied MILS to 203 patients, randomized to Macintosh DL or AWS[45]. They obtained the glottic view significantly earlier with the AWS, achieved better laryngeal exposure, had fewer failures (0/99 vs. 11/104) but the time to intubation was the same with both devices. They did not evaluate the cervical movement but assumed this to be minimal. Maruyama et al. used a commercial head immobilizer and performed continuous cervical fluoroscopy on 13 patients during Macintosh and AWS laryngoscopy and intubation[46]. Laryngoscopies were performed to achieve adequate, not optimal, glottic exposure, probably best approximating the clinical practice in a patient at risk of cervical injury. Although these patients lacked features generally associated with a difficult (direct) laryngoscopy, head and neck immobilization usually produces such an effect. Less cumulative upper cervical spine movement was needed with the AWS than the Macintosh DL. The C/L scores for AWS and Macintosh were 1 and 2 ($p<0.001$) suggesting that the head and neck position may not have created a sufficient challenge, immobilization may not have been complete, or too few patients participated in the study. In another study, the same group compared the AWS with Macintosh DL and the activated McCoy DL but without cervical stabilization[47]. Without restraint, cervical movement was least with the AWS, though intubation took longer. Furthermore, the bulkiness of the AWS PBlade necessitated greater mouth opening requiring more upper cervical manipulation. In both of these studies, all the laryngoscopies were performed by a single person, obviously not blinded to the technique and despite his experience, AWS intubation took longer to achieve in the latter study. Nonetheless, these patients lacked features associated with difficult (direct) laryngoscopy and did not in fact have cervical injuries. The variety of such injuries and their effects on soft and skeletal tissue necessitate caution in extrapolating these results to patients with or at risk of cervical spine injury.

In a study comparing the AWS with a combination Macintosh and StyletScope® (Nihon Kohden Corporation, Tokyo) in patients immobilized with a cervical collar, mucosal or lip injuries were noted in 7 of the 50 StyletScope subjects compared with 3 of the AWS patients.* Intubation success was slightly higher and intubation time significantly faster with the AWS[48]. One patient could not be intubated despite three attempts with the AWS. This resulted from unintended separation of the ETT from the channel. Seven patients experienced injuries during laryngoscopy with the AWS, including 3 mucosal and 4 lip traumas. These injuries occurred while attempting to introduce the device into the mouth. There were however, fewer injuries and failures with the AWS than the StyletScope. The authors also performed laryngoscopy in patients in a cervical collar using either the AWS or a Macintosh laryngoscope in combination with a gum elastic bougie[49]. Intubation was accomplished significantly faster using the AWS and there was a trend toward a higher success rate. As with the previous study, a single, experienced but unblinded laryngoscopist performed all the intubations. There was no difference in the incidence of minor mucosal and lip injuries between the AWS (9/48 patients) and the Macintosh/GEB group (11/48). There were no esophageal intubations in the AWS group but 8 in the DL/GEB cohort.

---

*This raises the question—relevant to other video laryngoscope devices—whether such injuries are a consequence of the operator paying more attention to the display than the insertion of the device into the mouth.

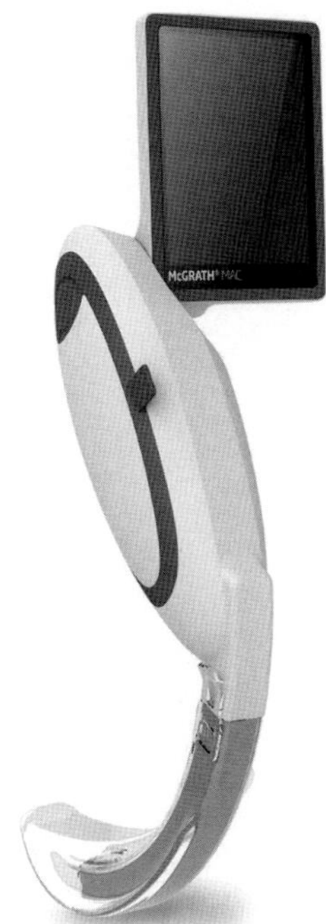

Figure 6.25 The McGrath MAC was introduced in 2010. Its camera stick is at a fixed length and while this reduces its versatility, it results in better image stability. The monitor articulates in only one plane. The battery is proprietary but its extended life expectancy is displayed on the screen. As of the time of publication, there is no literature on its performance, particularly in more challenging airways; however like the GlideScope Direct, it is useful for the supervision of trainees

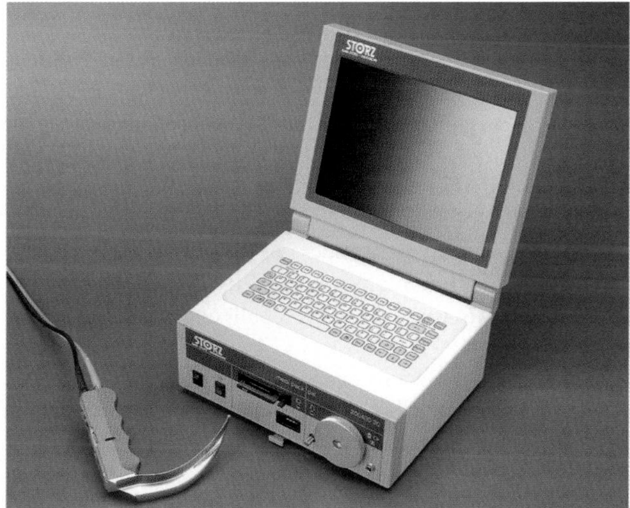

Figure 6.26. The second-generation Storz VL, the V-MAC, is shown with its proprietary monitor, processor, and light source (Telepak). The electronics are housed as a removable module within the blade handle. The blade can then be sent for sterilization. The device is used like a conventional Macintosh laryngoscope, with direct or indirect viewing possible. © 2011 Photo courtesy of Karl Storz Endoscopy-America, Inc.

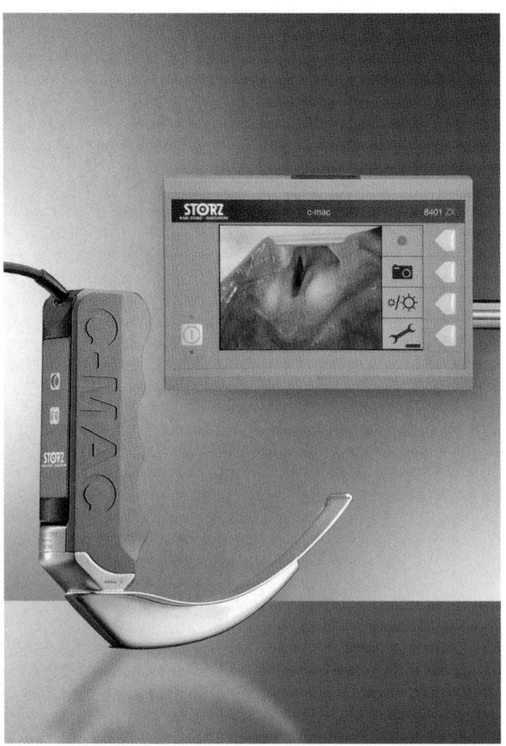

Figure 6.27 The third-generation Storz VL is the C-MAC which employs video chip (CMOS) technology. The camera is located distally and the image is displayed on a dedicated battery-operated monitor with on-board recording of still (jpeg) or video images (mpeg). Recordings can be initiated on the monitor or the handle itself. © 2011 Photo courtesy of Karl Storz Endoscopy-America, Inc.

The V-MAC was evaluated in a multicenter study involving 867 adults undergoing elective surgery[109]. All operators were trained on manikins and had performed at least ten intubations with the device prior to the study. The patients were neither consecutive nor randomized; the operators were not blinded and some centers recruited patients with more challenging airways. The laryngeal views[104] obtained by DL and indirect (VL) were compared using the same device. The view on the monitor (VL) was an improvement of at least one grade compared with DL in 41.5% of patients; it was worse in 23/865 (2.7%). In this study, 101/123 patients with a C/L grade 3 or 4 view by DL improved to a grade 1 or 2. In 3% of cases, fogging resulted in a worse view. In a previous study by Kaplan et al.[106] patients were divided into routine and more challenging airways. All but one of 235 patients was successfully intubated however ELM was required in 22/217 of the routine patients and all 18 of those with features generally associated with challenges. They concluded that the magnified view obtained from a distal vantage point facilitated laryngoscopic instruction and airway management. Because of its similarity to Macintosh DL, the learning curve was minimal and the device setup was simple.

More recently, Karl Storz (Tuttlingen, Germany) has introduced a video laryngoscope employing CMOS technology rather than a fiberoptic bridge to a processor[110] (Figure 6.27). The image sensor is recessed from the blade tip to provide a wide viewing perspective. The C-MAC is currently available in six sizes or configurations (Macintosh 2, 3, and 4, Miller 0 and 1) and recently introduced the D-BLADE, intended for the less easily visible larynx. Like the GVL and MVL, the D-BLADE has a more pronounced upward curve. Also, like the aforementioned VLs, a stylet is strongly recommended since direct viewing cannot be achieved. The blades are available with or without a suction channel, located to the left

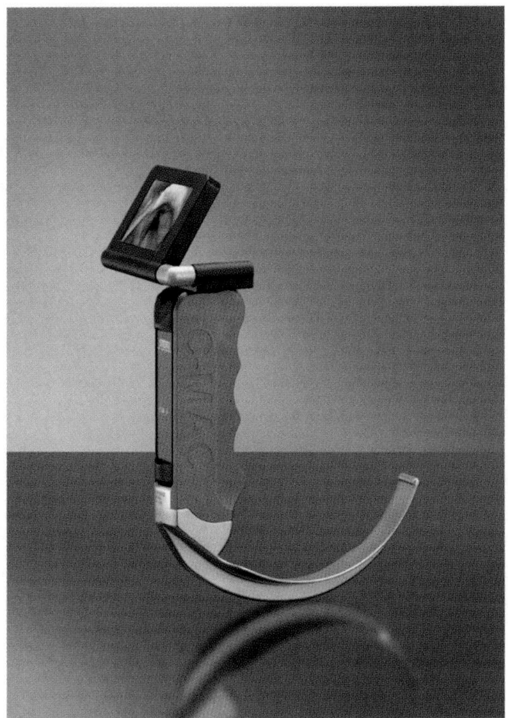

Figure 6.28 Two recent additions to the Storz line are shown in this photograph. This blade is a departure from the traditional Miller or Macintosh style and is referred to as the D-BLADE (difficult). It has a gentle upward curve intended to provide better views of more challenging anatomy. In addition, a small portable monitor displays the view in a manner similar to the McGrath. © 2011 Photo courtesy of Karl Storz Endoscopy-America, Inc.

of the sensor and light source. An intense white LED illuminates the field and the image is conveyed to a dedicated, rechargeable Li-ion battery-powered high-resolution (800 × 400), 7-in. LCD monitor. An electronic unit is plugged into the monitor and laryngoscope housing. The image can be recorded onto a secure digital (SD) card as a still image (jpeg) or a video (M-PEG 4) clip. The monitor is run off either the wall current or its stored charge. Image capture can be initiated and terminated on either the laryngoscope handle or the monitor console. Recently, a 2.7-in. LCD monitor has become available, which can be attached to the handle for portable viewing (Figure 6.28).

The C-MAC is prepared for use by inserting the electronic module into the appropriate laryngoscope blade, plugging the module into the charged monitor, inserting an SD memory card if an image is to be captured, and applying an antifogging solution to the image sensor. The use of a stylet is optional[111], though probably required for the D-BLADE (Alternatively, the ETT can be redirected using the Boedeker forceps.). The blade is introduced like a conventional Macintosh laryngoscope—along the right tongue margin—sweeping it to the left.

To date, there has been only one study evaluating the C-MAC[110], involving 60 adults requiring elective endotracheal intubation. The optimal modified laryngoscopic views[104] were assessed on the monitor with and without ELM. The use of a gum elastic bougie was permitted. Endotracheal intubation was achieved in all patients, on the first, second, and third attempts in 52, 6, and 2 patients, respectively. A gum elastic bougie was required in 8 (13%) patients. A C/L 1, 2a, or 2b view was obtained in 30, 22, and 6 patients prior to ELM; this increased to 52, 6, and 2 with applied pressure. Intubation was achieved in a mean of 16 s (range: 6–68).

Conclusion and Future Directions

Compared with fiberoptic laryngoscopes, these devices are easier to set up and incorporate into clinical practice. With the exception of the Bullard Laryngoscope and its very low profile, VL is likely to supersede the rigid fiberoptic laryngoscopes. Compared with line-of-sight methods (i.e. DL), VL offers better laryngeal exposure and permits a significantly higher percentage of visualized, controlled endotracheal intubations. Many clinicians, who have adopted VL into their practice, have no wish to revert to DL for either routine or challenging airways. Yet a recent meta-analysis, examining publications between 1997 and 2006, involving "alternative devices" concluded that there is insufficient evidence to support their routine use[112]. The authors looked at 189 publications, 57 of which met their criteria, involving 6,622 patients. They observed that the patient populations tended to be heterogeneous, definitions of difficulty varied—the authors rejected the notion that C/L 3 views represented a truly difficult intubation, though such a definition was the one most commonly used in the studies—some patients were merely predicted to be difficult (direct) laryngoscopies, and some of the devices considered had undergone modifications during the study period. They acknowledge that worldwide, many of these devices have been used to manage truly difficult airways but such data is frequently not reported and therefore lost. They concluded that existing evidence for these devices does not support a contention of superiority over DL and argue persuasively for a multicentered airway registry and more robust evaluations.*

Frerk observed that definitions of failure vary so widely that an assessment of whether devices and techniques are acceptable is highly problematic[113]. He suggested that the fundamental question is "how often can I intubate the trachea in a reasonable period of time?" and proposes that the evaluation of a device be subject to the same rules we apply to new pharmaceuticals.

Is it likely that manikin and cadaver studies are sufficiently validated to be reliable? Manikins vary greatly with regard to "tissue" compliance and anatomic fidelity[114,115]. Neither manikin nor cadaver causes fogging. Studies involving those unlikely to use these devices or involving insufficient training or practice prior to the evaluation probably do not contribute to useful assessment. If a device is proposed for routine as well as difficult airways, it should be evaluated under such conditions with meaningful outcomes[116].

It has been argued that the quality of the current evidence does not warrant the replacement of the Macintosh DL with a VL for routine airway management[112,113] yet given the poor sensitivity and specificity of our tools to predict a difficult DL, the demonstrable superiority of many of the indirect devices to visualize the larynx, the improved performance achieved by frequent use, the increasing maturation of several of these products and market place pressure, it is probable that the price gap between DL and VL will narrow. Many products and techniques have, correctly or otherwise, been introduced into practice based upon testimony rather than compelling evidence. Time, safety, or financial considerations have in some instances corrected inappropriate intrusions. The author suspects that time will select the better devices but these are more likely to involve indirect (VL) rather than direct (DL) techniques.

---

*A recent publication involving 2004 patients intubated with the GVL provides some of the required evidence. Among patients in whom DL failed, 224/239 patients were successfully intubated by GVL. Likewise, 8 of 10 patients were rescued by GVL when flexible bronchoscopic intubation failed. A 98% success rate was achieved when the GVL was used as a primary device for patients with features suggesting a difficult DL. Of equal interest was the observation that success differed between the two institutions. Increased availability and use were rewarded with greater success[72].

References

1. Prodol. Description of Airtraq benefits, sizes, optional video system, clinical data, tips & instructions,distribution, FAQs, video gallery. http://www.airtraq.com/airtraq/portal.portal.action. Accessed 23 Dec 2009.
2. Pott LM, Murray WB. Review of video laryngoscopy and rigid fiberoptic laryngoscopy. Curr Opin Anaesthesiol. 2008;21(6):750–8.
3. Thong SY, Lim Y. Video and optic laryngoscopy assisted tracheal intubation—the new era. Anaesth Intensive Care. 2009;37(2):219–33.
4. Missaghi SM, Krasser K, Lackner-Ausserhofer H, Moser A, Zadrobilek E. The Airtraq optical laryngoscope: experiences with a new disposable device for orotracheal intubation. Int J Airway Manage. 2007;4. http://www.adair.at/ijam/volume04/clinicalinvestigation02/default.htm. Accessed 1 Nov 2009.
5. Henderson JJ, Suzuki A. Rigid indirect laryngoscope insertion techniques. Anaesthesia. 2008;63(3):323–4.
6. Maharaj CH, O'Croinin D, Curley G, Harte BH, Laffey JG. A comparison of tracheal intubation using the Airtraq or the Macintosh laryngoscope in routine airway management: a randomised, controlled clinical trial. Anaesthesia. 2006;61(11):1093–9.
7. Woollard M. Use of the Airtraq laryngoscope in a model of difficult intubation by prehospital providers not previously trained in laryngoscopy. Anaesthesia. 2007;62(10):1061.
8. Savoldelli GL, Schiffer E, Abegg C, Baeriswyl V, Clergue F, Waeber JL. Comparison of the Glidescope, the McGrath, the Airtraq and the Macintosh laryngoscopes in simulated difficult airways. Anaesthesia. 2008;63(12):1358–64.
9. Maharaj CH, Higgins BD, Harte BH, Laffey JG. Evaluation of intubation using the AirtraqR or Macintosh laryngoscope by anaesthetists in easy and simulated difficult laryngoscopy—a manikin study. Anaesthesia. 2006;61(5):469–77.
10. Maharaj CH, Costello JF, Harte BH, Laffey JG. Evaluation of the Airtraq and Macintosh laryngoscopes in patients at increased risk for difficult tracheal intubation. Anaesthesia. 2008;63(2): 182–8.
11. Adnet F, Borron SW, Racine SX, et al. The intubation difficulty scale (IDS): proposal and evaluation of a new score characterizing the complexity of endotracheal intubation. Anesthesiology. 1997;87(6):1290–7.
12. Maharaj CH, Costello JF, McDonnell JG, Harte BH, Laffey JG. The Airtraq as a rescue airway device following failed direct laryngoscopy: a case series. Anaesthesia. 2007;62(6):598–601.
13. Savoldelli GL, Schiffer E, Abegg C, Baeriswyl V, Clergue FO, Waeber J-L. Learning curves of the Glidescope, the McGrath and the Airtraq laryngoscopes: a manikin study. Eur J Anaesthesiol. 2009;26(7):554–8.
14. Ndoko SK, Amathieu R, Tual L, et al. Tracheal intubation of morbidly obese patients: a randomized trial comparing performance of Macintosh and Airtraq™ laryngoscopes. Br J Anaesth. 2008;100(2):263–8.
15. Savoldelli GL, Schiffer E. Videolaryngoscopy for tracheal intubation: the guide channel or steering techniques for endotracheal tube placement? Can J Anaesth. 2008;55(1):59–60.
16. Dhonneur G, Abdi W, Amathieu R, Ndoko S, Tual L. Optimising tracheal intubation success rate using the Airtraq laryngoscope. Anaesthesia. 2009;64(3):315–9.
17. Dhonneur G, Ndoko S, Amathieu R, Housseini LE, Poncelet C, Tual L. Tracheal intubation using the Airtraq(R) in morbid obese patients undergoing emergency cesarean delivery. Anesthesiology. 2007;106(3):629–30.
18. Dhonneur G, Ndoko SK, Amathieu R, et al. A comparison of two techniques for inserting the Airtraq™ laryngoscope in morbidly obese patients. Anaesthesia. 2007;62(8):774–7.
19. Holst B, Hodzovic I, Francis V. Airway trauma caused by the Airtraq laryngoscope. Anaesthesia. 2008;63(8):889–90.
20. Turkstra TP, Pelz D, Jones P. Cervical spine motion: a fluoroscopic comparison of the AirTraq laryngoscope versus the Macintosh laryngoscope. Anesthesiology. 2009;111(1):97–101.
21. Hirabayashi Y, Fujita A, Seo N, Sugimoto H. A comparison of cervical spine movement during laryngoscopy using the Airtraq or Macintosh laryngoscopes. Anaesthesia. 2008;63(6): 635–40.
22. Santoni BGPD, Hindman BJMD, Puttlitz CMPD, et al. Manual in-line stabilization increases pressures applied by the laryngoscope blade during direct laryngoscopy and orotracheal intubation. Anesthesiology. 2009;110(1):24–31.

23. Maharaj C, Buckley E, Harte BH, Laffey JG. Endotracheal intubation in patients with cervical spine immobilization: a comparison of macintosh and airtraq laryngoscopes [article]. Anesthesiology. 2007;107(1):53–9.
24. Maharaj CH, Costello JF, Higgins BD, Harte BH, Laffey JG. Learning and performance of tracheal intubation by novice personnel: a comparison of the Airtraq and Macintosh laryngoscope. Anaesthesia. 2006;61(7):671–7.
25. Woollard M, Lighton D, Mannion W, et al. Airtraq vs standard laryngoscopy by student paramedics and experienced prehospital laryngoscopists managing a model of difficult intubation. Anaesthesia. 2008;63(1):26–31.
26. Hirabayashi Y, Seo N. Airtraq optical laryngoscope: tracheal intubation by novice laryngoscopists. Emerg Med J. 2009;26(2):112–3.
27. Maharaj CH, Costello J, Higgins BD, Harte BH, Laffey JG. Retention of tracheal intubation skills by novice personnel: a comparison of the Airtraq™ and Macintosh laryngoscopes. Anaesthesia. 2007;62(3):272–8.
28. Dimitriou VK, Zogogiannis ID, Liotiri DG. Awake tracheal intubation using the Airtraq laryngoscope: a case series. Acta Anaesthesiol Scand. 2009;53(7):964–7.
29. Suzuki A, Toyama Y, Iwasaki H, Henderson J. Airtraq™ for awake tracheal intubation. Anaesthesia. 2007;62(7):746–7.
30. Hirabayashi Y, Seo N. The Airtraq® laryngoscope for placement of double-lumen endobronchial tube. Can J Anaesth. 2007;54(11):955–7.
31. Mort TC. Tracheal tube exchange: feasibility of continuous glottic viewing with advanced laryngoscopy assistance. Anesth Analg. 2009;108(4):1228–31.
32. Koyama J, Aoyama T, Kusano Y, et al. Description and first clinical application of AirWay Scope for tracheal intubation. J Neurosurg Anesthesiol. 2006;18(4):247–50.
33. Suzuki A, Abe N, Sasakawa T, Kunisawa T, Iwasaki H. Pentax-AWS (Airway Scope) and Airtraq: big difference between two similar devices. J Anesth. 2008;22(2):191–2.
34. Malik MA, Hassett P, Carney J, Higgins BD, Harte BH, Laffey JG. A comparison of the Glidescope(R), Pentax AWS (R), and Macintosh laryngoscopes when used by novice personnel: a manikin study. Can J Anaesth. 2009;56(11):802–11.
35. Malik MA, O'Donoghue C, Carney J, Maharaj CH, Harte BH, Laffey JG. Comparison of the Glidescope, the Pentax AWS, and the Truview EVO2 with the Macintosh laryngoscope in experienced anaesthetists: a manikin study. Br J Anaesth. 2009;102(1):128–34.
36. Miki T, Inagawa G, Kikuchi T, Koyama Y, Goto T. Evaluation of the Airway Scope, a new video laryngoscope, in tracheal intubation by naive operators: a manikin study. Acta Anaesthesiol Scand. 2007;51(10):1378–81.
37. Koyama Y, Inagawa G, Miyashita T, et al. Comparison of the Airway Scope, gum elastic bougie and fibreoptic bronchoscope in simulated difficult tracheal intubation: a manikin study. Anaesthesia. 2007;62(9):936–9.
38. Hirabayashi Y, Seo N. Airway Scope: early clinical experience in 405 patients. J Anesth. 2008;22(1):81–5.
39. Cook TM. A new practical classification of laryngeal view. Anaesthesia. 2000;55(3):274–9.
40. Levitan RM, Hollander JE, Ochroch EA. A grading system for direct laryngoscopy. Anaesthesia. 1999;54(10):1009–10.
41. Suzuki A, Toyama Y, Katsumi N, et al. The Pentax-AWS(R) rigid indirect video laryngoscope: clinical assessment of performance in 320 cases. Anaesthesia. 2008;63(6):641–7.
42. Kurihara R, Inagawa G, Kikuchi T, Koyama Y, Goto T. The Airway Scope for difficult intubation. J Clin Anesth. 2007;19(3):240–1.
43. Asai T, Liu EH, Matsumoto S, et al. Use of the Pentax-AWS(R) in 293 patients with difficult airways. Anesthesiology. 2009;110(4):898–904.
44. Hirabayashi Y, Fujita A, Seo N, Sugimoto H. Cervical spine movement during laryngoscopy using the Airway Scope compared with the Macintosh laryngoscope. Anaesthesia. 2007;62(10):1050–5.
45. Enomoto Y, Asai T, Arai T, Kamishima K, Okuda Y. Pentax-AWS, a new videolaryngoscope, is more effective than the Macintosh laryngoscope for tracheal intubation in patients with restricted neck movements: a randomized comparative study. Br J Anaesth. 2008;100:544–8.
46. Maruyama K, Yamada T, Kawakami R, Hara K. Randomized cross-over comparison of cervical-spine motion with the AirWay Scope or Macintosh laryngoscope with in-line stabilization: a video-fluoroscopic study. Br J Anaesth. 2008;101(4):563–7.

47. Maruyama K, Yamada T, Kawakami R, Kamata T, Yokochi M, Hara K. Upper cervical spine movement during intubation: fluoroscopic comparison of the AirWay Scope, McCoy laryngoscope, and Macintosh laryngoscope. Br J Anaesth. 2008;100(1):120–4.
48. Komatsu R, Kamata K, Hamada K, Sessler DI, Ozaki M. Airway scope and StyletScope for tracheal intubation in a simulated difficult airway. Anesth Analg. 2009;108(1):273–9.
49. Komatsu R, Kamata K, Hoshi I, Sessler DI, Ozaki M. Airway scope and gum elastic bougie with Macintosh laryngoscope for tracheal intubation in patients with simulated restricted neck mobility. Br J Anaesth. 2008;101(6):863–9.
50. Suzuki A, Terao M, Fujita S, Henderson JJ. Tips for intubation with the Pentax-AWS rigid indirect laryngoscope in morbidly obese patients. Anaesthesia. 2008;63(4):442–4.
51. Osborn IPMD, Behringer ECMD, Kramer DCMD. Difficult airway management following supratentorial craniotomy: a useful maneuver with a new device [letter]. Anesth Analg. 2007;105(2):552–3.
52. Jones P, Turkstra T, Armstrong K, Armstrong P, Harle C. Comparison of a single-use GlideScope® Cobalt videolaryngoscope with a conventional GlideScope® for orotracheal intubation. Can J Anaesth. 2010;57:18–23.
53. Cooper RM, Pacey JA, Bishop MJ, McCluskey SA. Early clinical experience with a new videolaryngoscope (GlideScope). Can J Anaesth. 2005;52(2):191–8.
54. Jones PM, Turkstra TP, Armstrong KP, et al. Effect of stylet angulation and endotracheal tube camber on time to intubation with the GlideScope(R): [Effet de l'angulation du mandrin et de la cambrure de la sonde endotracheale sur le temps requis pour l'intubation avec le GlideScope(R)]. Can J Anaesth. 2007;54(1):21–7.
55. Doyle DJ, Zura A, Ramachandran M. Videolaryngoscopy in the management of the difficult airway. Can J Anaesth. 2004;51(1):95.
56. Dow WA, Parsons DG. 'Reverse loading' to facilitate Glidescope(R) intubation. Can J Anaesth. 2007;54(2):161–2.
57. Turkstra TP, Harle CC, Armstrong KP, et al. The GlideScope(R)-specific rigid stylet and standard malleable stylet are equally effective for GlideScope(R) use: [Le mandrin rigide specifique au GlideScope(R) et le mandrin flexible standard sont tous deux aussi efficaces pour l'utilisation avec le GlideScope(R)]. Can J Anaesth. 2007;54(11):891–6.
58. Turkstra TP, Jones PM, Ower KM, Gros ML. The Flex-It(TM) stylet is less effective than a malleable stylet for orotracheal intubation using the GlideScope(R) [miscellaneous article]. Anesth Analg. 2009;109(6):1856–9.
59. Krasser K, Moser A, Missaghi-Berlini SM, Lackner-Ausserhofer H, Zadrobilek E. Experiences with the Lo Pro adult GlideScope video laryngoscope for orotracheal intubation. Int J Airway Manage. 2007;4. http://www.ijam.at/volume04/clinicalinvestigation01/default.htm.
60. Cooper RM. Complications associated with the use of the glidescope videolaryngoscope. Can J Anaesth. 2007;54(1):54–7.
61. Choo MKF, Yeo VST, See JJ. Another complication associated with videolaryngoscopy. Can J Anaesth. 2007;54(4):322–4.
62. Williams D, Ball DR. Palatal perforation associated with McGrath videolaryngoscope. Anaesthesia. 2009;64(10):1144–5.
63. Krasser K, Moser A, Missaghi SM, Lacner- Ausserhofer H, Zadrobilek E. Evaluation with the Lo Pro Adult GlideSope Video Laryngoscope for protracheal intubation. Internet Journal of Airway Management 4, 2006–2007. Date accessed: December 31, 2007 http://www.adair.at/ijam/volume04/clinicalinvestigation01/default.htm.
64. Cortellazzi P, Minati L, Falcone C, Lamperti M, Caldiroli D. Predictive value of the El-Ganzouri multivariate risk index for difficult tracheal intubation: a comparison of Glidescope(R) videolaryngoscopy and conventional Macintosh laryngoscopy. Br J Anaesth. 2007;99(12):906–11.
65. Cooper RM. Videolaryngoscopy in the management of the difficult airway: reply. Can J Anaesth. 2004;51(1):95–6.
66. Jones PM, Harle CC. Avoiding awake intubation by performing awake GlideScope laryngoscopy in the preoperative holding area. Can J Anaesth. 2006;53:1264–5.
67. Doyle DJ. Awake intubation using the GlideScope video laryngoscope: initial experience in four cases. Can J Anaesth. 2004;51(5):520–1.
68. el Ganzouri AR, McCarthy RJ, Tuman KJ, Tanck EN, Ivankovich AD. Preoperative airway assessment: predictive value of a multivariate risk index. Anesth Analg. 1996;82(6): 1197–204.
69. Xue F, Zhang G, Liu J, et al. A clinical assessment of the Glidescope videolaryngoscope in nasotracheal intubation with general anesthesia. J Clin Anesth. 2006;18(8):611–5.

70. Jones PM, Turkstra TP. Nasotracheal intubation, direct laryngoscopy and the GlideScope(R). Anesth Analg. 2009;108(2):674.
71. Cooper RM. Use of a new videolaryngoscope (GlideScope(R)) in the management of a difficult airway. Can J Anaesth. 2003;50(6):611–3.
72. Aziz MF, Healy D, Kheterpal S, Fu RF, Dillman D, Brambrink A. Routine clinical practice effectiveness of the glidescope in difficult airway management: an analysis of 2,004 glidescope intubations, complications, and failures from two institutions. Anesthesiology. 2011;114(1): 34–41.
73. Serocki G, Bein B, Scholz J, Dorges V. Management of the predicted difficult airway: a comparison of conventional blade laryngoscopy with video-assisted blade laryngoscopy and the GlideScope [miscellaneous article]. Eur J Anaesthesiol. 2010;27(1):24–30.
74. Seal RF. Pediatric and neonatal patients. In: Alberta U, editor. Anesthesiology news, vol. PG093. New York: McMahon Publishing; 2009. p. 21–4.
75. Hirabayashi Y, Otsuka Y. Early clinical experience with GlideScope video laryngoscope in 20 infants. Paediatr Anaesth. 2009;19(8):802–4.
76. Kim JT, Na HS, Bae JY, et al. GlideScope(R) video laryngoscope: a randomized clinical trial in 203 paediatric patients. Br J Anaesth. 2008;101(4):531–4.
77. Redel A, Karademir F, Schlitterlau A, et al. Validation of the GlideScope video laryngoscope in pediatric patients. Paediatr Anaesth. 2009;19(7):667–71.
78. Griffiths S, Graham B, Brooks P. Use of the neonatal GlideScope in the management of acute upper airway obstruction. Anaesthesia. 2010;65(1):111–2.
79. Bishop S, Clements P, Kale K, Tremlett MR. Use of GlideScope Ranger in the management of a child with Treacher Collins syndrome in a developing world setting. Paediatr Anaesth. 2009;19(7):695–6.
80. Milne AD, Downer AM, Hackmann T. Airway management using the pediatric GlideScope®; in a child with Goldenhar syndrome and atypical plasma cholinesterase. Paediatr Anaesth. 2007;17(5):484–7.
81. Taub PJ, Silver L, Gooden CK. Use of the GlideScope for airway management in patients with craniofacial anomalies. Plast Reconstr Surg. 2008;121(4):237e–8.
82. Xue FS, Tian M, Liao X, Xu YC. Safe and successful intubation using the glidescope videolaryngoscope in children with craniofacial anomalies. Plast Reconstr Surg. 2009;123(3):1127–9.
83. Eaton J, Atiles R, Tuchman JB. GlideScope for management of the difficult airway in a child with Beckwith-Wiedemann syndrome. Paediatr Anaesth. 2009;19(7):696–8.
84. Gooden CK. Successful first time use of the portable GlideScope(R) videolaryngoscope in a patient with severe ankylosing spondylitis. Can J Anaesth. 2005;52(7):777–8.
85. Smith MP, Khodadadi O, Doyle DJ. Use of GlideScope video laryngoscope in morbidly obese patients (>45 BMI): a retrospective review. Anesthesiology. 2007;107:A926.
86. Bustamante S, Alfirevic A, O'Connor M. Two-operator approach to improve eye–hand coordination using the GlideScope® videolaryngoscope. Can J Anaesth. 2009;56:984–5.
87. Practice Guidelines for Management of the Difficult Airway. An updated report by the American society of anesthesiologists task force on management of the difficult airway. Anesthesiology. 2003;98(5):1269–77.
88. Crosby ET, Cooper RM, Douglas MJ, et al. The unanticipated difficult airway with recommendations for management. Can J Anaesth. 1998;45(8):757–76.
89. Cooper RM, Hagberg CA. Extubation and changing endotracheal tubes. In: Benumof JL, editor. Benumof's airway management, vol. 2. Philadelphia: Mosby Elsevier; 2007. p. 1146–80.
90. Peral D, Porcar E, Bellver J, Higueras J, Onrubia X, Barbera M. Glidescope video laryngoscope is useful in exchanging endotracheal tubes. Anesth Analg. 2006;103(4):1043–4.
91. Mort TC. Emergency tracheal intubation: complications associated with repeated laryngoscopic attempts. Anesth Analg. 2004;99(2):607–13.
92. Mort TC. The incidence and risk factors for cardiac arrest during emergency tracheal intubation: a justification for incorporating the ASA Guidelines in the remote location. J Clin Anesth. 2004;16(7):508–16.
93. Katz SH, Falk JL. Misplaced endotracheal tubes by paramedics in an urban emergency medical services system. Ann Emerg Med. 2001;37(1):32–7.
94. Latifi R, Weinstein RS, Porter JM, et al. Telemedicine and telepresence for trauma and emergency care management. Scand J Surg. 2007;96(4):281–9.

95. Sakles JC, Mosier J, Hadeed G, Hudson M, Valenzuela T, Latifi R. Telemedicine and telepresence for prehospital and remote hospital tracheal intubation using a GlideScope videolaryngoscope: a model for tele-intubation. Telemed J E Health. 2011;17(3):185–8.
96. Kaplan MB, Ward D, Hagberg CA, Berci G, Hagiike M. Seeing is believing: the importance of video laryngoscopy in teaching and in managing the difficult airway. Surg Endosc. 2006;20 Suppl 2:S479–83.
97. Howard-Quijano KJ, Huang YM, Matevosian R, Kaplan MB, Steadman RH. Video-assisted instruction improves the success rate for tracheal intubation by novices. Br J Anaesth. 2008;101(4):568–72.
98. Shippey B, Ray D, McKeown D. Case series: the McGrath(R) videolaryngoscope—an initial clinical evaluation: [Serie de cas: Le videolaryngoscope McGrath(R)—une premiere evaluation clinique]. Can J Anaesth. 2007;54(4):307–13.
99. Shippey B, Ray D, McKeown D. Use of the McGrath videolaryngoscope in the management of difficult and failed tracheal intubation. Br J Anaesth. 2008;100(1):116–9.
100. Budde AO, Pott LM. Endotracheal tube as a guide for an Eschmann gum elastic bougie to aid tracheal intubation using the McGrath(R) or GlideScope(R) videolaryngoscopes. J Clin Anesth. 2008;20(7):560.
101. Thong SY, Shridhar IU, Beevee S. Evaluation of the airway in awake subjects with the McGrath videolaryngoscope. Anaesth Intensive Care. 2009;37(3):497–8.
102. McGuire BE. Use of the McGrath video laryngoscope in awake patients. Anaesthesia. 2009;64(8):912–4.
103. O'Leary AM, Sandison MR, Myneni N, Cirilla DJ, Roberts KW, Deane GD. Preliminary evaluation of a novel videolaryngoscope, the McGrath series 5, in the management of difficult and challenging endotracheal intubation. J Clin Anesth. 2008;20(4):320–1.
104. Yentis SM, Lee DJ. Evaluation of an improved scoring system for the grading of direct laryngoscopy. Anaesthesia. 1998;53(11):1041–4.
105. Walker L, Brampton W, Halai M, et al. Randomized controlled trial of intubation with the McGrath(R) Series 5 videolaryngoscope by inexperienced anaesthetists. Br J Anaesth. 2009;103(3):440–5.
106. Kaplan MB, Ward DS, Berci G. A new video laryngoscope—an aid to intubation and teaching. J Clin Anesth. 2002;14(8):620–6.
107. Jungbauer A, Schumann M, Brunkhorst V, Brgers A, Groeben H. Expected difficult tracheal intubation: a prospective comparison of direct laryngoscopy and video laryngoscopy in 200 patients. Br J Anaesth. 2009;102(4):546–50.
108. Shiga T, Wajima Z, Inoue T, Sakamoto A. Predicting difficult intubation in apparently normal patients: a meta-analysis of bedside screening test performance. Anesthesiology. 2005;103(2):429–37.
109. Kaplan MB, Hagberg CA, Ward DS, et al. Comparison of direct and video-assisted views of the larynx during routine intubation. J Clin Anesth. 2006;18(5):357–62.
110. Cavus EMD, Kieckhaefer JMD, Doerges VMD, Moeller TMD, Thee CMD, Wagner KMD. The C-MAC videolaryngoscope: first experiences with a new device for videolaryngoscopy-guided intubation [article]. Anesth Analg. 2010;110(2):473–7.
111. van Zundert AMDPF, Maassen RMD, Lee RBE, et al. A macintosh laryngoscope blade for videolaryngoscopy reduces stylet use in patients with normal airways [miscellaneous article]. Anesth Analg. 2009;109(3):825–31.
112. Mihai R, Blair E, Kay H, Cook TM. A quantitative review and meta-analysis of performance of non-standard laryngoscopes and rigid fibreoptic intubation aids. Anaesthesia. 2008;63(7): 745–60.
113. Frerk C, Lee G. Laryngoscopy: time to change our view. Anaesthesia. 2009;64(4):351–4.
114. Cook TM, Green C, McGrath J, Srivastava R. Evaluation of four airway training manikins as patient simulators for the insertion of single use laryngeal mask airways. Anaesthesia. 2007;62(7):713–8.
115. Lee C., et al. "Variablility of force during direct laryngoscopy: A comparision of four airway training manikins: 19AP6–2." Eur J Anaesthesiol 2010;27(47):258–259.
116. Benumof JL. Intubation difficulty scale: anticipated best use. Anesthesiology. 1997;87(6): 1273–4.

7 The Role of the Supraglottic Airway

Irene P. Osborn

Introduction

The supraglottic airway (SGA) is a device designed for upper airway management, serving as a bridge, with respect to invasiveness, between facemask ventilation and endotracheal intubation. Most devices consist of an inflatable silicone or polyvinyl chloride mask and connecting tube. When blindly inserted into the pharynx, it forms a low-pressure

I.P. Osborn (✉)
Department of Anesthesiology, Mount Sinai Medical Center, One Gustave L. Levy Place, Box 1010, New York, NY 10029, USA
e-mail: Irene.Osborn@mountsinai.org

D.B. Glick et al. (eds.), *The Difficult Airway: An Atlas of Tools and Techniques for Clinical Management*, DOI 10.1007/978-0-387-92849-4_7, © Springer Science+Business Media New York 2013

Table 7.1. Advantages of the LMA.
Allows rapid access
Does not require laryngoscope
Relaxants not needed
Provides airway for spont/controlled ventilation
Tolerated at lighter anesthetic planes

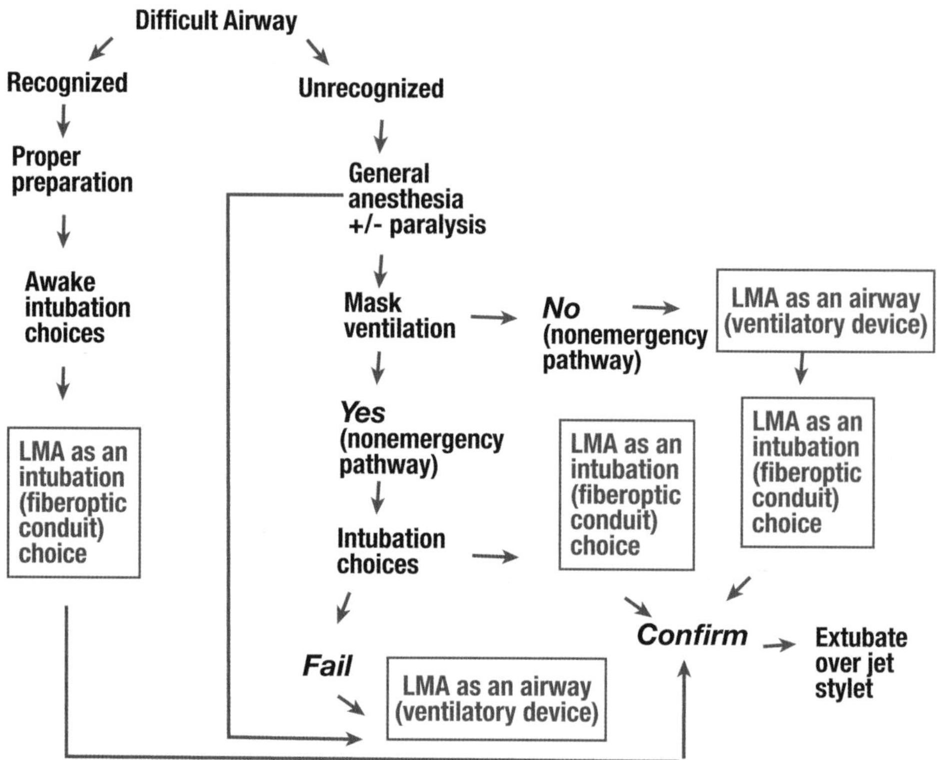

Figure 7.1. Role of the supraglottic airway (SGA) in the ASA Difficult Airway Algorithm.

seal around the laryngeal inlet. The SGA allows ventilation and oxygenation with less stimulation than laryngoscopy and intubation. The laryngeal mask airway (LMA) is the most commonly used SGA and has the largest body of experience and literature. The LMA was invented by Dr. Archie Brain and became commercially available in the UK in 1988[1]. Dr. Brain remains involved in its continued development and evolution. The device has allowed for the advancement of anesthetic techniques for ambulatory and other types of surgery. It is particularly useful when intubation is difficult, hazardous, or unsuccessful (see Table 7.1).

If successfully placed, the SGA can provide rescue ventilation or serve as a conduit for flexible bronchoscopic (FB) intubation. It has also been used to provide temporary ventilation between laryngoscopy attempts or while a surgical airway is being performed. With multiple applications, the SGA is an important option within the ASA and other difficult airway algorithms (Figure 7.1). The device has undergone an evolution over time with adaptations to provide for safer use, greater ease of insertion, and greater intubation success. And yet while SGAs are in widespread use, there is evidence that this approach is sometimes not used appropriately, with poor patient selection, inappropriate device selection, and failure to pay attention to details relating to insertion, fixation, or removal techniques[2]. This discussion will describe its role in management of the difficult airway. The LMA was the first widely used supraglottic device and later devices were designed to emulate or improve upon its success. The techniques described in this chapter are applicable to all supraglottic devices, except where otherwise stated.

Basic Use

The LMA provides an adequate airway choice for many outpatient procedures and is most commonly used in ambulatory surgery. While its use and applications continue to expand, it is important to be aware of its principal limitations, which are: (1) the potential for regurgitation and/or aspiration, (2) possible gastric inflation, and (3) the potential for displacement. The device is contraindicated for *elective* use in patients with known or suspected full stomach. In addition, the device may not seat properly in patients with abnormal or obstructive lesions of the oropharynx and may produce inadequate ventilation. Furthermore, conditions characterized by increased airway resistance or diminished compliance may not be successfully managed with a supraglottic device[3], particularly the "first generation" devices, such as the LMA Classic™.

The insertion technique for most SGAs is best accomplished with the patient's head in the sniffing position or with slight extension. Using the dominant hand, the device is pushed along the roof of the mouth and the posterior wall of the pharynx until it stops, much as a bolus of food being swallowed. The correctly positioned SGA tip lies at, and partially blocks, the upper esophagus (Figure 7.2). It is important to avoid over-inflation of the cuff of any SGA device. This happens commonly in an effort to achieve a better seal and is sometimes the source of postoperative discomfort or unintended displacement. The first generation LMA (the LMA Classic™) was manufactured using medical grade silicone and was reusable. It could be autoclaved up to 50 times (Figure 7.3). The proper insertion technique was important to avoid folding of the mask or downfolding of the epiglottis[4]. Subsequently, disposable masks (e.g. LMA Unique™) have become popular and more economical, the efficacy generally assumed to be comparable to their reusable counterparts. While important, insertion technique has been de-emphasized because of the inherent stiffness of polyvinyl chloride and other newer materials.

Following successful placement, it is important not to exceed the maximum cuff inflation volumes. If the maximum inflation volume is necessary to maintain a seal, the use of a larger size mask should be considered. Clinical studies have shown that a better seal is obtained using a larger size with less air[5]. Using an over-inflated smaller mask will exert more pressure on the hypopharyngeal mucosa, impairing local blood flow and producing a poor fit within the pharyngeal space. Increased leak, gastric insufflation, and malpositioning are more likely when the maximum cuff volume is exceeded and may be associated with adverse events.

Many clinicians prefer to utilize spontaneous ventilation with SGAs as this allows for monitoring of respiratory rate and facilitates an assessment of anesthetic depth. This technique essentially provides a "hands free" alternative to facemask ventilation and is used commonly in short anesthetic procedures.

Positive pressure ventilation (PPV) with a SGA is a useful technique for longer procedures or may be utilized when spontaneous ventilation is inadequate. PPV with a SGA may be achieved with or without muscle relaxants. When a relaxant technique is chosen, the relaxant drug may be given either before or after insertion. Leaks during PPV may be attributable to light anesthesia, use of too small a SGA, a reduction in lung/chest wall compliance related to the surgical or diagnostic procedure, patient factors, or displacement of the device by head turning or traction[6]. It is important to monitor the peak inspiratory pressures during ventilation, as this is often an indication of adequate placement, appropriate anesthetic depth, and lack of obstruction to ventilation. Placement of a bite block adjacent to the SGA, if one is not integrated into the device, is helpful in avoiding airway obstruction during emergence. Prior to emergence from anesthesia, the muscle relaxant should be reversed or allowed to wear off before discontinuing the anesthetic agent. With

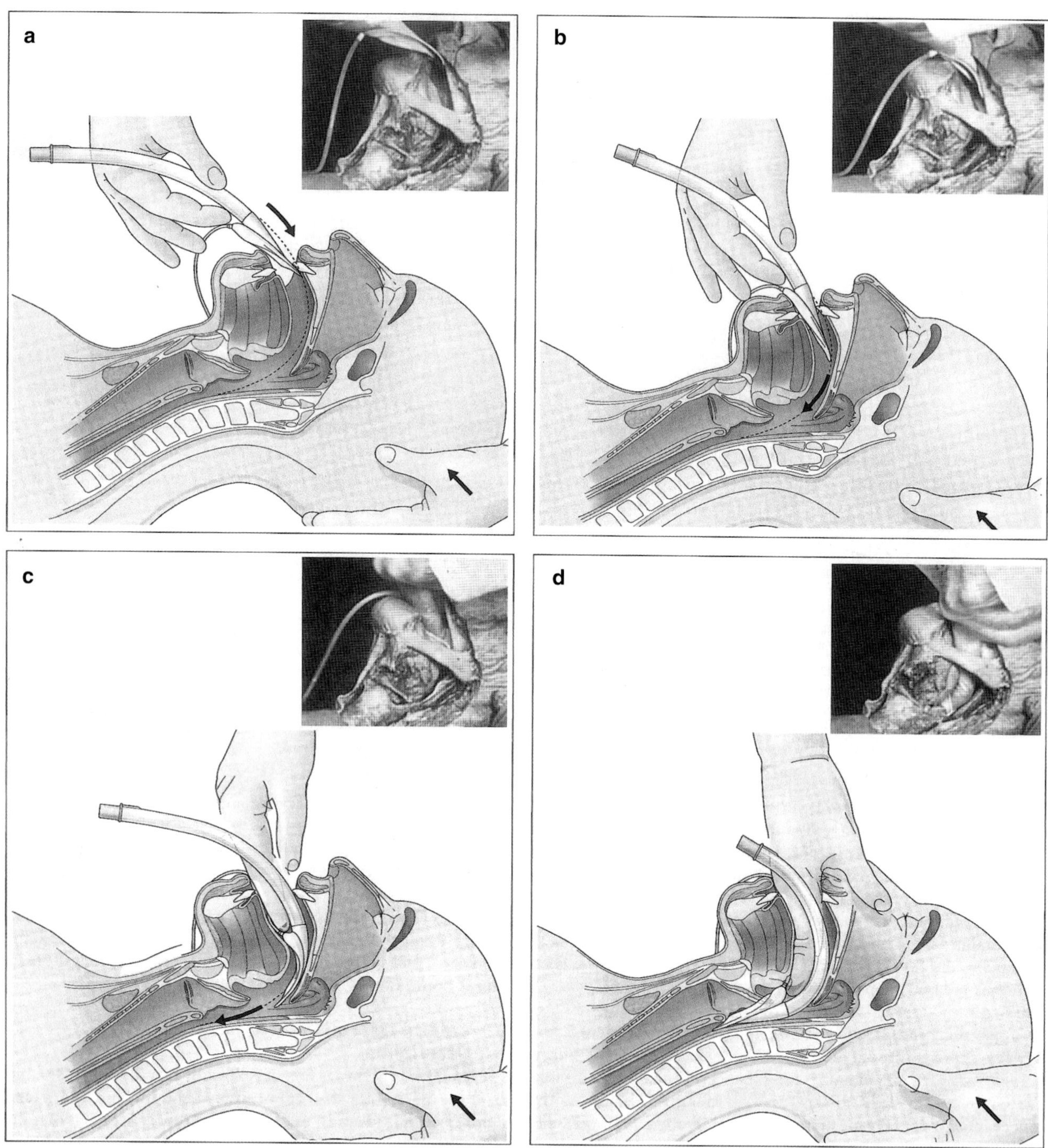

Figure 7.2. Insertion technique for the LMA classic (reproduced with permission from Brimacombe JR. Laryngeal mask anesthesia, Chapter 8: placement phase. Philadelphia: Saunders; 2005).

gentle, assisted ventilation, the patient should be allowed to resume normal spontaneous ventilation. The SGA is removed, usually without deflation, as the patient begins to swallow and demonstrates a return of airway reflexes. Current recommendations suggest a maximum duration of 6–8 h with frequent evaluation and adjustment of intracuff pressure, particularly in the presence of nitrous oxide. The true limits, however, are unknown. When intracuff pressure was maintained at 60-cm H_2O, less sore throat was reported by patients[7]. Prolonged use has been associated with potential nerve injury, dislodgement, or mucosal injury.

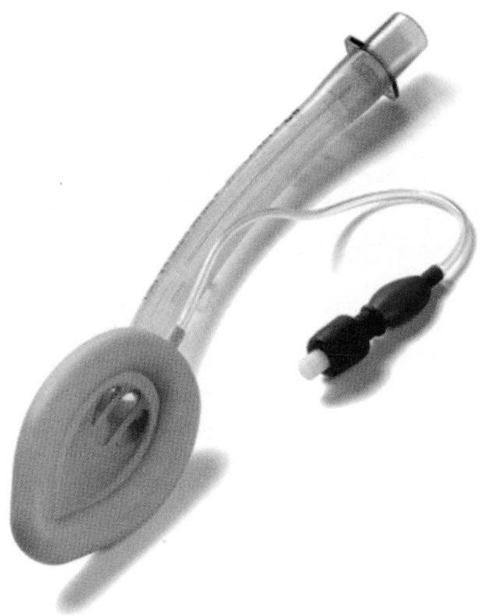

Figure 7.3. The LMA Classic™.

The LMA as a Rescue Device

In the setting of a failed intubation, if adequate mask ventilation cannot be obtained or maintained, urgent placement of a familiar SGA should be considered. Generally, insertion of the LMA is not more difficult in patients with Mallampati class III or IV airways or in those patients in whom laryngoscopy reveals Cormack-Lehane Grade 3 or 4 views[8]. It is unclear whether this is equally true for all other SGAs. Following numerous reports of successful LMA use in failed intubation and ventilation, the LMA was incorporated into the "Practice Guidelines for management of the difficult airway" in 1993[9]. In the 2003 ASA Difficult Airway Practice guidelines, the LMA (specifically) moved up to the first position in the "Can't Intubate, Can't Ventilate" portion of the algorithm[10]. In patients whose lungs cannot be ventilated because of supraglottic obstruction and whose trachea cannot be intubated due to unfavorable anatomy (but not periglottic pathology), the LMA should be immediately available and considered as the first treatment choice[11] (Figure 7.1).

Case reports detail the successful use of the LMA in a variety of congenital and acquired syndromes associated with difficult airway management. The LMA has been successfully used as a rescue airway device after failed intubation in patients with lingual tonsillar hyperplasia, but more difficult and traumatic insertion of the LMA has been reported in that situation[12]. The placed LMA (and likely other SGAs) can be (1) left in place, (2) removed for intubation attempts with a flexible bronchoscope (FB), or (3) used as a conduit for intubation (see below).

In the patient with a full stomach, cricoid pressure may interfere with correct placement of the SGA[13]. A reasonable alternative between competing concerns of continuously maintaining cricoid pressure in a patient at risk for aspiration and failure to properly insert the SGA is to momentarily release cricoid pressure as the distal tip of the SGA reaches the hypopharynx. This maximizes the chance of correct SGA placement while minimizing risk of aspiration. Once the LMA (and possibly other SGAs) is in situ, it probably does not interfere with the efficacy of cricoid pressure[14].

Flexible Bronchoscopic Intubation Via the SGA

The SGA is useful in failed intubations as a rescue airway, and it can also serve as a conduit for endotracheal intubation. The aperture bars of the LMA were intended to prevent the epiglottis from obstructing the shaft (Figure 7.3). If adequate ventilation is possible through

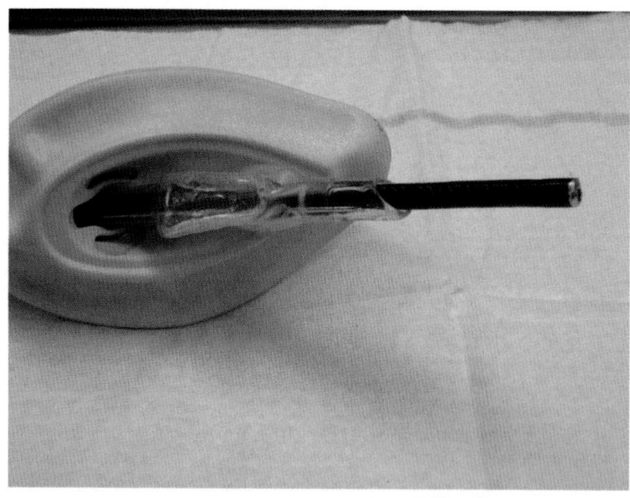

Figure 7.4. Fiberoptic bronchoscope via the LMA Classic™.

the LMA, it is probable that the bowl of the LMA surrounds the larynx and FB-guided tracheal intubation will be successful. Endotracheal intubation through the LMA was first described in 1989 by Allison and McCrory using a gum-elastic bougie (GEB)[15], but their initial success could not be easily duplicated. While it is tempting to consider blindly placing an endotracheal tube through the LMA, this is not recommended. First, the LMA must be properly seated to ventilate the patient. In patients with distorted airway anatomy and when proper seating and ventilation are suboptimal, it is less likely that a GEB or blind passage through the LMA will result in tracheal placement.

Lim and co-workers evaluated three types of ETTs and three head and neck positions finding a significant difference with both variables. Although the best head and neck position for blind intubation through the LMA-C was the sniffing position, this was only successful in approximately half the cases[16]. Conversely, intubation over a FB passed through the LMA is highly successful in most series. Thus, if the difficulty during conventional intubation was due to unfavorable anatomical alignment and not periglottic pathology and one can ventilate through a SGA, it provides a suitable conduit to the trachea[17]. If ventilation is poor after SGA insertion, because of poor apposition to the laryngeal aperture, or there is major periglottic pathology, FB-guided tracheal intubation may be difficult.

Bronchoscopic intubation through the SGA may be performed electively or as a rescue maneuver. It has been described in numerous clinical situations and is the cornerstone for management of failed intubation in pediatric patients[18]. Advantages of this technique include the ability to oxygenate the patient effectively before and between attempts at ETT placement and the ability to inspect the airway above the glottis. It may also be a good choice in the patient unwilling or unable to cooperate with awake intubation.

When using the LMA C, the aperture bars may dictate the size of the ETT unless an Aintree Intubation Catheter (AIC) is used (see below). The ETT is loaded onto a lubricated FB. The endoscope is passed through the LMA aperture bars and under the epiglottis, until a clear view of the glottis is obtained. The FB is advanced well into the trachea until the carina is in view. The FB is then stabilized as the lubricated ETT is advanced over the FB, through the LMA and into the trachea. If resistance is encountered, the ETT may have to be withdrawn a few centimeters, rotated 90°, and re-advanced one or more times to move the tip past the glottis. The ETT and the LMA are held fixed and the FB is withdrawn (Figure 7.4). Inflation of the ETT cuff, ventilation through the ETT, and confirmation with $ETCO_2$ and bilateral breath sounds should then proceed. The LMA is deflated and the ETT is secured to the shaft of the device. The entire unit (ETT and LMA) can remain in place until exchanged.

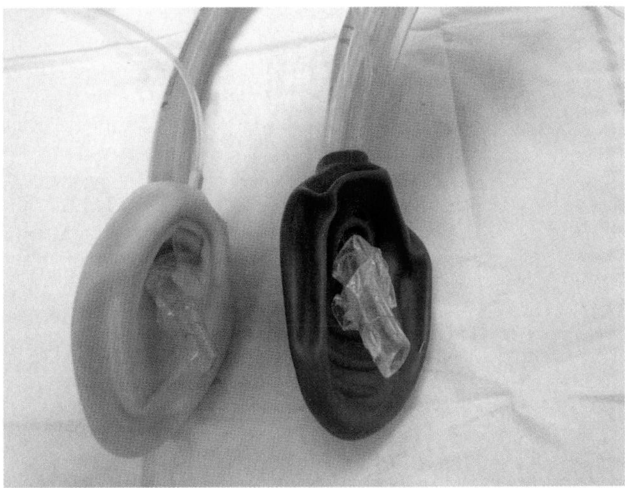

Figure 7.5. Endotracheal tubes via LMA Excel™ and ILA™.

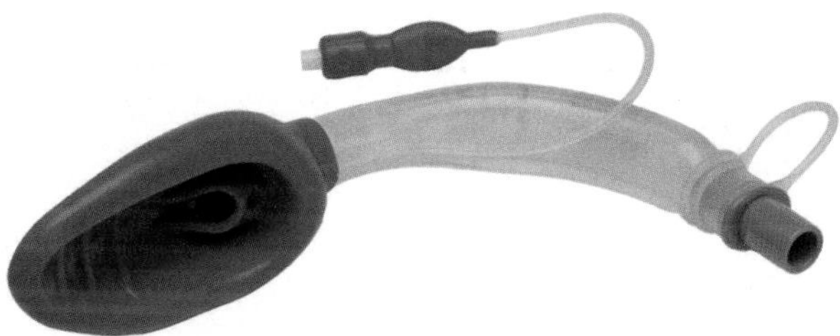

Figure 7.6. Intubating laryngeal airway (ILA™).

A 6.0 mm-ID cuffed ETT may be passed over the FB and through the shaft of a size #3 or #4 LMA and a 7.0 mm-ID cuffed ETT may be passed over the FB and through the shaft of a size #5 LMA. If a larger ETT is desired, the LMA and the ETT can be exchanged for a larger ETT over a tube exchanger or an AIC (see below).

Other Supraglottic Airways for Intubation

The SGA for intubation is primarily used as an airway intubator in adults with difficult airways, but can also be used as an alternative to routine laryngoscopy. (Care must be taken to avoid the use of a SGA to avoid intubating the patient if no backup plan exists.) These devices can facilitate airway management in patients who *may* be difficult to ventilate and intubate such as morbidly obese patients, patients with sleep apnea, or patients with limited neck movement. Furthermore, SGAs can be very helpful in the unanticipated difficult airway. A properly performed insertion causes less hemodynamic response; therefore it could be a less stimulating alternative to rigid laryngoscopy for patients with cardiovascular comorbidities. The Intubating Laryngeal Airway (ILA, Mercury Medical, Clearwater, FL) was introduced as an alternative device for airway management. It features a modified cuff, wider shaft, and lacks the aperture bars characteristic of the LMA (Figs. 7.5 and 7.6). The disposable version is called the Air-Q®.

The Air-Q® is inserted using the same technique as standard SGAs and inflated. Blind insertion of an ETT is not recommended and flexible or rigid endoscopes (air-VU®, Mercury Medical) are used. After intubation, the device can be easily removed using the manufactured stylet or the device can remain in place to facilitate a smooth extubation (Figure 7.7a, b).

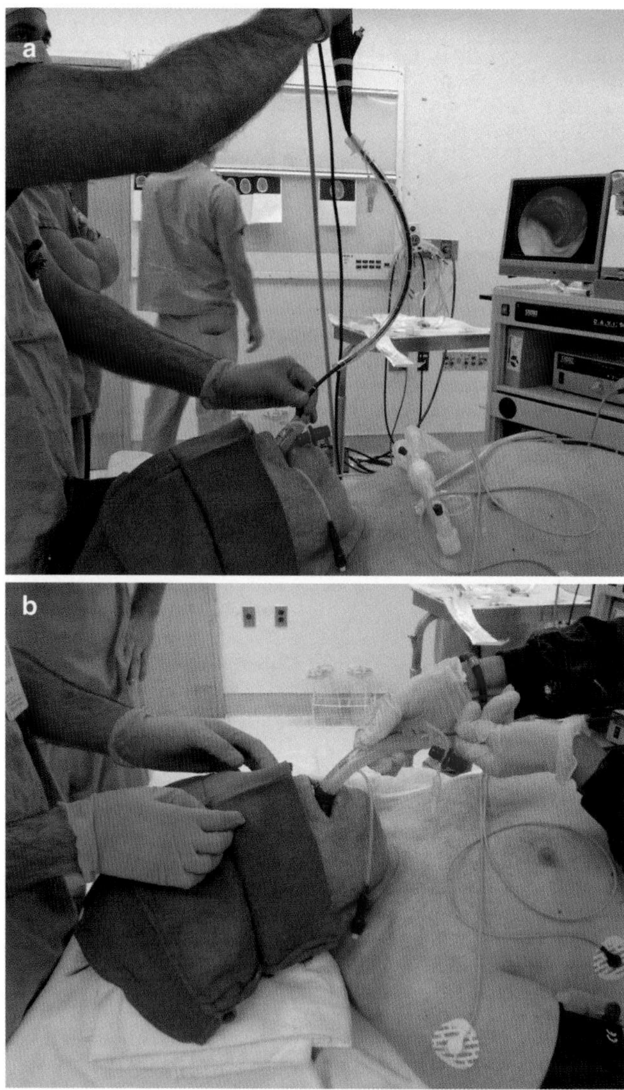

Figure 7.7. (**a**) Fiberoptic intubation via the ILA™. (**b**) Removal of the ILA™ using the removal stylette.

Awake Placement of the Laryngeal Mask

There are numerous descriptions of using the LMA in properly prepared awake patients as a conduit for fiberoptic intubation[19]. There are several reasons why this technique is suitable when the preoperative evaluation indicates the patient should be intubated awake. First, even though awake tracheal intubation can be performed by many techniques in a properly prepared patient, insertion of a SGA is generally tolerated producing little hemodynamic change. The relative lack of stimulation in passing an LMA reduces the amount of preparation (topicalization, sedation) that a semi-conscious patient may require for the procedure. Lighter sedation also facilitates the act of swallowing which aids in the insertion of the LMA. Second, when the SGA is in good position, the shaft of the device is directed toward the larynx, and visualization of the laryngeal aperture with a FB is easy. Third, the patient who maintains spontaneous breathing is less likely to become hypoxemic than if ventilation ceases or intubation is prolonged. Fourth, and perhaps most importantly, with the patient awake, no options are eliminated, and risk remains low even if there is difficulty in inserting the SGA or the FB.

Proper placement of the SGA into an awake patient also allows the device to be used as a primary means of airway control in patients whose airways are potentially difficult, but who may not require endotracheal intubation. The topicalization technique is similar to that required for awake FB intubation (see Chap. 3), with perhaps more emphasis on the oropharynx to block the glossopharyngeal nerves. This technique is particularly useful in patients with obstructive sleep apnea as the SGA can rapidly overcome the cause(s) of obstruction and allow unimpeded spontaneous ventilation. Whether performed in awake or asleep patients, the SGA allows for opening of the laryngeal space, which is beneficial in the bloodied or soiled airway.

The Intubation LMAs (Fastrach™ and CTrach™)

The Intubating LMA (Fastrach™)

The intubating LMA (ILMA) was developed to allow for endotracheal intubation via the laryngeal mask as well as provide for efficient ventilation of the patient[20,21]. Introduced in 1997, the ILMA was designed to overcome the shortcomings of FB techniques through the LMA classic and to improve the success rate of blind intubation. The limitations of the FB techniques included reduced ETT size, LMA tube length and inner diameter, aperture bars, and the frequent need to replace the entire apparatus, which included the LMA. The ILMA consists of a mask attached to an anatomically shaped rigid stainless steel shaft, which aligns with the glottis. The angle of the metal shaft was specially designed to fit into the oral and pharyngeal space while maintaining the head and neck in neutral position (Figure 7.8)[22].

The ILMA has a 13-mm internal shaft diameter that can accommodate an 8.0-mm cuffed endotracheal tube, which can be advanced into the larynx either blindly or with FB guidance. The shaft is short enough to ensure that the tracheal tube cuff extends beyond the vocal cords. The mask of the ILMA is similar to the classic LMA, however, the aperture bars are replaced by an epiglottic-elevating bar, which facilitates tube placement. The device is best utilized with special tubes, which have soft, blunt tips and flexible shafts (Figure 7.9).

These ILMA-ETTs have blunt tips and low-compliance cuffs, requiring careful cuff inflation to avoid tracheal mucosal injury. Until recently, these were only available as expensive reusable tubes, often inadvertently discarded. Alternatively, a standard ETT can be inserted using the ILMA. This mostly requires softening the tube in warm water and/or turning the ETT 180° prior to insertion into the ILMA. This maneuver reduces the natu-

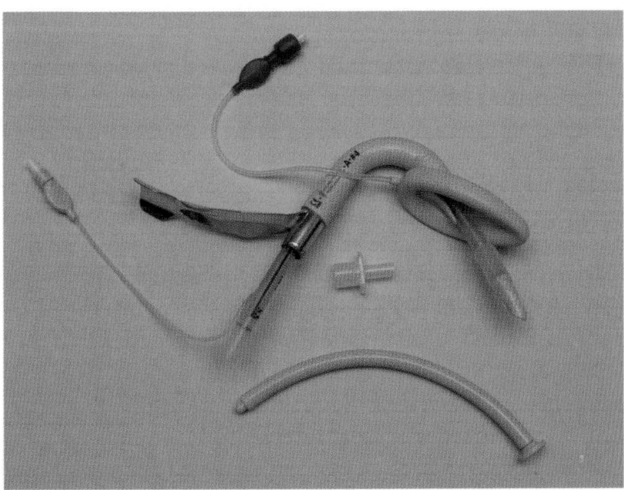

Figure 7.8. The LMA Fastrach™ and its parts.

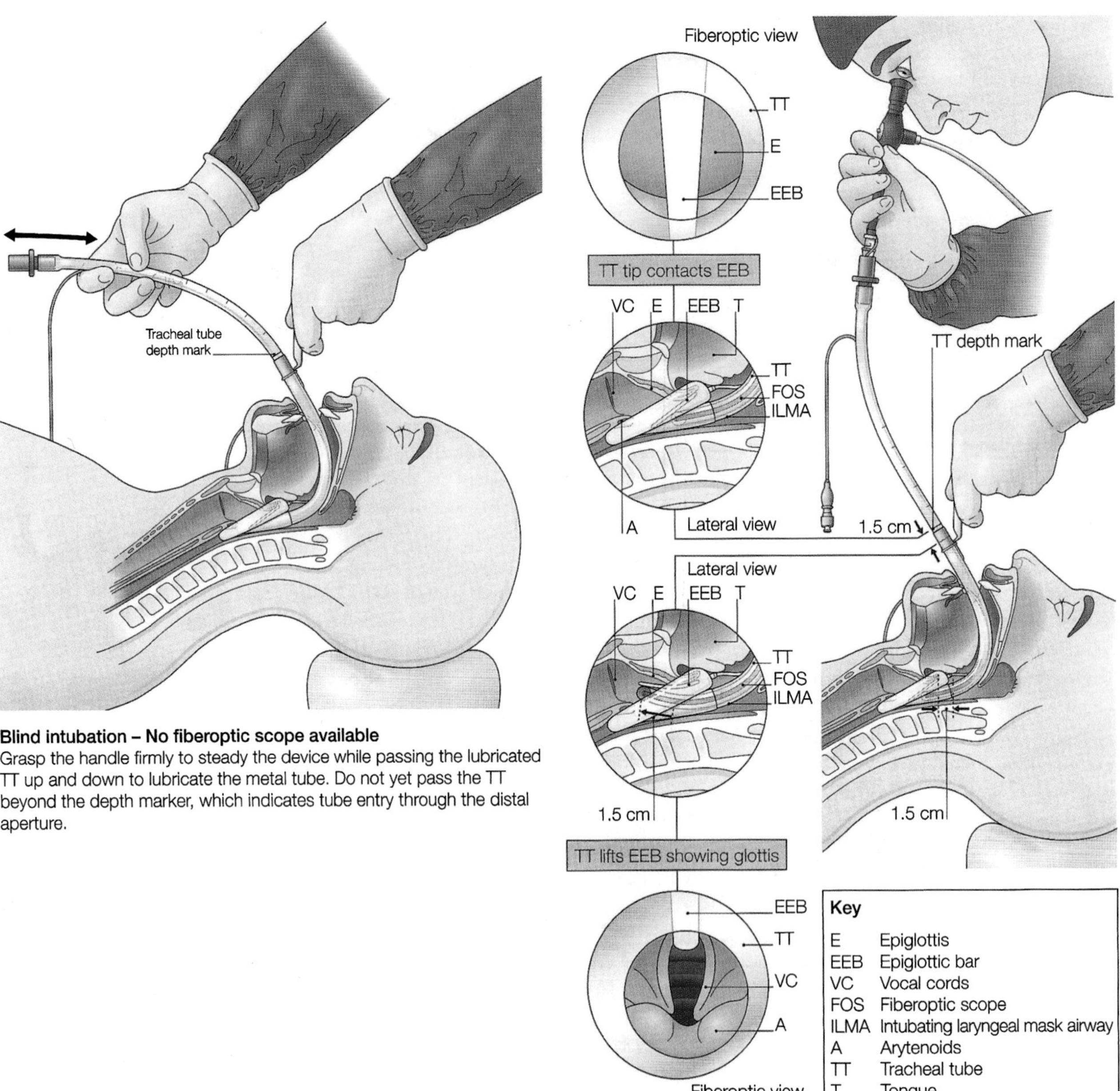

Figure 7.9. The LMA Fastrach™ showing blind and fiberoptic insertion techniques (reproduced with permission from Brimacombe JR. Laryngeal mask anesthesia, Chapter 18: Intubating LMA for airway intubation. Philadelphia: Saunders; 2005).

ral curve of most polyvinylchloride tubes and allows placement (Figure 7.10)[21]. The ILMA can be used electively in patients with normal airways as an intubating tool. It can also be utilized to prevent excessive hemodynamic response in patients with cardiovascular compromise. Early clinical reports described its benefits in patients with reduced or immobilized cervical spine disease because of the neutral insertion technique. A multi-centered survey by Ferson et al. described use of the ILMA in 254 patients with difficult-to-manage airways and reported an overall success rate for blind and FB-guided intubations of 97 % and 100 %, respectively[23]. The classic LMA as well as the ILMA can be inserted in a variety of patient positions (lateral, prone, sitting) when required for rescue ventilation[24].

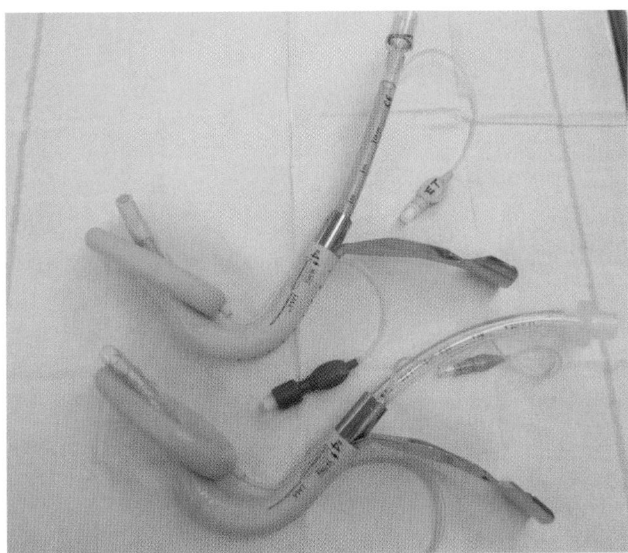

Figure 7.10. Placement of the Euromedical ETT and standard polyvinylchloride ETT, with 180° curve.

While the ILMA has been used extensively as a device for airway management in patients with limited neck movement, Combes et al. initially demonstrated its role in the failed ventilation/intubation scenario. In a prospective study involving over 11,000 patients, difficult ventilation was encountered in only 6 patients and intubation using the ILMA was attempted in 15 failed intubations. Success was achieved on the first attempt in 9 and the second attempt in 3 with failure occurring in 2[25]. Like other airway techniques, the ILMA should be practiced in normal airways to gain proficiency. The device is most successful following failed intubation in patients with seemingly normal airways. It can, however, be placed in awake patients with topical anesthesia when FB-guided intubation fails or is unavailable. Shung et al. in South Africa described successful awake intubation through an ILMA in 15 patients with difficult airways[26].

For successful intubation in the anesthetized patient with the ILMA and CTrach™ (see below), the "Chandy maneuver" is extremely helpful[23] (Figure 7.11). Before insertion of these devices, an adequate depth of anesthesia must be confirmed and muscle relaxants (or tracheal topicalization) should be administered. After insertion in the neutral position followed by ventilation, the "Chandy maneuver" should be performed, which consists of two steps performed sequentially. The first step, which is important for establishing optimal ventilation, is to rotate the ILMA slightly in the sagittal plane using the metal handle to optimize chest compliance during bag ventilation. The second step, performed just before blind intubation, consists of using the metal handle to slightly lift (but not tilt) the ILMA away from the posterior pharyngeal wall. This facilitates the smooth passage of the ETT into the trachea. It is recommended that one remove the ILMA after intubation, using the stabilizing rod to keep the ETT in place as the ILMA is removed.

Frappier et al. studied the use of the ILMA in 118 consecutive morbidly obese patients for elective surgery with a success rate of 96.3 %. In their hands the ILMA was an effective and safe ventilatory device associated with a high success rate for blind intubation in morbidly obese patients[27]. Nevertheless, the choice of the primary technique (laryngoscopy or ILMA) for tracheal intubation of an adult obese patient remains to be determined. The ILMA has been included in the difficult airway algorithms in the United Kingdom[28] and Europe and has gained acceptance in pre-hospital use in many regions. Despite its success in these patients, many continue to have concerns about use of the ILMA in unstable cervical spine injuries based on cadaver studies[29]. In multi-trauma situations, the risk of cervical spine injury must sometimes be balanced against the need for timely oxygenation and ventilation.

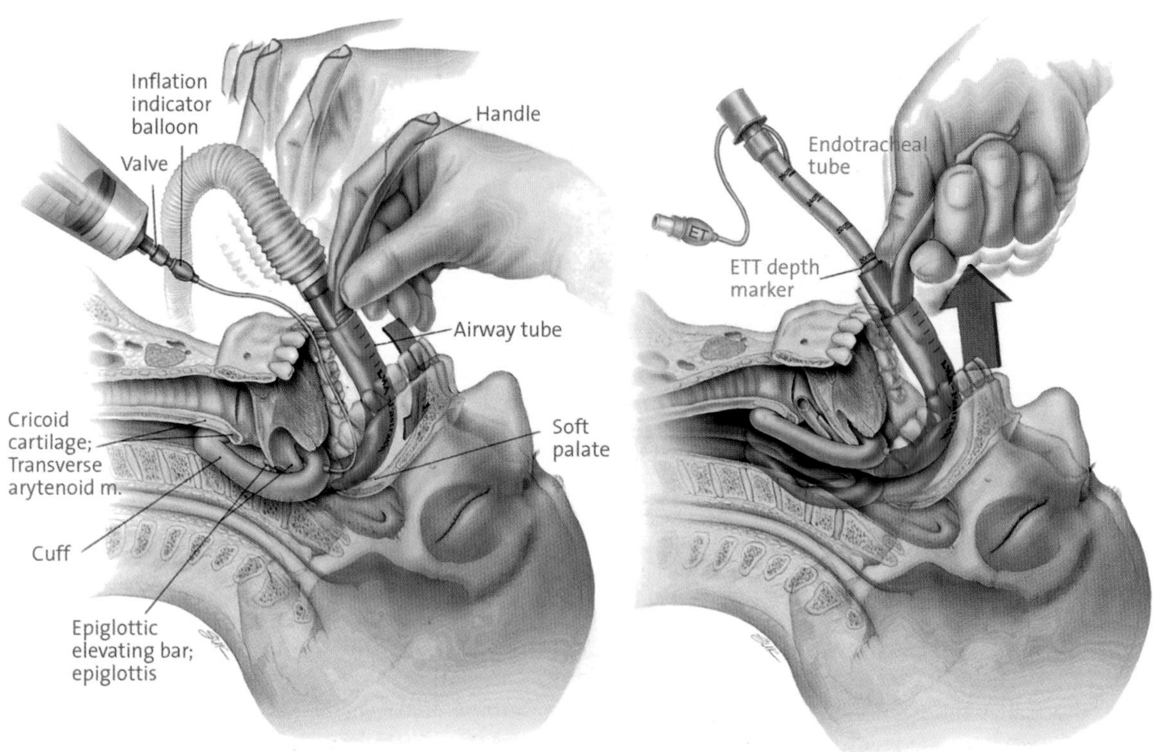

Figure 7.11. The "Chandy maneuver" (reproduced with permission from Ferson et al.[23]).

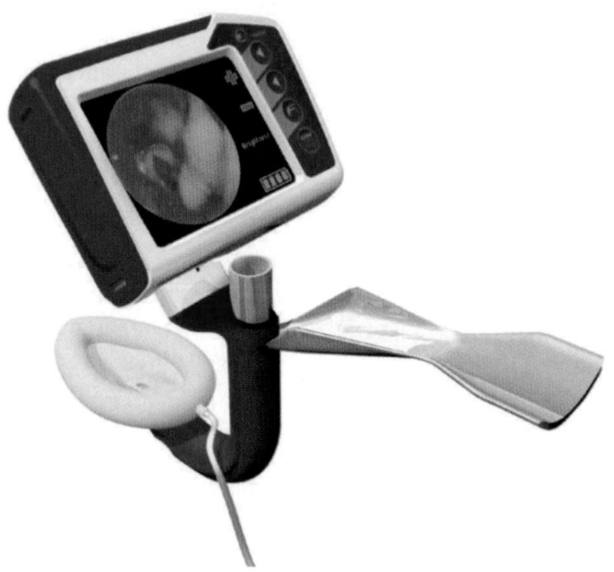

Figure 7.12. The LMA C-Trach™.

The ILMA C-Trach™ is a modification of the ILMA that combines the features of the ILMA with a fiberoptic system and a detachable LCD screen. The device was released in 2005, but was recently discontinued. A detachable screen provided a video image, acquired from a video sensor located in the epiglottic elevator. This facilitates alignment of device and ETT advancement through the laryngeal inlet[30] (Figure 7.12). Liu and associates described 48 patients with difficult airways managed electively or following failed laryngoscopy using the LMA CTrach™. Their report detailed the importance of optimizing ventilation, which was not possible in two of their patients[31]. Awake placement of the LMA CTrach™ has been successfully accomplished and described in morbidly obese patients with difficult airways[32].

LMAs with Gastric Access

The LMA ProSeal™

The ProSeal LMA (PLMA) is a laryngeal mask device that features a larger cuff and a drainage tube, allowing access to the gastrointestinal tract. This device was the first of the "second generation" SGAs, significantly addressing the limitations of the LMA C (and other first generation SGAs): (1) the potential for gastric inflation and (2) the risk of aspiration of gastric contents (Figure 7.13). Brain's design goal was to construct a laryngeal mask with improved ventilatory characteristics that also offered protection against regurgitation and gastric inflation[33]. The PLMA was introduced into clinical practice in 2000 and was designed primarily for elective use. Its silicone construction is allegedly softer than that of the LMA-C and is better designed to conform to the contours of the hypopharynx. This device incorporates a second lumen, arising from the distal end of the laryngeal mask and terminating outside of the patient airway. This lumen, termed the gastric drain, has been demonstrated to passively vent regurgitated esophageal contents[34]. A gastric tube can also be placed down this lumen to empty the stomach.

The PLMA is designed for advanced clinical uses such as prolonged operative procedures, surgical procedures in the lateral or prone position, and to extend SGA benefits to a greater number of patients. While the PLMA may be used with spontaneous ventilation, it is well suited for PPV, with and without muscle relaxants. The design of the PLMA permits PPV at higher peak pressures. It has been used electively as an alternative to endotracheal intubation for laparoscopic surgery in a number of reports[35,36] though some question the wisdom of this practice[37]. The advantages have primarily been the ease of insertion, lack of hemodynamic and airway reflex stimulation, and smooth emergence from anesthesia with minimal coughing and hypertension. While these are features of the LMA C™, the PLMA extends these benefits to larger patients or those with mild or controlled gastric

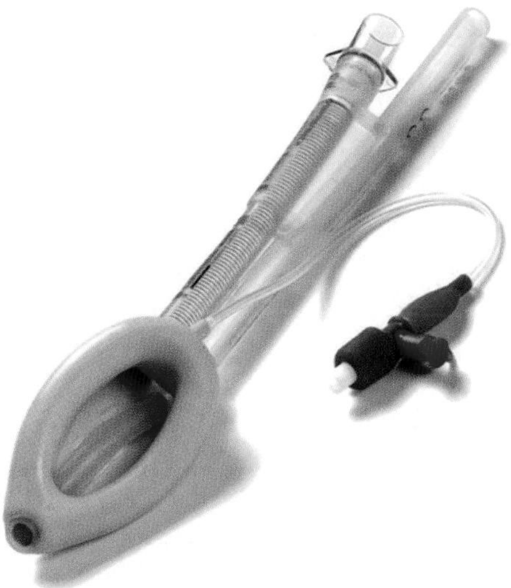

Figure 7.13. The LMA ProSeal™.

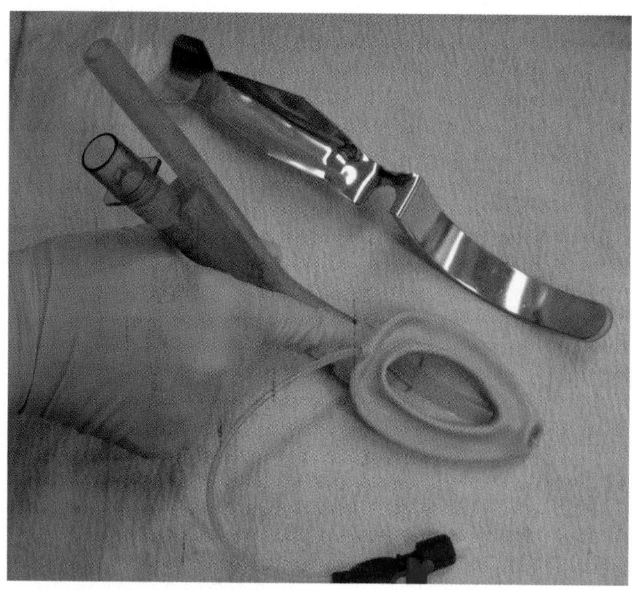

Figure 7.14. The LMA ProSeal™ with finger cuff and optional insertion tool.

reflux. Studies comparing the PLMA to the LMA Classic™ have demonstrated higher airway sealing pressure with the PLMA without an increase in mucosal pressure[33]. There are isolated case reports of its use in failed intubation and ventilation emergency situations[38]. Rosenblatt reported a case where the PLMA was used to decompress the abdomen after repeated attempts at intubation had failed and mask ventilation had caused extensive gastric inflation[39].

A pocket-like opening for the index finger, which helps to maintain proper insertion technique, facilitates insertion of the PLMA. The PLMA can also be inserted using an optional insertion tool, which obviates the need of the operator inserting fingers into the patient's mouth (Figure 7.14). The PLMA was the first SGA that provided a sequence of steps and tests to assure proper placement. These are important points for use because the device has a larger surface area and potentially can fold-over in the hypopharynx[40,41]. This might provide ventilation, but may not permit optimal positioning or gastric decompression. Brimacombe reported on the technique of using an Eschmann intubation guide and laryngoscope for successful placement of the PLMA. This insertion technique had a high success rate and was of particular advantage when PLMA placement proved challenging[42,43]. This would be recommended in the event that laryngoscopy and intubation failed and it was deemed necessary to place the device in patients with possible gastric contents (Figure 7.15). There are no aperture bars in the PLMA, but there is a bite block to protect the patient from biting the shaft and occluding the airway. The PLMA was designed for effective and efficient ventilation. It was not designed to be a conduit for endotracheal intubation though this is possible with a fiberoptic bronchoscope using an AIC (see below).

LMA Supreme™

The LMA Supreme™ (SLMA), released in 2007, combines the integrated bite block and gastric drainage tube of the PLMA and the preconfigured shape of the ILMA Fastrach™. This single-use plastic device has a high-volume/low-pressure cuff providing a higher seal pressure and fixation tab to help secure the airway[44] (Figs. 7.16 and 7.17). The device is intended for elective use as well as potential use in pre-hospital and resuscitative scenarios. Like the PLMA, the gastric drainage tube reduces the risk of regurgitation and aspiration if properly seated.

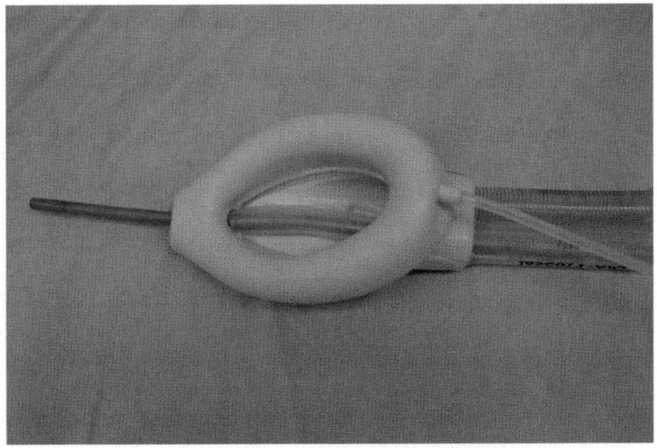

Figure 7.15. A gum-elastic bougie may be used to facilitate placement of the LMA ProSeal™.

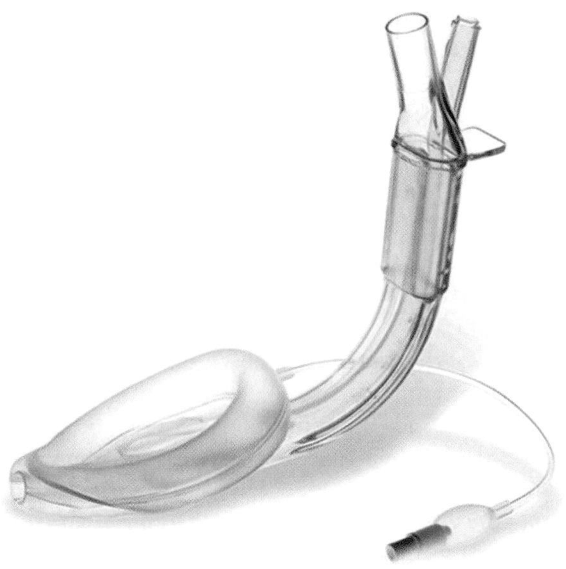

Figure 7.16. The LMA Supreme™.

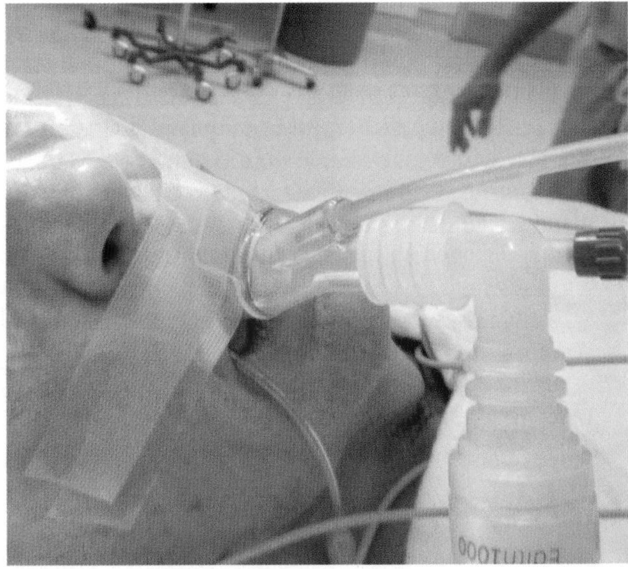

Figure 7.17. Aspiration of contents from the gastric port of the LMA Supreme™.

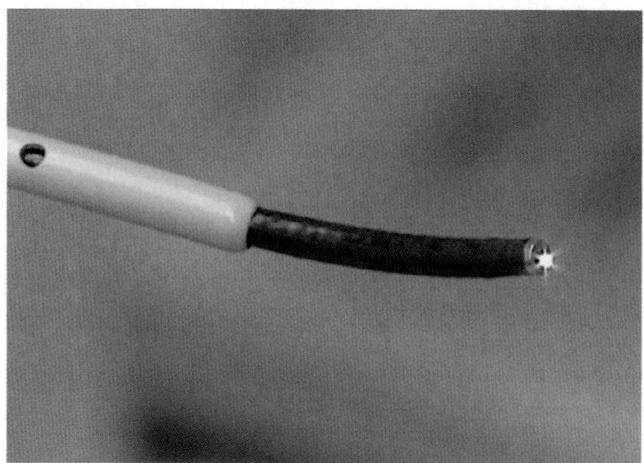

Figure 7.18. Aintree catheter with fiberoptic bronchoscope.

Several studies have compared the SLMA and PLMA. The SLMA has slightly lower oropharyngeal leak pressures than the PLMA[45]. The success of the first attempt insertion was higher for the SLMA and this is to be expected because of its design. The device appears to be efficacious and easy-to-use in elective ambulatory procedures. The higher rate of success on first attempt insertion may make it more suitable as an airway rescue device[46]. It is also intended for use in cardiopulmonary resuscitation procedures as well as in the failed intubation and the "can't intubate-can't ventilate" situation[47].

The ease of insertion of the SLMA™ has been one of its most attractive features. It has been described for insertion in the prone position. This approach may be utilized in the stressful circumstance of accidental extubation of a patient in the prone or lateral position. Some expert users describe elective SLMA placement when the patient is induced and the airway secured in the prone position[48].

The SLMA should not be used for the resuscitation of patients who are not profoundly unconscious unless adequate topical anesthesia has been provided.

Intubating Through LMAs (Classic, Supreme, and ProSeal: Using the Aintree Intubation Catheter)

The AIC (Cook Medical, Bloomington IN) is similar in concept to the Cook Airway Exchange Catheter® (see Chap. 16). Its larger internal diameter (4.8 mm) will accommodate a lubricated FB of 4.0 mm OD or smaller (Figure 7.18)[49]. The AIC's external diameter (6.5 mm) allows its use with endotracheal tubes 7.0 mm and larger. The AIC facilitates the placement of a larger endotracheal tube, otherwise precluded by the inner diameter of the SGA shaft or the aperture bars. It should be noted that the AIC is 56 cm in length, leaving a relatively limited amount of flexible scope to protrude beyond the catheter distally (Figure 7.19). After introducing the SGA and establishing successful ventilation, the FB is introduced into the AIC. This FB-AIC assembly is introduced through the shaft of the SGA and into the trachea. When the FB is within the trachea, the AIC is advanced

(a) The bronchoscope is withdrawn
(b) The SGA is removed over the AIC
(c) An ETT is advanced over the AIC
(d) A Rapi-Fit™ connector can be attached to the AIC to permit PPV between maneuvers (Figure 7.20)

This technique is suitable for use with a wide range of SGAs. It has a role in elective management of the patient in whom bag mask ventilation is difficult or in whom intubation difficulties are anticipated or have been encountered[50,51].

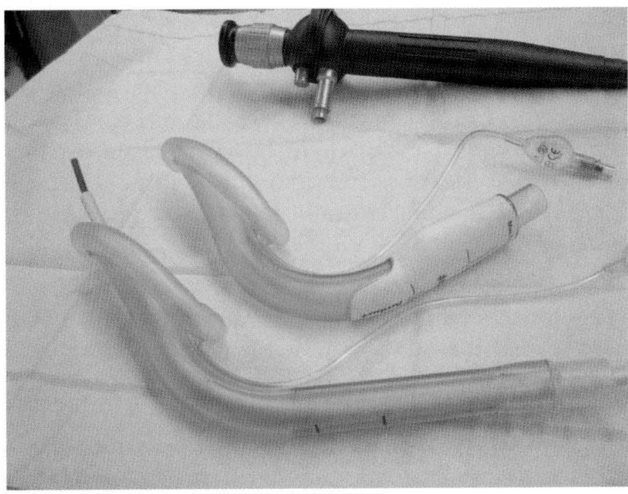

Figure 7.19. Aintree catheter with Ambu SGA.

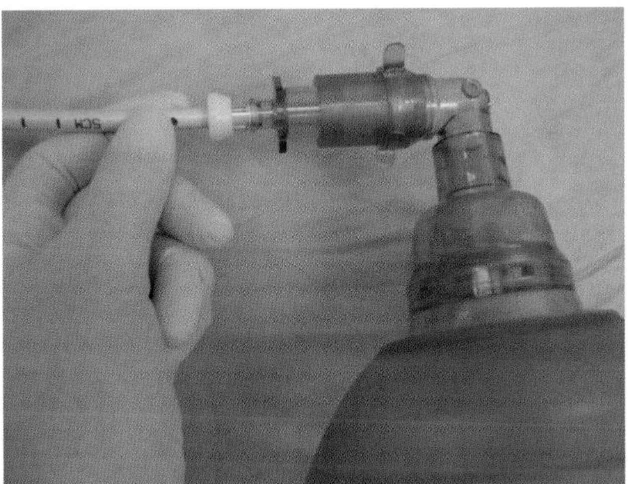

Figure 7.20. Aintree catheter with "Rapi-fit" connector.

Conclusion

SGAs represent a considerable advancement in the management of routine and complex airways. This chapter has devoted disproportionate attention to the LMA because it has been used more widely and more has been written about it than all the other SGAs combined; however as of this writing, over 70 varieties of SGAs are available. For some of these devices, there is limited evidence, but others such as the igel™ (Intersurgical, Wokingham UK) and air-Q™ (Mercury Medical, Clearwater FL) are generating interest and clinical support. "First generation" SGAs represented a better mask; "second generation" SGAs separated the respiratory and gastrointestinal tract, at least theoretically reducing the risk of aspiration while at the same time providing a more effective seal for PPV. All can be used as conduits for endotracheal intubation, particularly when combined with a flexible bronchoscope and an AIC.

For all their advantages, a number of issues remain. In a prospective study involving nearly three million general anesthetics in the U.K., SGAs were used in 56 % of cases and were involved in 33/133 of major airway complications resulting in death, brain injury, surgical airway, or unintended ICU admission[2,52,53]. These complications occurred as a result of aspiration, airway trauma, failure to establish or loss of the airway, and extubation-related complications. Improper insertion technique, inadequate confirmation, poor patient selection, inappropriate device selection with excessive reliance on first-generation SGAs, and the use of SGA in a patient with a difficult airway, without an adequate backup plan in the event of failure, were the emerging themes. The SGAs represent an advance in airway management, but patient safety will only be enhanced if the user has acquired proficiency through frequent use and critical self-assessment. In a patient with a known or presumed difficult airway, reliance upon a SGA to avoid tracheal intubation without an adequate backup plan does not advance patient safety.

References

1. Brain AI. The laryngeal mask—a new concept in airway management. Br J Anaesth. 1983;55(8):801–5.
2. Cook TM, Woodall N, Frerk C. Major complications of airway management in the UK: results of the Fourth National Audit Project of the Royal College of Anaesthetists and the Difficult Airway Society. Part 1: anaesthesia. Br J Anaesth. 2011;106(5):617–31.
3. Benumof JL. Laryngeal mask airway. Indications and contraindications. Anesthesiology. 1992;77(5):843–6.
4. Brain A. Proper technique for insertion of the laryngeal mask. Anesthesiology. 1990;73(5):1053.
5. Gaitini LA, Vaida SJ, Somri M, Yanovski B, Ben-David B, Hagberg CA. A Randomized controlled trial comparing the ProSeal™ laryngeal mask airway with the laryngeal tube suction in mechanically ventilated patients. Anesthesiology. 2004;101(2):316–20.
6. Brimacombe J, Berry A, Verghese C. The laryngeal mask airway: its uses in anesthesiology. Anesthesiology. 1994;80(3):706.
7. Seet E, Yousaf F, Gupta S, Subramanyam R, Wong DT, Chung F. Use of manometry for laryngeal mask airway reduces postoperative pharyngolaryngeal adverse events: a prospective, randomized trial. Anesthesiology. 2010;112(3):652–7.
8. Brimacombe J, Berry A. Mallampati classification and laryngeal mask airway insertion. Anaesthesia. 1993;48(4):347.
9. American Society of Anesthesiologists Task Force on Management of the Difficult Airway. Practice guidelines for management of the difficult airway. A report by the American Society of Anesthesiologists Task Force on Management of the Difficult Airway. Anesthesiology. 1993;78(3):597–602.
10. Practice Guidelines for Management of the Difficult Airway. An updated report by the American Society of Anesthesiologists Task Force on Management of the Difficult Airway. Anesthesiology. 2003;98(5):1269–77.
11. Benumof JL. Laryngeal mask airway and the ASA difficult airway algorithm. Anesthesiology. 1996;84(3):686–99.
12. Ovassapian A, Glassenberg R, Randel GI, Klock A, Mesnick PS, Klafta JM. The unexpected difficult airway and lingual tonsil hyperplasia: a case series and a review of the literature. Anesthesiology. 2002;97(1):124–32.
13. Asai T, Morris S. The role of the laryngeal mask for failed tracheal intubation in the patient with a "full stomach". Anesth Analg. 1994;78(4):817–9.
14. Brimacombe J, Berry A, White A. An algorithm for use of the laryngeal mask airway during failed intubation in the patient with a full stomach. Anesth Analg. 1993;77(2):398–9.
15. Allison A, McCrory J. Tracheal placement of a gum elastic bougie using the laryngeal mask airway. Anaesthesia. 1990;45(5):419–20.
16. Lim SL, Tay DHB, Thomas E. A comparison of three types of tracheal tube for use in laryngeal mask assisted blind orotracheal intubation. Anaesthesia. 1994;49(3):255–7.
17. Benumof JL. Use of the laryngeal mask airway to facilitate fiberscope-aided tracheal intubation. Anesth Analg. 1992;74(2):313–5.
18. Rabb MF, Minkowitz HS, Hagberg CA. Blind intubation through the laryngeal mask airway for management of the difficult airway in infants. Anesthesiology. 1996;84(6):1510–1.
19. Asai T. Fiberoptic tracheal intubation through the laryngeal mask in an awake patient with cervical spine injury. Anesth Analg. 1993;77(2):404.
20. Parr M, Baskett GM. The intubating laryngeal mask. Anaesthesia. 1998;53:343.

21. Gerstein NS, Braude DA, Hung O, Sanders JC, Murphy MF. The Fastrach(TM) intubating laryngeal mask Airway(R): an overview and update. Can J Anaesth. 2010;57(6):588.
22. Brain AI, Verghese C, Addy EV, Kapila A. The intubating laryngeal mask. I: development of a new device for intubation of the trachea. Br J Anaesth. 1997;79(6):699–703.
23. Ferson DZ, Rosenblatt WH, Johansen MJ, Osborn I, Ovassapian A. Use of the intubating LMA-Fastrach in 254 patients with difficult-to-manage airways. Anesthesiology. 2001;95(5):1175–81.
24. Dimitriou V, Iatrou C, Brimacombe J, Voyagis GS. Intubating laryngeal mask airway in lateral position. Anesthes Analg. 2004;99(6):1877; author reply.
25. Combes X, Le Roux B, Suen P, Dumerat M, Motamed C, Sauvat S, et al. Unanticipated difficult airway in anesthetized patients: prospective validation of a management algorithm. Anesthesiology. 2004;100(5):1146–50.
26. Shung J, Avidan MS, Ing R, Klein DC, Pott L. Awake intubation of the difficult airway with the intubating laryngeal mask airway. Anaesthesia. 1998;53(7):645–9.
27. Frappier J, Guenoun T, Journois D, Philippe H, Aka E, Cadi P, et al. Airway management using the intubating laryngeal mask airway for the morbidly obese patient. Anesthesh Analg. 2003;96(5):1510–5, table of contents.
28. Henderson JJ, Popat MT, Latto IP, Pearce AC. Difficult Airway Society guidelines for management of the unanticipated difficult intubation. Anaesthesia. 2004;59(7):675–94.
29. Brimacombe J, Keller C, Kunzel KH, Gaber O, Boehler M, Puhringer F. Cervical spine motion during airway management: a cinefluoroscopic study of the posteriorly destabilized third cervical vertebrae in human cadavers. Anesth Analg. 2000;91(5):1274–8.
30. Timmermann A, Russo S, Graf BM. Evaluation of the CTrach—an intubating LMA with integrated fibreoptic system. Br J Anaesth. 2006;96(4):516–21.
31. Liu EH, Goy RW, Lim Y, Chen FG. Success of tracheal intubation with intubating laryngeal mask airways: a randomized trial of the LMA Fastrach and LMA CTrach. Anesthesiology. 2008;108(4):621–6.
32. Wender R, Goldman AJ. Awake insertion of the fibreoptic intubating LMA CTrach in three morbidly obese patients with potentially difficult airways. Anaesthesia. 2007;62(9):948–51.
33. Brimacombe J, Keller C. The ProSeal laryngeal mask airway: a randomized, crossover study with the standard laryngeal mask airway in paralyzed, anesthetized patients. Anesthesiology. 2000;93(1):104–9.
34. Keller C, Brimacombe J, Kleinsasser A, Loeckinger A. Does the ProSeal laryngeal mask airway prevent aspiration of regurgitated fluid? Anesth Analg. 2000;91(4):1017–20.
35. Maltby JR, Beriault MT, Watson NC. Use of the laryngeal mask is not contraindicated for laparoscopic cholecystectomy. Anaesthesia. 2001;56(8):799.
36. Maltby JR, Beriault MT, Watson NC, Liepert DJ, Fick GH. LMA-Classic and LMA-ProSeal are effective alternatives to endotracheal intubation for gynecologic laparoscopy. Can J Anaesth. 2003;50(1):71–7.
37. Cooper RM. The LMA, laparoscopic surgery and the obese patient—can vs should. Can J Anesth. 2003;50(1):5–10.
38. Baxter S, Brooks A, Cook T. Use of a proseal LMA for maintenance after failed intubation during a modified rapid sequence induction. Anaesthesia. 2003;58(11):1132–3.
39. Rosenblatt WH. The use of the LMA-ProSeal in airway resuscitation. Anesth Analg. 2003;97(6):1773–5.
40. O'Connor Jr JCJ, Borromeo CJ, Stix MS. Assessing ProSeal laryngeal mask positioning: the suprasternal notch test. Anesth Analg. 2002;94(5):1374–5.
41. Osborn IP, Behringer EC, Cooper RM, Verghese C. Detecting the etiologies of acute airway obstruction associated with the laryngeal mask airway supreme(TM). Anesthesiology. 2009;111(2):451–2. doi:10.1097/ALN.0b013e3181adf285.
42. Brimacombe J, Howath A, Keller C. A more 'failsafe' approach to difficult intubation with the gum elastic bougie. Anaesthesia. 2002;57(3):292.
43. Brimacombe J, Keller C. Aspiration of gastric contents during use of a ProSealTM laryngeal mask airway secondary to unidentified foldover malposition. Anesth Analg. 2003;97(4): 1192–4.
44. Verghese C, Ramaswamy B. LMA-Supreme—a new single-use LMA with gastric access: a report on its clinical efficacy. Br J Anaesth. 2008;101(3):405–10.
45. Tan BH, Chen EG, Liu EH. An evaluation of the laryngeal mask airway supreme' in 100 patients. Anaesth Intensive Care. 2010;38(3):550–4.

46. Seet E, Rajeev S, Firoz T, Yousaf F, Wong J, Wong DT, et al. Safety and efficacy of laryngeal mask airway Supreme versus laryngeal mask airway ProSeal: a randomized controlled trial. Eur J Anaesthesiol. 2010;27(7):602–7.
47. Abdi W, Dhonneur G, Amathieu R, Adhoum A, Kamoun W, Slavov V, et al. LMA supreme versus facemask ventilation performed by novices: a comparative study in morbidly obese patients showing difficult ventilation predictors. Obes Surg. 2009;19(12):1624–30.
48. Lopez AM, Valero R, Brimacombe J. Insertion and use of the LMA Supreme in the prone position. Anaesthesia. 2010;65(2):154–7.
49. Bogdanov A, Kapila A. Aintree intubating bougie. Anesth Analg. 2004;98(5):1502.
50. Blair EJ, Mihai R, Cook TM. Tracheal intubation via the classic and proseal laryngeal mask airways: a manikin study using the aintree intubating catheter. Anaesthesia. 2007;62(4):385–7.
51. Micaglio M, Ori C, Parotto M, Feltracco P. Three different approaches to fibreoptic-guided intubation via the Laryngeal Mask Airway Supreme. J Clin Anesth. 2009;21(2):153–4.
52. Woodall N, Frerk C, Cook TM. Can we make airway management (even) safer?—lessons from national audit. Anaesthesia. 2011;66 Suppl 2:27–33.
53. Woodall NM, Cook TM. National census of airway management techniques used for anaesthesia in the UK: first phase of the Fourth National Audit Project at the Royal College of Anaesthetists. Br J Anaesth. 2011;106(2):266–71.

8

The Role of Flexible Bronchoscopy

David B. Glick

D.B. Glick (✉)
Department of Anesthesia & Critical Care, University of Chicago Hospitals, 5841S Mary land Ave, MC 4028, Chicago, IL 60615, USA
e-mail: dglick@dacc.uchicago.edu

D.B. Glick et al. (eds.), *The Difficult Airway: An Atlas of Tools and Techniques for Clinical Management*, DOI 10.1007/978-0-387-92849-4_8, © Springer Science+Business Media New York 2013

Introduction

Over the past 45 years flexible bronchoscopy has become the "gold standard" for managing the expected and unexpected difficult airway[1,2]. Unlike rigid laryngoscopy, intubation using a flexible bronchoscope does not require that an unobstructed straight view from the upper incisors to the larynx be created for intubation. Thus, patients with limited oral apertures, a mobile cervical spine, upper airway abnormalities (tumors, lingual tonsils, etc.), and redundant pharyngeal tissue are some of the classes of difficult airways that are better managed with fiberoptic intubations than with classic direct laryngoscopy.

The first fiberoptic intubation was performed by Murphy using a choledochoscope in 1967[3]. Though the technique was initially slow to be adopted, the flexible bronchoscope is now used routinely in airway management. Because of its flexible character and small diameter, the fiberoptic bronchoscope can be used for either nasal or oral intubations, and because it has been shown to cause less hemodynamic stimulation and moderately sedated patients find it less irritating than direct laryngoscopy, fiberoptic bronchoscopy has become the most widely used technique for awake intubations.

Equipment Necessary for Fiberoptic Intubation

Preparing for fiberoptic intubations requires more equipment than most other intubating techniques. The bronchoscope itself is relatively complex compared to other intubating devices (Figure 8.1). It is composed of an eyepiece, a control section, a flexible insertion tube that is manipulated with an angulation controller, a universal cord containing the light fiber bundles and electrical wiring, and the light guide connector section. In addition to the camera and light fibers, the larger sized insertion tubes may also contain a channel for suctioning at the tip and/or a working channel that can be used to introduce catheters or instruments at the tip of the bronchoscope or to deliver fluids (e.g., saline flushes or local anesthesia) at the tip. The insertion tube used for adult intubations is usually about 4 mm in diameter. Larger diameter insertion tubes are available with larger working channels. Obviously, larger insertion tubes require that larger endotracheal tubes be used since the internal diameter of the endotracheal tube must be large enough to accommodate the bronchoscope (Table 8.1). One common example of the need to balance insertion tube size

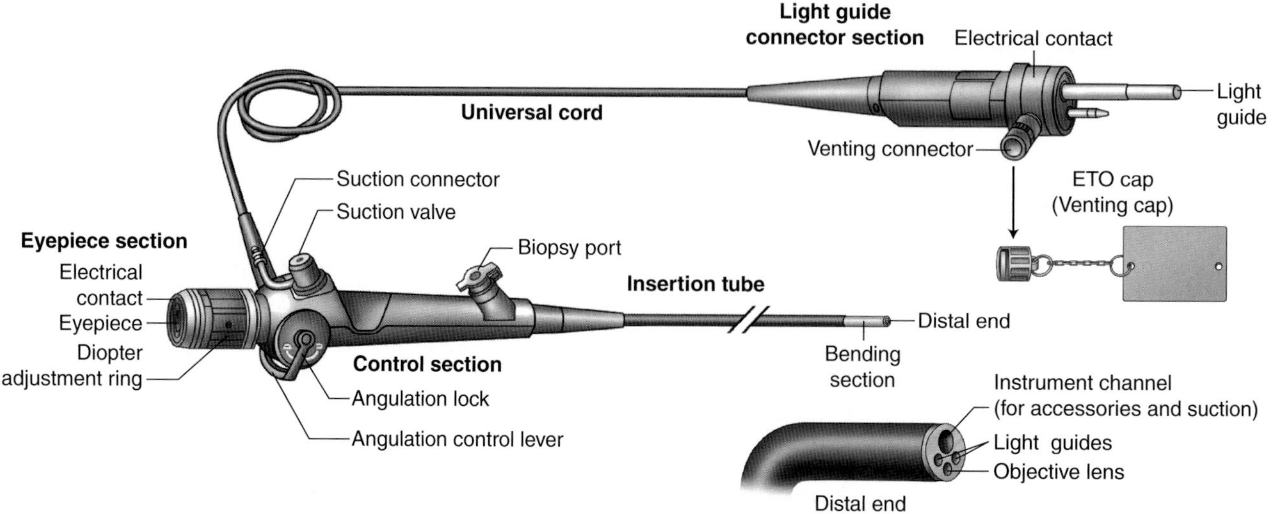

Figure 8.1. Schematic diagram of a flexible bronchoscope.

Table 8.1. Insertion tube diameters, minimum ETT IDs, and lengths of commonly used bronchoscopes.

	Insertion tube size (mm)	Min size ETT ID (mm)	Length (mm)
Olympus			
BF-P160	4.9	6.0	600
BF-P40	5.0	6.5	600
BF-3C160	3.8	5.0	600
LF-V	4.0	5.0	600
LF-GP	4.1	5.0	600
LF-TP	5.2	6.5	600
LF-2	4.0	5.0	600
LF-P	2.2	2.5	600
LF-DP	3.1	3.5	600
Storz			
11301-ABN1	2.8	3.5	500
11301-AB1	2.8	3.5	500
11302-BDN1	3.7	4.5	650
11302-BD1	3.7	4.5	650
1131-BNN1	5.2	6.0	650
1131-BN1	5.2	6.0	650
Pentax			
FB-8V	2.8	3.5	600
FB-10V	3.4	4.0	600
FB-15V	4.9	5.5	600
EB-1570	5.1	6.0	600
FI-13BS	4.1	5.0	600
EB-1170K	3.8	4.5	600
Ambu			
aScope2[a]	5.4	6.0	630

[a]The Ambu aScope2 is a single use (disposable) intubating scope. ETT= endotracheal tube, ID = internal diameter

against the size of the endotracheal tube is in the pediatric patient. Thus, flexible bronchoscopes with very small insertion tubes are available (as small as 2.2 mm in diameter) to permit fiberoptic intubations in small children (including neonates). However, because the insertion tube is so small, it is not possible to accommodate a working channel or a suction channel in these scopes.

In addition to the bronchoscope itself, a light source is also required. Portable bronchoscopes are available that have a light source built into the control section; unfortunately, these light sources do not provide the same light intensity as the external light source units. The external light sources are quite large and, as a result, are usually placed on a cart to permit the user to push the light source around the operating room or to offsite locations. Additionally, a cart can be rigged to carry the fiberoptic scope and intubation supplies discussed below. A typical cart setup is shown in Figure 8.2.

Classically, the person performing a fiberoptic procedure looks through the eyepiece of the control section. Teaching adapters (Figure 8.3) were developed to allow a second person to watch the procedure with the same view as the individual performing the procedure. Now, many flexible bronchoscope carts include a video monitor to which the bronchoscope can be attached to allow the image to be displayed on a larger format, and one which the entire team can see. This allows the assistant to offer more useful help and allows an experienced bronchoscopist to better see and explain the technique to the novice/trainee. Many contemporary bronchoscopes have no eyepiece at all and require a video monitor for image display. These systems often allow for still and video image capture, as well.

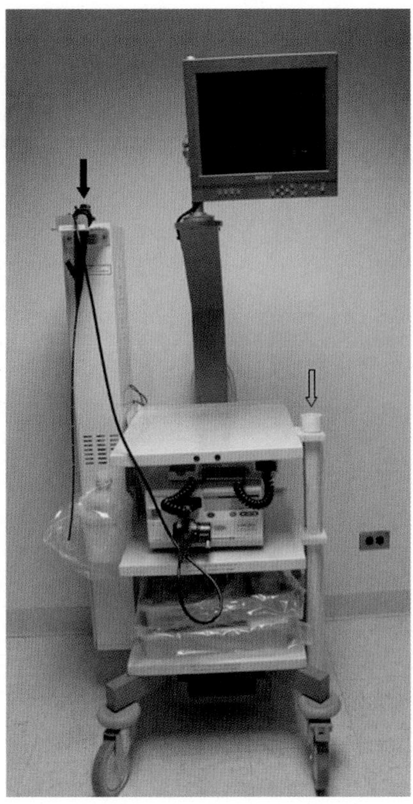

Figure 8.2. A bronchoscope cart with a light source and video hook-up on the middle shelf, and trays with commonly used drugs and airway equipment on the bottom shelf. The video screen is attached to a pole at the back of the cart and there is a protective case containing clean scopes on the *left* of the cart (marked with a *solid black arrow*) and a protective tube (marked with a *black outlined arrow*) on the *right* for the safe storage of used/dirty scopes.

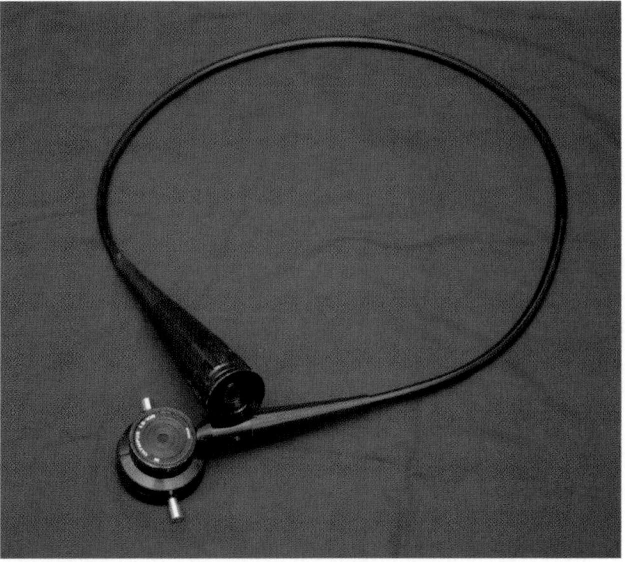

Figure 8.3. The teaching attachment allows a second person (e.g., a more experienced bronchoscopist) to see what the bronchoscopist is seeing to help guide the intubation.

Additional Supplies Necessary for Flexible Bronchoscopy

In addition to the bronchoscope and light source, the cart often contains other useful drugs and supplies to facilitate intubations.

The Intubating Airway

There are a number of intubating airways available. Unlike standard oral airways, these devices have open channels on top or along their sides to permit the midline introduction of the bronchoscope and endotracheal tube while allowing for passage of a relatively large caliber tube and easy removal of the airway after successful intubation. While the Ovassapian airway was developed specifically for use during fiberoptic intubations, many of the other devices were initially developed to facilitate blind oral intubations but worked effectively for fiberoptic intubations as well. Several of these devices are shown in Figure 8.4.

Other Common Contents of the Cart

It is useful to have 4 × 4 gauze pads available both to facilitate the assistant's grasping of the tongue (when an intubating airway is not being used) and to apply surgical lubricant to the insertion tube to ease the passage of the endotracheal tube off of the scope and into the airway. The cart can also store surgical lubricant, local anesthetics (usually lidocaine 4 % liquid and 5 % jelly), an atomizer (or other aerosolizing device to spray the liquid lidocaine into the oropharynx), and tongue depressors to facilitate intubating airway placement and to apply 5 % lidocaine jelly to the base of the tongue.

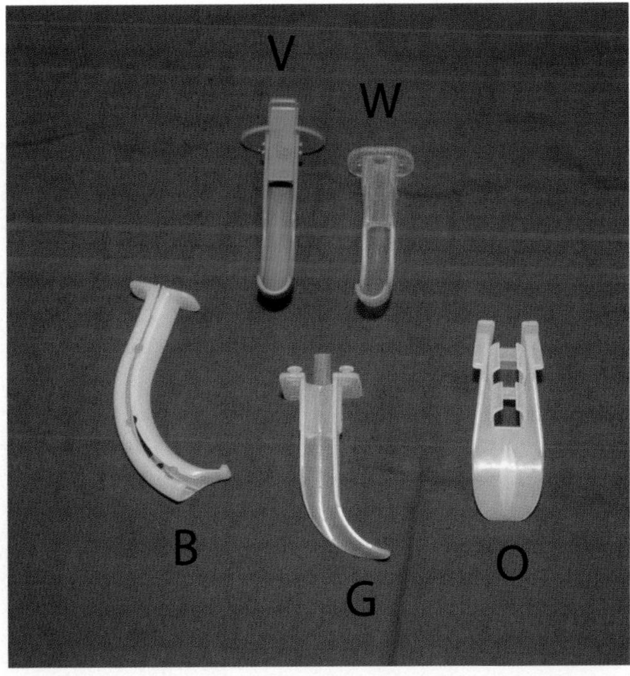

Figure 8.4. Several popular intubating airways are shown. *V* the VAMA (Valentin Andres Madrid airway) airway; *W* the Williams airway intubator; *B* the Berman airway; *G* the VBM Guedel airway; *O* the Ovassapian airway.

Setting up for Fiberoptic Intubation

Before beginning the procedure, it is important to be sure that all of the equipment is in good working order. The bronchoscope should be plugged into the light source and the video monitor (if one is being used) and powered up to be sure the light is shining at the bronchoscope's tip and that the image is focused and clear. The tip of the scope should then be placed in a container with warm water (not saline!) along with the endotracheal tube that is to be used (Figure 8.5). The bronchoscope is kept in the warm water to keep the lens from fogging when it is placed into the warm, moist atmosphere of the airway, and the endotracheal tube is placed in the water to soften it up so that it can pass more easily along the curved length of the insertion tube into the trachea. The presence of working suction and the availability of a reliable supply of oxygen should also be confirmed before starting.

Whether the patient is to be intubated awake or asleep a dose of glycopyrrolate, unless it is contraindicated, is given to dry the patient's airway. Standard premedicants including midazolam and fentanyl are also usually given as are famotidine, metoclopramide, and sodium citrate/citric acid (bicitra) if the patient is at risk for aspiration. The desired endotracheal tube is loaded on the lubricated insertion tube of the flexible bronchoscope before starting the procedure so that it is ready for use. To keep the tube from sliding down the insertion tube, the endotracheal tube can be secured by holding the pilot balloon with your fifth finger or the adapter end of the endotracheal tube can be taped to the control section (Figure 8.6).

Techniques for Fiberoptic Intubation

Asleep Oral Intubation

For oral intubations the bronchoscopist can stand either at the head of the bed in the traditional intubating position or to the patient's side looking towards the patient's chin. In either case, it is important that the insertion tube is kept as straight as possible. This can

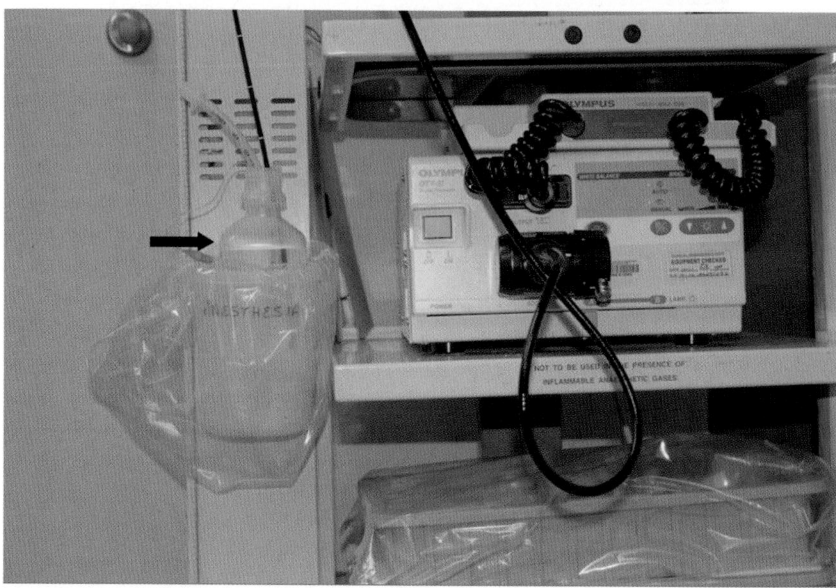

Figure 8.5. The *arrow* indicates the endotracheal tube and the tip of the insertion tube in a bottle of warm water in a basket attached to the bronchoscope cart.

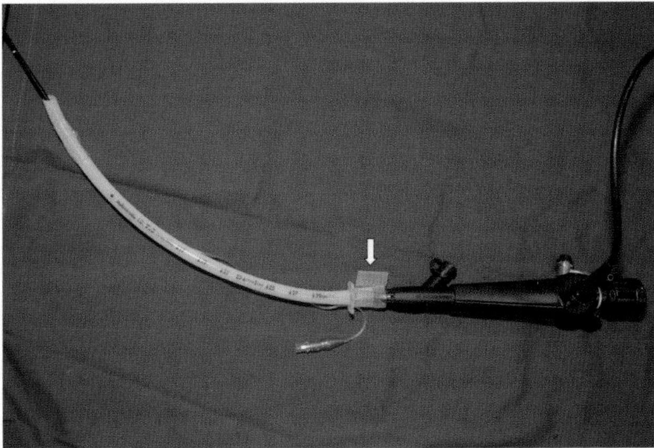

Figure 8.6. The endotracheal tube attached to the hub of the bronchoscope control section with a piece of tape.

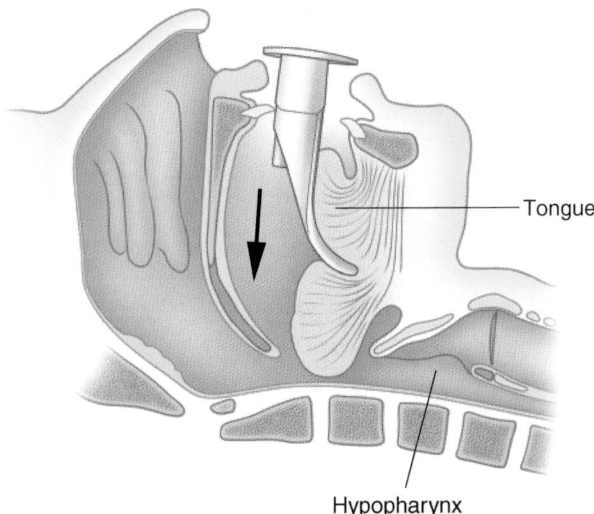

Figure 8.7. The phalange of the airway is caught along the superior surface of the tongue and posterior force on the plastic airway pushes the base of the tongue into the posterior oropharynx obstructing the channel to the hypopharynx.

often be facilitated by lowering the height of the operating room bed. Prior to induction, the patient is given glycopyrrolate, midazolam, and/or fentanyl as described above. Once the patient has been induced and the ability to bag-mask ventilate has been confirmed, the patient can be given a muscle relaxant (I usually prefer succinylcholine unless there is a contraindication to this drug because it's short duration of action allows the patient to resume spontaneous respirations in the rare instance when intubation proves impossible and bag-mask ventilation becomes ineffective). Oxygen via nasal cannula at 3–5 L/min can also be used to provide apneic oxygenation[4]. This can be especially useful in obese patients and others with diminished functional residual capacity.

Once the muscle relaxants have taken effect, an intubating airway is inserted over the tongue with the phalange running along the base of the tongue. The placement of the airway is extremely important because improper placement can actually make intubation much harder, or impossible. Specifically, improper placement of the intubating airway can lead to obstruction of the posterior oropharynx by either the base of the tongue or the airway itself. If the airway is placed with the tip of the phalange on the tongue and then pushed straight posteriorly, the tongue can get pushed back into the posterior oropharynx and block the inlet to the hypopharynx (Figure 8.7). On the other hand, if the airway is placed too far into the mouth, its distal phalange can narrow the posterior oropharynx

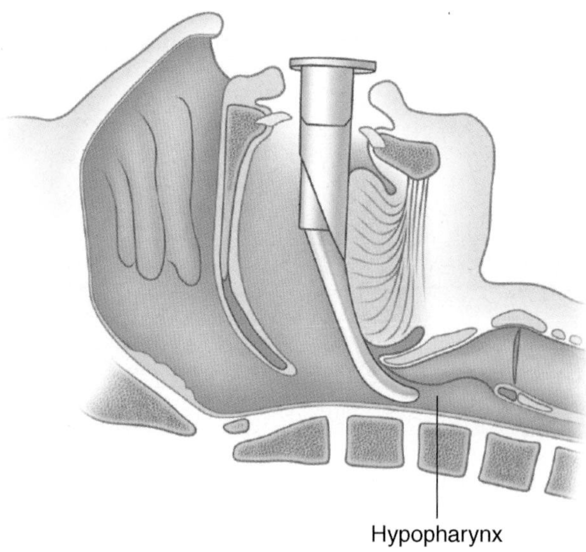

Figure 8.8. The airway is inserted too deeply into the mouth and the phalange obstructs the channel to the hypopharynx.

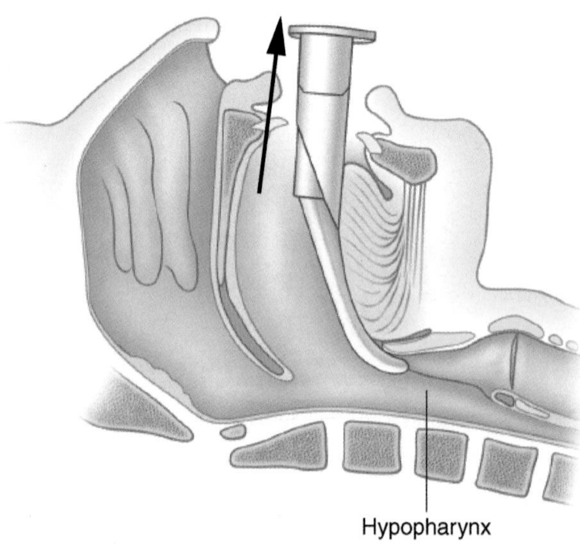

Figure 8.9. The airway is pulled back (outward) enough to bring it against the base of the tongue and open the channel to the hypopharynx.

(Figure 8.8). Either of these errors can make the bronchoscopic entry into the hypopharynx harder, or impossible.

To avoid this problem, either of two intubating airway placement techniques can be used. Either a tongue depressor can be used to flatten the tongue and allow the bronchoscopist to see directly into the posterior oropharynx and place the distal phalange along the base of the tongue without pushing the airway in too far or pushing the base of the tongue into the posterior oropharynx. Alternatively, the intubating airway can be placed about two thirds of the way into the mouth and then lower jaw thrust can be applied while pushing the airway in further. The jaw thrust maneuver opens the posterior oropharynx and allows the tip of the airway to drop into the now widely opened posterior space. Jaw thrust can then either be maintained by the assistant and fiberoptic bronchoscopy initiated or the airway can be pulled back gently until the phalange settles along the posterior aspect of the base of the tongue (Figure 8.9).

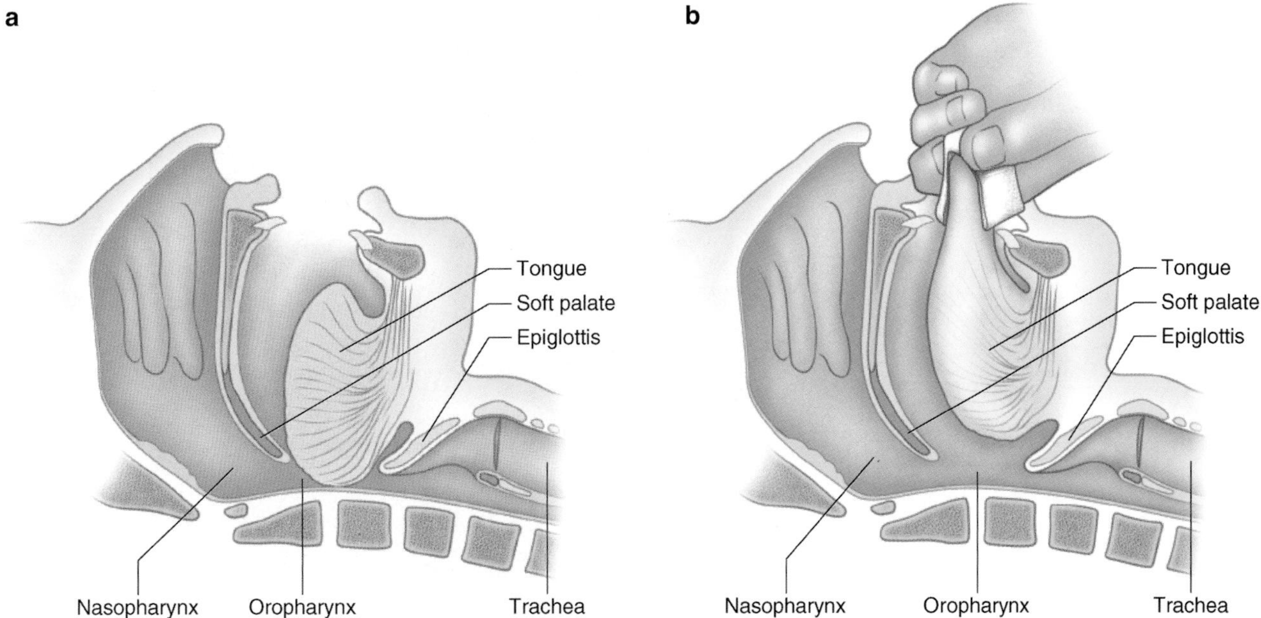

Figure 8.10. (**a**) The base of the tongue obstructs passage through the oropharynx. (**b**) An assistant grasps the tongue and exerts outward pressure to pull the base of the tongue forward out of the posterior oropharynx.

It is important to note that it is not as easy to perform bag-mask ventilation when the intubating airway is in place. Thus, if the patient desaturates and positive pressure ventilation becomes necessary during the procedure, it is often best to remove the intubating airway and replace it with a standard airway until the patient's hypoxia has been corrected and you are ready to resume efforts at intubation.

Once the intubating airway is in place (or, alternatively, if your assistant is providing direct outward pressure on the tongue to open up the oropharyngeal space—Figure 8.10), you are ready to start the procedure. First the eyepiece must be oriented so that the triangular reference marker is at the 12 o'clock position. Prior to inserting the bronchoscope into the mouth, it is very important to have your assistant provide firm lower jaw thrust to facilitate the passage of the tip of the bronchoscope through the oropharynx. The tip of the bronchoscope should be tilted at 45° (upward if you are intubating from the head of the bed, or downward if you are intubating from the side of the bed) as shown in Figure 8.11. Then, using the hand you will be using to control the insertion tube, hold the insertion tube 6–8 in. from the tip firmly between your thumb and index finger. The tip of the insertion tube can then be introduced into the mouth under direct vision (Figure 8.12). Hold the insertion tube so that the tip is looking directly over the phalange of the intubating airway and down towards the larynx (Figure 8.13). In this way you can avoid the struggle of finding your way from the teeth to the posterior oropharynx, and your first view through the scope is often looking directly onto the laryngeal structures.

Once the tip of the scope has passed the intubating airway, the tip can be directed toward the cords. Normally, the tip of the insertion tube must be directed slightly downward to get under the tip of the epiglottis (this is facilitated by the jaw thrust or tongue pulling of your assistant) and then up over the arytenoid cartilages and through the cords into the trachea where the cartilaginous rings become apparent anteriorly (Figure 8.14). If it is necessary to steer the tip to the left or right (e.g., to avoid tumors or to navigate an airway that deviates from the midline due to previous external beam radiation or surgical scarring), the scope tip is tilted slightly up or down and small wrist movements of the hand holding the control section into mild pronation or supination permit fine adjustments in direction at the scope tip to steer the scope towards and through the vocal cords. This part of the procedure undoubtedly requires the most practice as the direction of tip movement

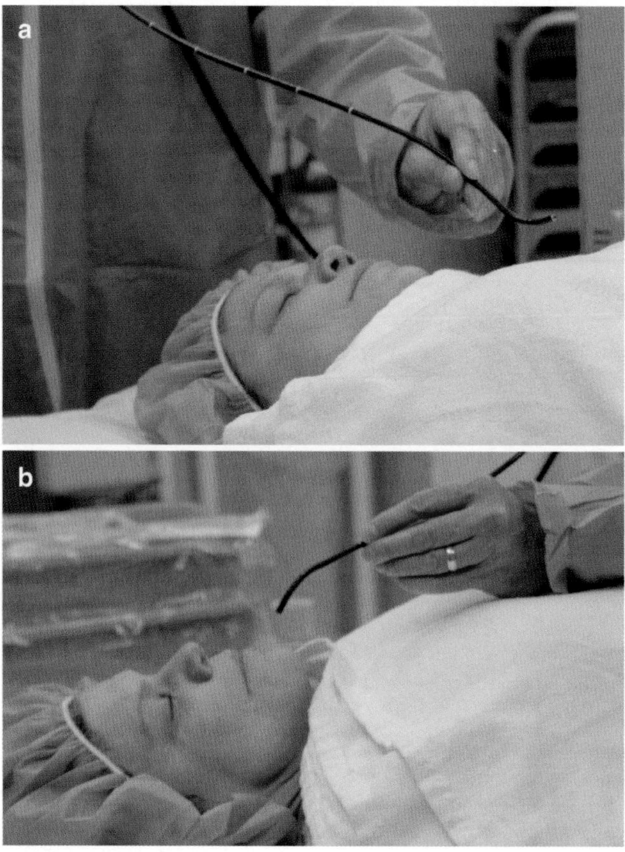

Figure 8.11. (**a**) When intubating from the head of the bed the tip of the bronchoscope is tilted *up* at a 45° angle, and the insertion tube is held firmly approximately 7 in. from the tip. (**b**) When intubating from the side of the bed the scope is tipped *down* at a 45° angle prior to insertion into the mouth.

with elevation or depression of the lever and pronation and supination of the wrist takes time to get used to since significant angular motion occurs even with small changes in wrist orientation.

Once the tip of the scope enters the trachea, it is advanced into the level of the mid-trachea. It is important not to push the scope in too far because contact of the scope tip with the carina can cause significant irritation of the airway leading to tachycardia, hypertension, and severe laryngospasm. When the tip of the scope reaches the level of the mid-trachea, the bronchoscopist can look away from the eyepiece (or video screen) and use the insertion tube to "blindly" guide the endotracheal tube into the trachea. First the tape (or fifth finger) holding the hub of the endotracheal tube in place is released. Then the tube is passed down the lubricated insertion tube. Often passage of the endotracheal tube through the oral cavity is easier if the intubating airway is removed first. If the tip of the endotracheal tube becomes stuck as it passes the base of the tongue, the jaw thrust maneuver by the assistant used earlier can open the passage into the larynx. If the tip seems to be getting stuck at the level of the larynx, the endotracheal tube can be turned gently clockwise or counterclockwise to free the tip from the epiglottis or the arytenoid cartilages and then advanced into the trachea. The likelihood of the endotracheal tube getting hung up on the laryngeal structures is markedly decreased if the internal diameter of the endotracheal tube is close in size to the diameter of the insertion tube. A snugger fit of the endotracheal tube on the insertion tube allows less freedom for the endotracheal tube tip to become caught on the epiglottis or at the arytenoid cartilages (Figure 8.15). Obviously, if the diameter of the endotracheal tube is too small, it will not pass smoothly onto or off of the insertion tube and the airway established will be smaller with a higher resistance to

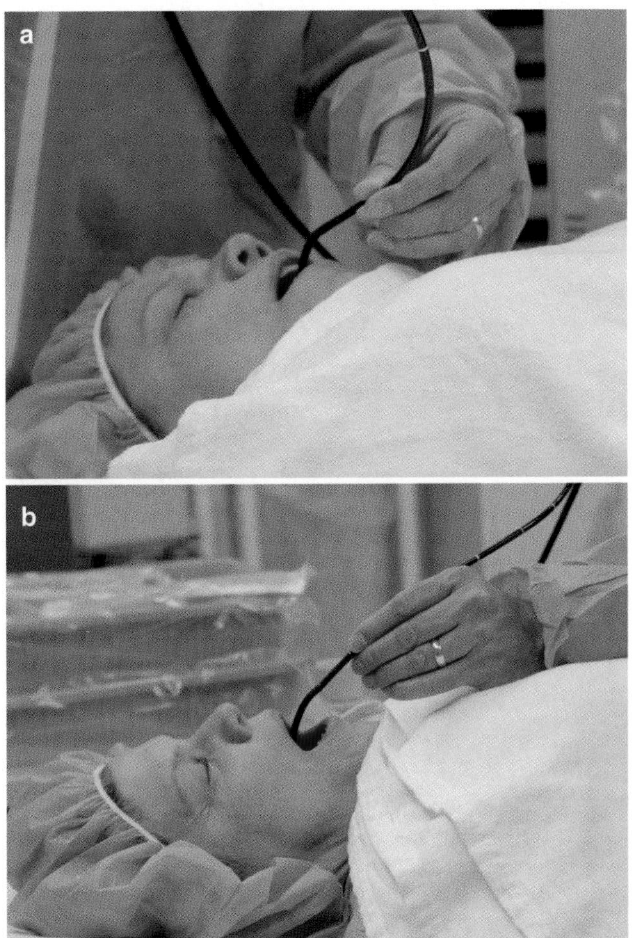

Figure 8.12 While looking directly into the mouth (not through the scope), the tip of the bronchoscope is introduced into the mouth and advanced until it is beyond the base of the tongue. (**a**) From the head of the bed, (**b**) from the side of the bed.

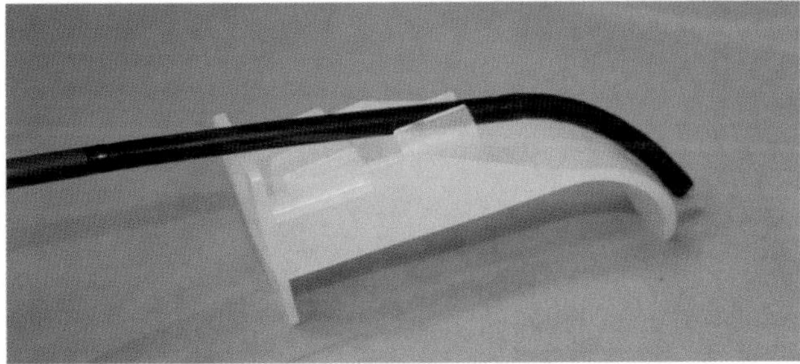

Figure 8.13. The tip of the scope is shown as it would follow the curve of the plastic airway into the hypopharynx.

airflow. So, a balance between endotracheal tube size and the challenge caused by play along the insertion tube must be reached for each patient.

Once the tube is in place, a quick look through the bronchoscope should allow you to establish how far above the carina the tip of the endotracheal tube lies (2–3 cm is usually optimal in an adult patient), and then the insertion tube is removed. The distance from the carina to the tip of the endotracheal tube can be determined by advancing the bronchoscope to just above the carina, marking the position on the bronchoscope with

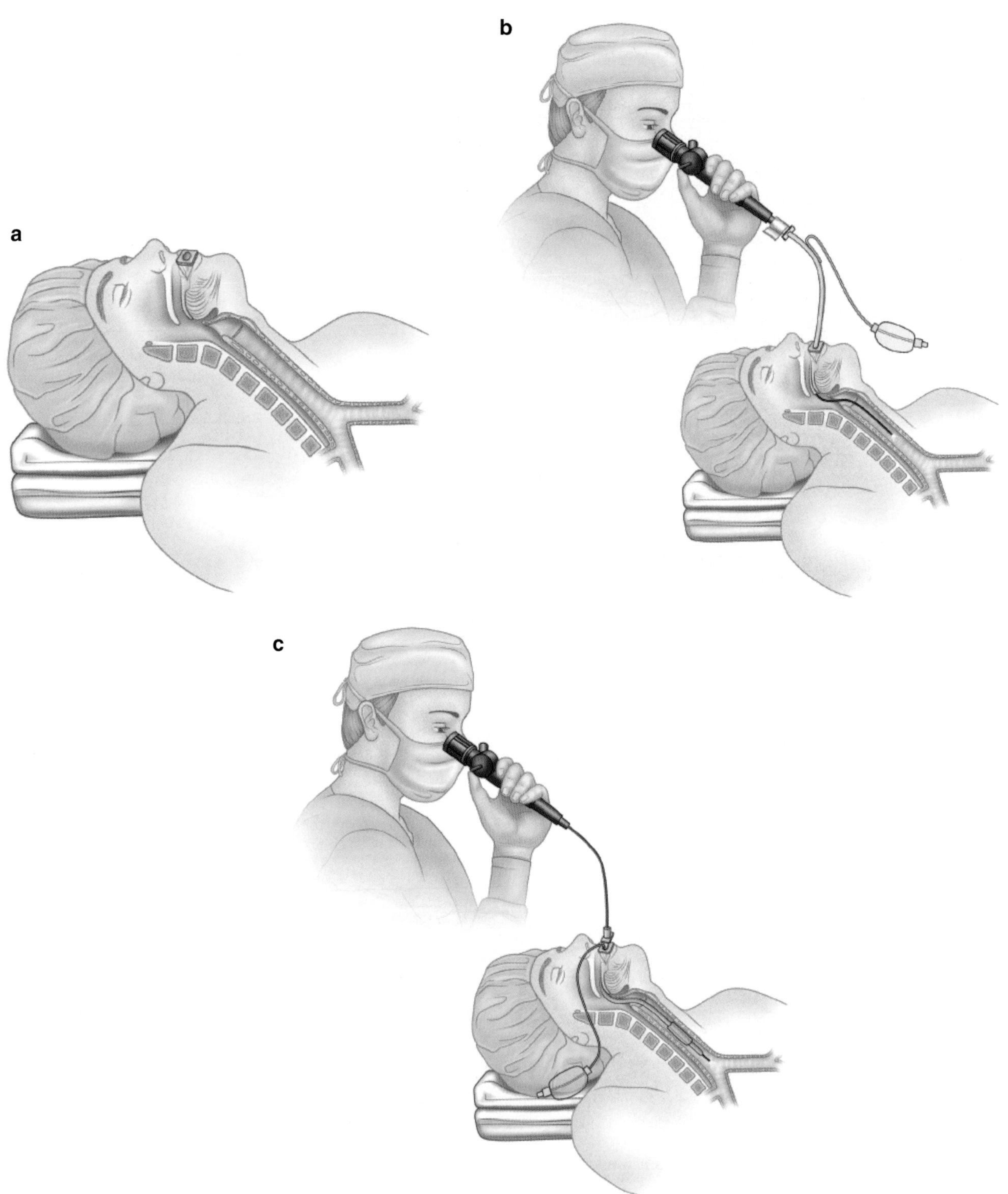

Figure 8.14. Standard technique for bronchoscopic orotracheal intubation. (**a**) The Ovassapian airway in place. (**b**) The bronchoscope with the endotracheal tube loaded on it is advanced into the mid-trachea. (**c**) The endotracheal tube is advanced over the bronchoscope into the trachea.

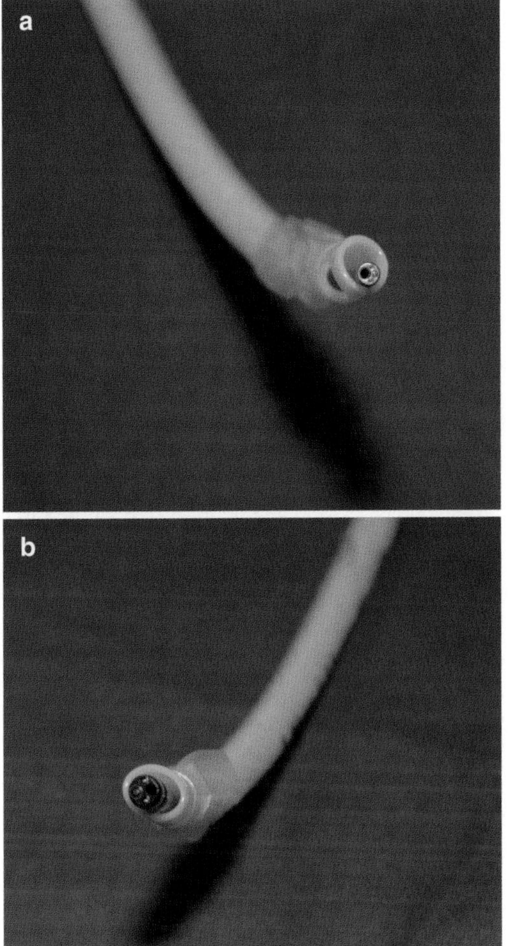

Figure 8.15. (**a**) Poor size match between the bronchoscope and the endotracheal tube is shown. The amount of play between scope and tube this permits increases the risk that the leading edge of the endotracheal tube will become caught on glottic structures as the endotracheal tube is passed towards the trachea over the bronchoscope. (**b**) Here there is better size-matching between the scope and the endotracheal tube so there is less risk of entrapment of the endotracheal tube tip at the level of the glottis.

the thumb and forefinger, withdrawing the scope to the tip of the bevel of the endotracheal tube, and measuring the difference between these[5] (Figure 8.16). The endotracheal tube is then attached to the anesthesia circuit, and the endotracheal tube is secured. Auscultation for breath sounds bilaterally is prudent to be sure that the left or right mainstem bronchus has not been intubated (as the lobar bronchial divisions can be mistaken for the carina).

Asleep Nasal Intubation

The preparatory setup for an asleep nasal fiberoptic intubation is the same as listed above in the section titled "Setting up for Fiberoptic Intubation." Once the equipment has been checked and the premedicants administered, an assessment of the nares is made and a determination as to whether one or the other nare is more widely patent is made. Generally, the nostril with greater patency should be selected. This can be established prior to induction by asking the patient to occlude each nostril in turn and sniff rapidly; however, it is wise to prepare both nostrils with a vasoconstrictor to shrink the nasal mucosal vasculature (this increases the size of the nasal channels to make passage of the endotracheal tube

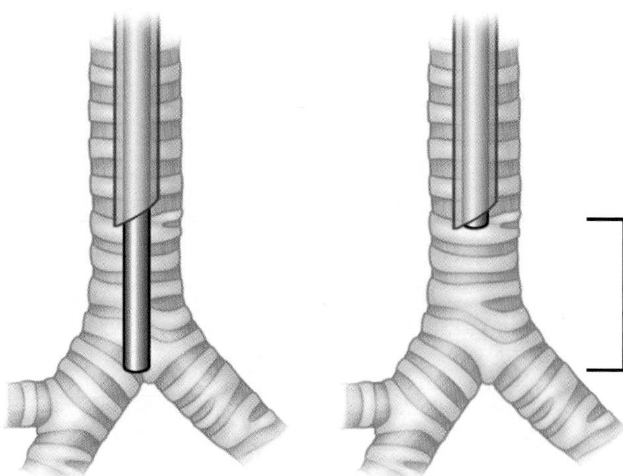

Figure 8.16. Using a bronchoscope to measure the distance from the carina to the tip of the endotracheal tube.

easier and decreases the blood flow through the nares thereby decreasing the risk of bleeding). General anesthesia is then induced as outlined above, ensuring that bag-mask ventilation is possible prior to giving the muscle relaxant.

A well-lubricated appropriately sized endotracheal tube (usually a size 7.0 or smaller) is then placed into the preferred nostril and pushed gently medially and posteriorly (as if placing a nasogastric tube). The endotracheal tube should be inserted approximately 2 1/2 to 3 in. (6–8 cm) into the nostril. The objective is to place the tip of the tube into the posterior oropharynx. It is important to recognize increased resistance to the advancement of the nasotracheal tube as it is advanced. (If this is a problem with both nares, the bronchoscope may be introduced prior to the nasotracheal tube in an effort to navigate around the turbinates.) The assistant then applies a firm lower jaw thrust (Figure 8.17) that is intended to draw the base of the tongue forward and open up the inlet to the larynx. Alternatively, the tip of the tongue can be grasped and pulled forward to drag the base of the tongue out of the oropharynx. A lubricated bronchoscope is then passed through the end of the endotracheal tube protruding from the nostril and advanced through the tube. Upon emerging from the endotracheal tube, the bronchoscopist should be looking directly onto the vocal cords. The bronchoscope is then advanced past the cords to the level of the mid-trachea and the endotracheal tube is gently advanced over the insertion tube of the bronchoscope into the trachea. To reach the mid-tracheal level, the endotracheal tube normally needs to be pushed all the way into the nostril such that the adapter at the end of the endotracheal tube is flush with the nostril (Figure 8.18). Alternatively, a pre-formed nasal RAE tube (Covidien) can be used for nasal intubations. These longer tubes are shaped in a way that permits placement of the endotracheal tube tip into the mid-trachea while leaving the bent segment of the tube outside the nostril. This makes it possible to connect the anesthesia circuit to the endotracheal tube above the patient's head instead of across their face (Figure 8.19). This arrangement is particularly helpful when the surgery is taking place below the level of the nose. Fiberoptic insertion of a nasal RAE tube is slightly more difficult than insertion of a standard endotracheal tube because the nasal RAE tube is longer and has a severe bend midway along its length. As with a standard tube, warming the nasal RAE tube can make it easier to slide it along the insertion tube. In addition, it is often necessary to hold the bent segment straight during the initial insertion of the bronchoscope into the nasal RAE tube to permit the passage of the insertion tube past the bend (Figure 8.20). Prior to removing the bronchoscope the distance to the carina can be noted, and then the scope is removed and the endotracheal tube is connected to the anesthesia circuit and end-tidal CO_2 is documented as are bilateral breath sounds. When securing the nasotracheal tube, it is very important to avoid any pressure on the nasal ala as this can result in very painful ulcers.

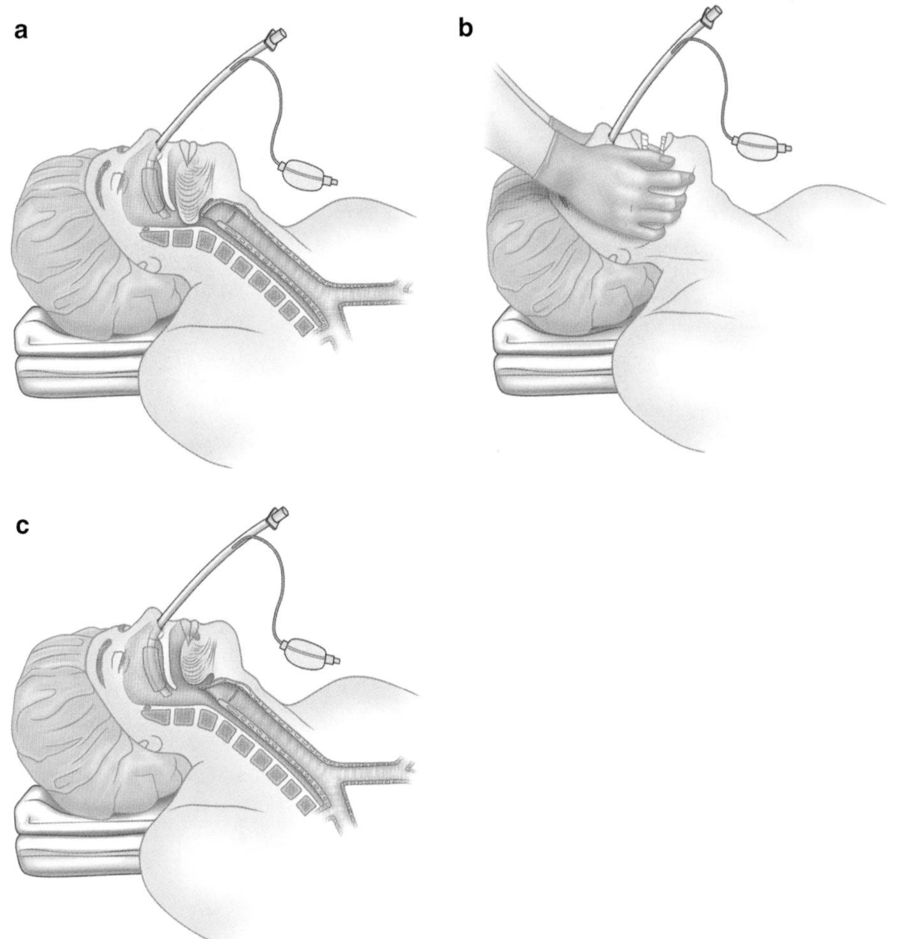

Figure 8.17. The jaw thrust maneuver is used to move the base of the tongue out of the posterior oropharynx and ease passage of the endotracheal tube into the hypopharynx during a bronchoscopic-assisted nasal intubation. (**a**) the base of the tongue obstructs the view to the larnyx (**b**) jaw thrust is applied by an assistant (**c**) while jaw thrust is applied the base of the tongue moves anteriorly allowing visualization of the larnyx.

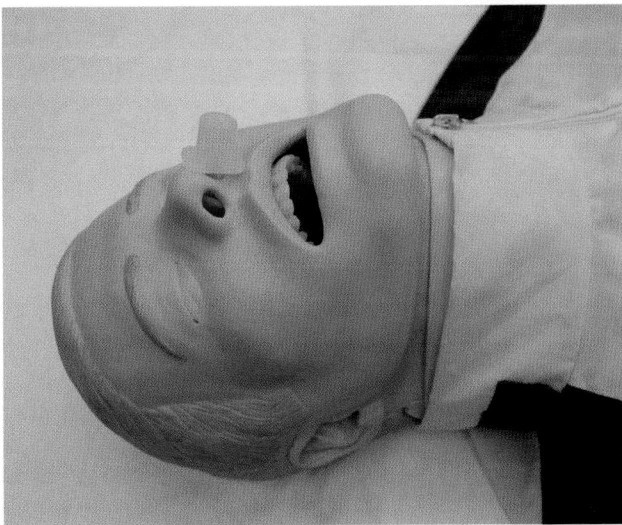

Figure 8.18. The standard endotracheal tube is inserted all the way to the adapter hub at the completion of a nasal intubation.

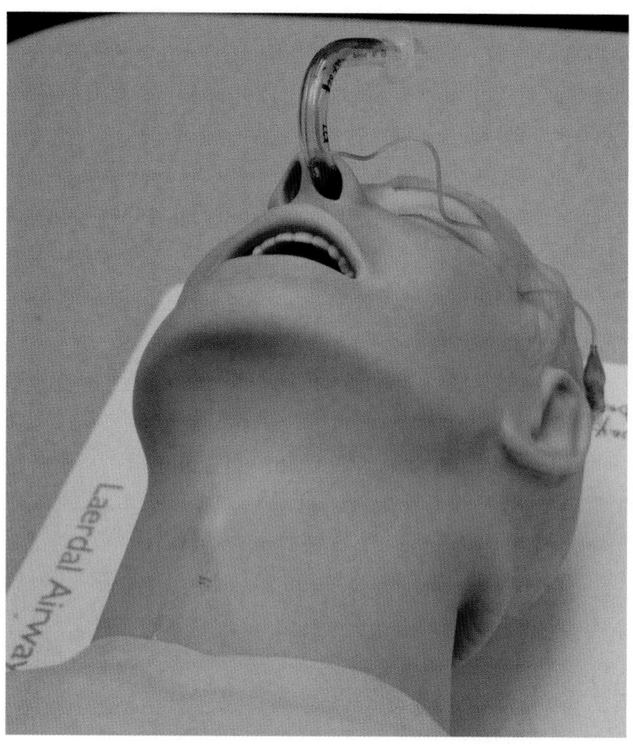

Figure 8.19. A nasal RAE tube in place leaving the face below the nostrils free of airway connections.

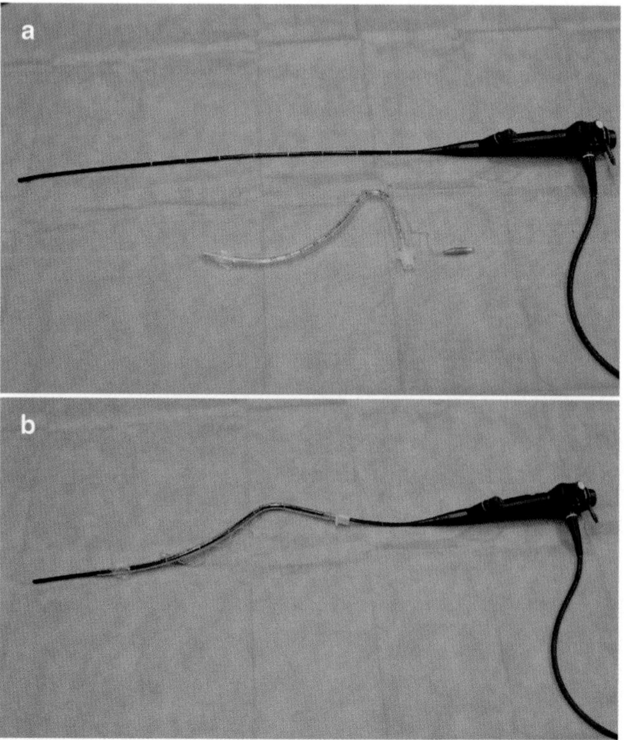

Figure 8.20. (**a**) The nasal RAE tube has a severe curve and requires firm straightening pressure applied at both ends to allow passage of the bronchoscope's insertion tube through it (**b**).

There are three significant advantages to inserting the endotracheal tube into the nostril prior to introducing the bronchoscope (the "tube first" technique). First, passing the relatively large and stiff endotracheal tube through the nostril into the oropharynx avoids the potential challenge of navigating the nasal passage with the relatively floppy insertion tube of the bronchoscope (this is especially beneficial for the novice bronchoscopist whose steering skills are still relatively limited). Second, prior insertion of the endotracheal tube avoids a situation where the bronchoscope has been successfully directed into the mid-trachea, but the endotracheal tube loaded on the insertion tube is too large to pass through the nasal canal requiring that the scope be removed and the procedure started anew. Finally, placing the tip of the nasotracheal tube into the oropharynx prior to performing bronchoscopy keeps the scope midline upon insertion and generally permits the first view to be a straight shot along the posterior wall of the oropharynx onto the cords. If the endotracheal tube cannot be advanced blindly from the nostril into the oropharynx, then the bronchoscope can be inserted through the tube and the scope can be used to direct the tip of the endotracheal tube into and through the oropharynx (the "scope first technique").

Awake Fiberoptic Intubation

The indications and basic setup for awake intubations are discussed in Chap. 3. Here we will concentrate on issues with awake intubations that are unique to the fiberoptic approach.

In addition to the high quality optics and maneuverability of the bronchoscope, another advantage of this device for awake intubations is the ability to "spray-as-you-go" to provide topical anesthesia to the airway all the way to the cords (or even below). As previously noted, the larger insertion tubes have suction ports and/or working channels. Epidural catheters can be inserted through either of these ports and advanced to the tip of the insertion tube. Lidocaine can then be sprayed over the airway and directed evenly over the cords (Figure 8.21). This technique allows the bronchoscopist to avoid the translaryngeal approach to the cords and more reliably delivers the local anesthetic to the laryngeal structures.

Awake Oral Fiberoptic Intubation

As always, the patient is given glycopyrrolate if it is not contraindicated. Then the patient can either be seated up in the bed (if they are not able to lie flat and/or to help open the channel through the oropharynx) or can be laid down, usually with a blanket ramp (Figure 4.9) to optimize the view. If possible, a surgical towel is placed over the patient's eyes to keep local anesthetic and other secretions from spraying into the eyes. Sedation and topical anesthesia as discussed in Chap. 3 can then proceed. Once the patient is adequately sedated and topical anesthesia has been achieved intubation can be performed. If the patient is sitting up or requires a very steep blanket ramp, it is usually easiest to approach the patient from the side of the bed looking up towards the patient's chin (Figure 8.22). If the patient can comfortably lie flat, intubating from the head of the bed is also possible. Nasal cannula oxygen is delivered at 4–5 L/min to decrease the risk of hypoxia during sedation and intubation. The oral airway is inserted as previously described making sure that neither the base of the tongue nor the phalange of the airway obstruct the route through the posterior oropharynx. A gentle jaw thrust is then provided by an assistant and the insertion tube with the endotracheal tube loaded on it is introduced with a 45° bend at the tip to the back of the oral cavity (Figure 8.11). If the view is clear, advance the insertion tube into the trachea and then pass the tube into the trachea. If the view is obstructed by redundant airway tissue, ask the patient to take a deep breath (this is why it is important to titrate the sedation to a level that still permits the patient to follow commands). With deep inspiration the epiglottis and laryngeal structures should become apparent and the insertion tube can be advanced into the trachea. Whether the initial view was clear or

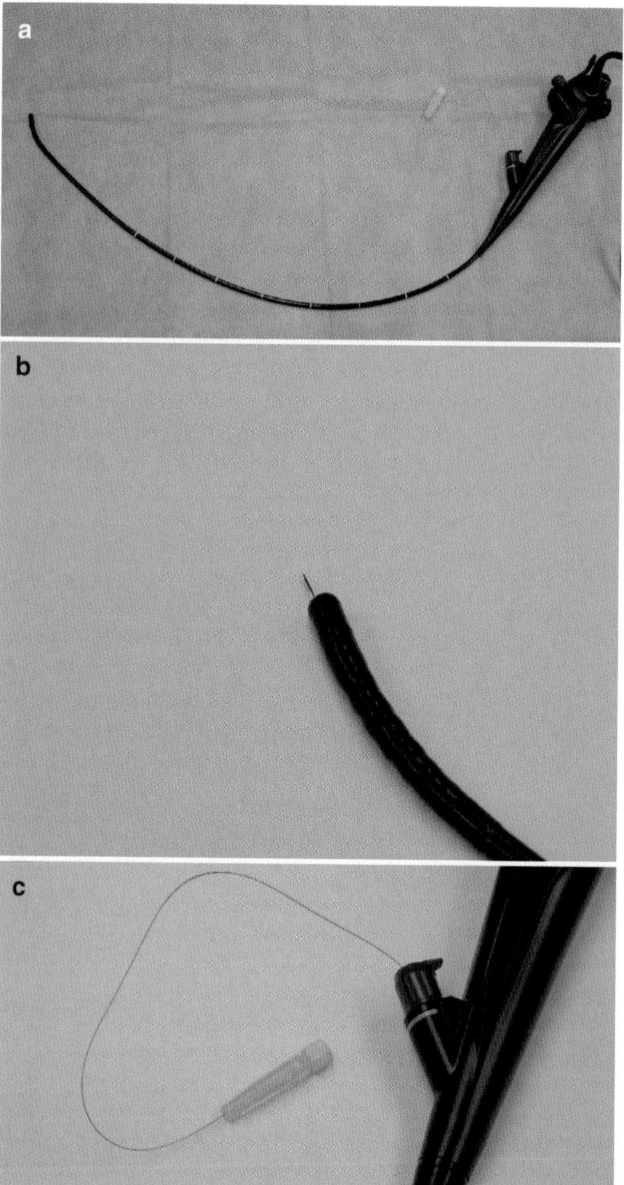

Figure 8.21. (a) An epidural catheter is shown entering the working channel port on the control section and exiting the tip of the insertion tube. (b) The epidural catheter is seen extending only a centimeter or so beyond the tip of the insertion tube. (c) Detail of the epidural catheter entering the port of the working channel.

obstructed, once the insertion tube is in the trachea, if the endotracheal tube does not pass easily over the insertion tube and into the trachea, another deep breath by the patient usually facilitates the passage of the endotracheal tube. Alternatively, gentle jaw thrust or tongue pulling by the assistant can also make endotracheal tube passage easier.

Once the endotracheal tube is in the trachea, a quick look through the bronchoscope to confirm the location is prudent (to be sure the bronchoscope had not become dislodged and delivered the endotracheal tube into the esophagus) prior to administering any intravenous sedative/hypnotic. If the intubation was difficult, it is reasonable to keep the bronchoscope nearby in case there are problems with the endotracheal tube during the case or in case the patient needs to be urgently reintubated after extubation at the end of the case.

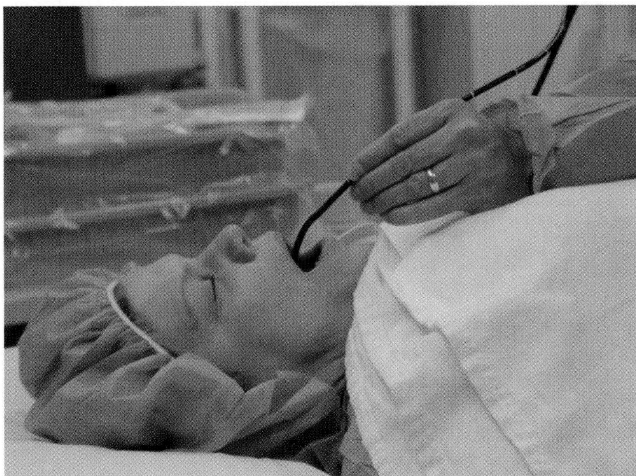

Figure 8.22. Bronchoscopic intubation from the side of the patient's bed.

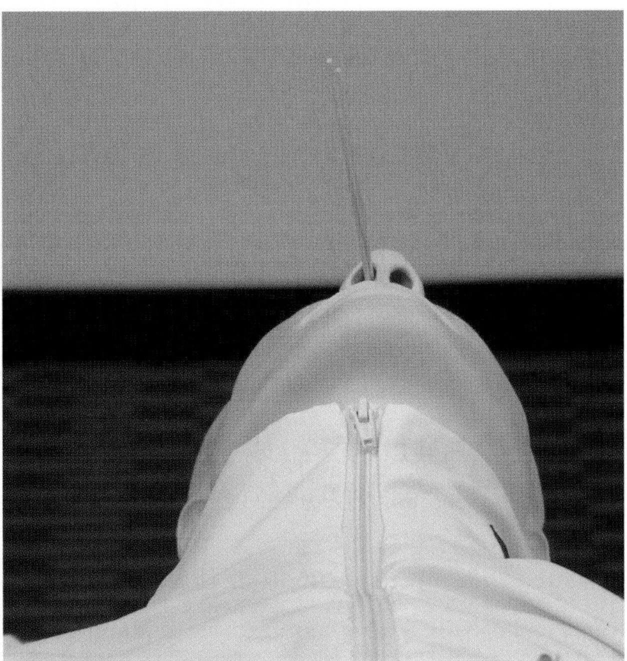

Figure 8.23. Cotton-tipped swabs coated with lidocaine jelly are placed into the nostril to anesthetize the nostril prior to awake nasal intubation.

Awake Nasal Fiberoptic Intubation

The most significant difference between awake and asleep nasal intubations is the need for topicalization of the nares prior to awake nasal intubation. This can be achieved using lidocaine jelly on cotton-tipped swaps gently placed into the nostrils (Figure 8.23). Alternatively, a nasal trumpet coated with lidocaine jelly can be inserted into the nostrils to spread the local anesthesia over the mucosal surfaces. As for the asleep nasal intubations, phenylephrine (or cocaine 4 %) should be applied to the nostrils to open the nasal canals and shrink the mucosal vasculature. Once the patient is sedated and sufficient topical anesthesia has been provided, the endotracheal tube is inserted into the nostril and intubation proceeds just as in an asleep nasal fiberoptic intubation. Often the laryngeal structures come immediately into view upon passing the insertion tube beyond the tip of the endotra-

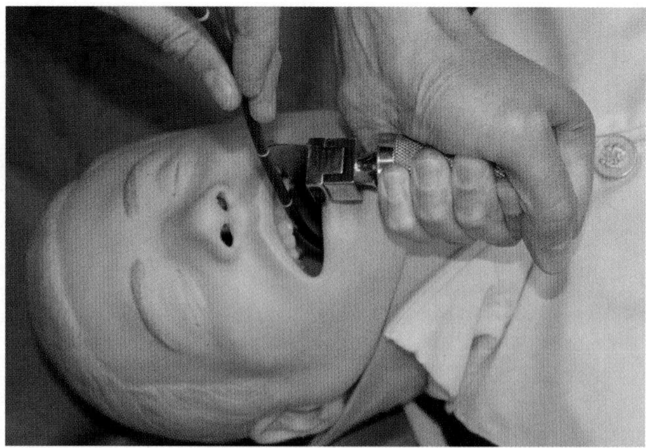

Figure 8.24. A laryngoscope is used to displace the tongue and facilitate bronchoscopic orotracheal intubation.

cheal tube, if not, a deep breath by the patient can open the glottis and permit passage of the insertion tube and the endotracheal tube into the trachea. Once the position of the endotracheal tube tip in the trachea is confirmed, a general anesthetic can be induced.

Fiberoptic Bronchoscopy in Combination with Other Airway Management Techniques

Fiberoptic Bronchoscopy Facilitated with Direct or Video Laryngoscopy

If the tongue cannot be adequately kept out of the way by an intubating airway or traction on the tip of the tongue, an assistant can insert a laryngoscope (either a direct laryngoscope[6] or a video laryngoscope like the GlideScope) into the mouth to retract the base of the tongue (Figure 8.24). The insertion tube of the bronchoscope can then be directed beyond the tip of the laryngoscope towards the glottic structures. Using this combination of techniques, the video laryngoscope helps retract the tongue and also permits indirect viewing of the endotracheal tube as it passes between the vocal cords.

Retrograde-Assisted Fiberoptic Intubation (Figure 8.25)

When tumor, redundant airway tissue, or scarring make it difficult to steer the tip of the bronchoscope to and through the larynx, it is sometimes useful to pass a wire through the cricothyroid membrane into the oropharynx over which the bronchoscope can be advanced[7]. For details of the retrograde technique see Chap. 11. When using the retrograde technique to facilitate fiberoptic intubation, there are three unique and important considerations. First, the insertion tube must have an open channel (suction or working) at the tip that runs up to the control handle. Second, the wire passed through the cricothyroid membrane and directed cephalad to the mouth must be long enough to pass all the way through the insertion tube with room to spare since it will have to reach from the insertion site in the airway all the way through the insertion tube. Finally, the wire must be small enough to fit through the open channel at the tip of the insertion tube yet sufficiently stiff to provide it with guidance (e.g. Amplatz wire, Cook Medical).

To perform retrograde-assisted intubations, after the patient is induced (or sedated and adequate topical anesthesia provided if an awake intubation is to be performed) a needle or catheter large enough to accommodate the guidewire is inserted through the cricothyroid cartilage and angled cephalad. The guidewire is then passed through the needle or catheter until it is identified at the back of the mouth. The wire can then be grasped and pulled out of the mouth and secured at the insertion site with a clamp.

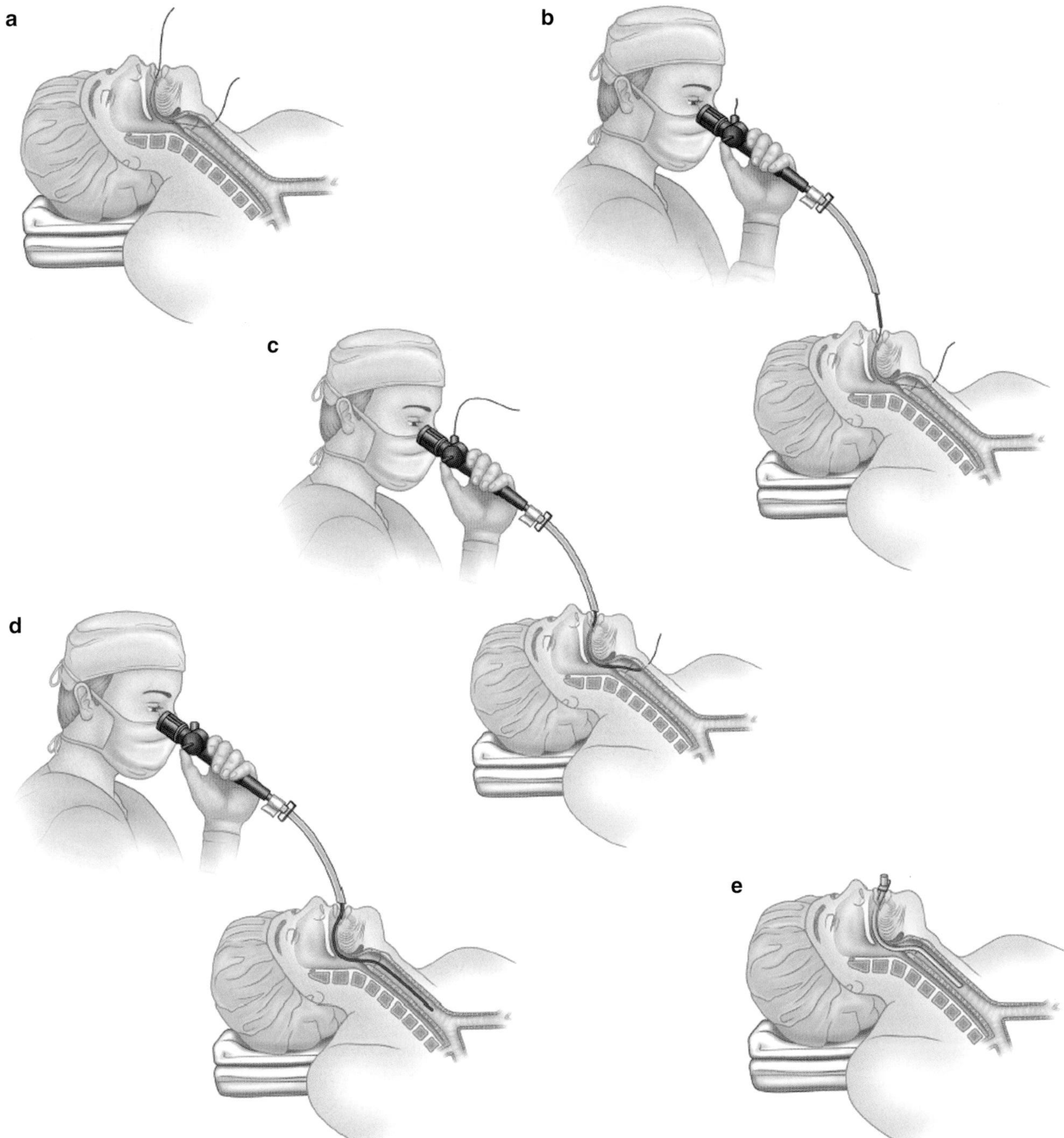

Figure 8.25. Retrograde-assisted fiberoptic intubation. (**a**) The guidewire is placed through the cricothyroid membrane and directed up the trachea and out the mouth. (**b**) The guidewire is inserted through the suction channel at the tip of the insertion tube of a bronchoscope with an endotracheal tube mounted on it. (**c**) The bronchoscope is advanced over the guidewire into the larynx. (**d**) The guidewire is released at the insertion site in the neck and pulled out through the proximal port of the suction channel, and the bronchoscope is advanced into the trachea. (**e**) The endotracheal tube is then passed over the bronchoscope's insertion tube into the trachea and the scope is removed.

The end of the wire protruding from the mouth is then introduced into the open channel at the tip of a bronchoscope with an endotracheal tube loaded on it (a size-appropriate Fastrach type tube might work best here because its floppy composition makes it easier to pass the tube around tight curves). The wire is then advanced through the insertion tube and out the port on the control handle (Figure 8.26). Gentle traction is applied to both

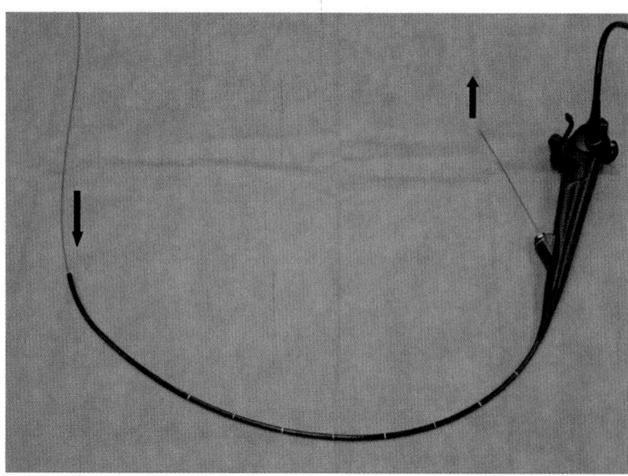

Figure 8.26. The guidewire is shown entering the tip of the insertion tube and exiting the working channel port on the control section.

ends of the wire by assistants, and the bronchoscope is carefully run along the guidewire into the trachea. Once the tracheal rings come into view and the scope tip meets the wire at its insertion point, the clamp at the insertion site can be released and the wire removed through the proximal port site. Then the insertion tube can be advanced to the mid-trachea and the endotracheal tube can be run over the insertion tube into the trachea.

Fiberoptic Intubation Through the Laryngeal Mask Airways

Fiberoptic bronchoscopy can be used to convert an LMA™ (Classic or Unique) managed airway to an endotracheal tube or to facilitate the placement of the endotracheal tube through an intubating supraglottic airway such as the Fastrach™ (LMA North America).

Converting a Classic/Unique LMA to an Endotracheal Tube

As discussed in Chap. 7, the laryngeal mask airway (LMA) can be used as an emergency airway device when other techniques fail. Thus, it may be necessary to convert an LMA to an endotracheal tube in a patient who has a challenging airway. In these circumstances, the bronchoscope can be used to exchange an endotracheal tube for the LMA.

With the LMA in place, an endotracheal tube small enough to fit through the tube of the LMA is selected[8]. The endotracheal tube is then loaded onto the bronchoscope and the well-lubricated bronchoscope is then directed through the LMA, under the epiglottis and between the cords (Figure 8.27). The endotracheal tube is then passed off the bronchoscope and through the LMA. The location of the endotracheal tube tip in the mid-trachea is confirmed, and then the cuff on the endotracheal tube is inflated. Depending on the plans for the patient going forward, the LMA can either be left in place and used to facilitate extubation or it can be removed. Removing the LMA requires that the adapter on the endotracheal tube be disconnected. Then a second endotracheal tube (usually one size smaller than the endotracheal tube in the airway) with its adapter removed is placed tip first into the tube in the airway and the LMA is removed over the tubes[9]. In this way the second tube keeps the first tube in the airway during the removing of the LMA (Figure 8.28).

A new device called an Aintree catheter (Cook Medical, Bloomington IN) has been developed to facilitate the fiberoptic-guided exchange of an endotracheal tube for an LMA already in the airway. The Aintree catheter is a 56-cm long plastic tube exchanger with a 4.8-mm inner diameter. The larger inner diameter permits the passage of an appropriately sized bronchoscope's insertion tube through the catheter (Figure 8.29). To perform the exchange from LMA to endotracheal tube, the Aintree catheter is loaded on a

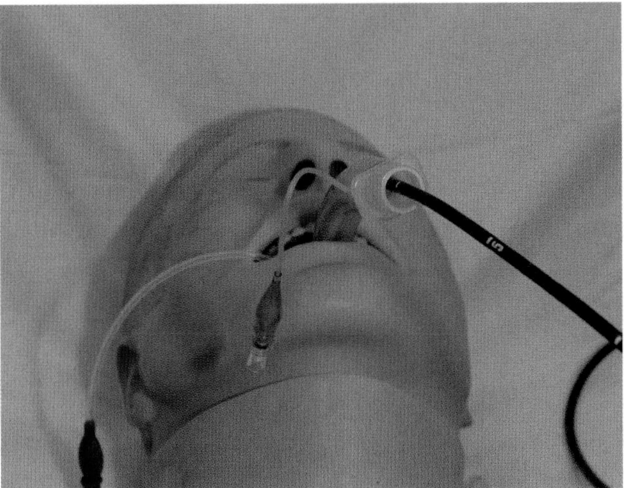

Figure 8.27. The bronchoscope is inserted through an endotracheal tube placed into the tube section of an LMA.

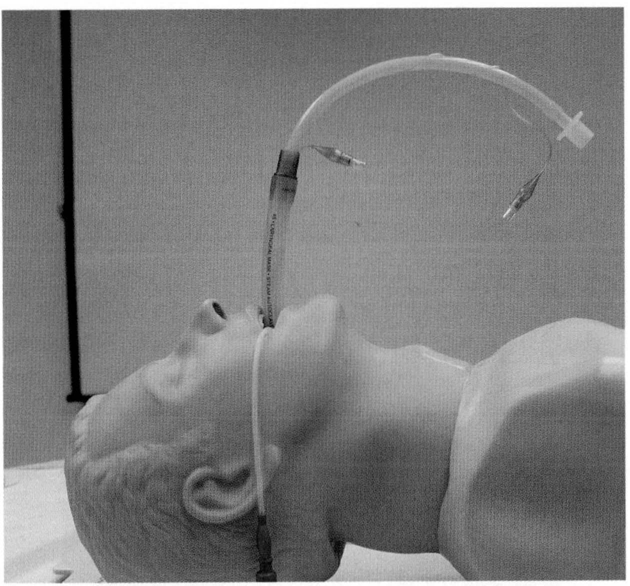

Figure 8.28. A second endotracheal tube is used to hold the first tube securely in place as the LMA is removed over the tubes.

well-lubricated bronchoscope and the insertion tube is then passed through the LMA into the trachea. The bronchoscope is then removed, leaving the Aintree catheter in place in the LMA (Figure 8.30). The Aintree catheter is then held in place while the LMA is removed (Figure 8.31). An endotracheal tube is then passed over the Aintree catheter into the trachea. The catheter is then removed from the endotracheal tube, and the location of the endotracheal tube's tip in the mid-trachea can be confirmed.

Fiberoptic-Assisted Use of the Fastrach (ILMA)

The Fastrach (Intubating LMA—ILMA, LMA North America, San Diego CA) was developed to permit blind passage of a flexible endotracheal tube through a customized supraglottic airway device and into the trachea. There are times that blind passage of the endotracheal tube through this device is either risky (e.g., when friable tumors or fresh suture lines lie along the path to the trachea) or impossible. In these situations, fiberoptic-assisted placement of the endotracheal tube might be desirable.

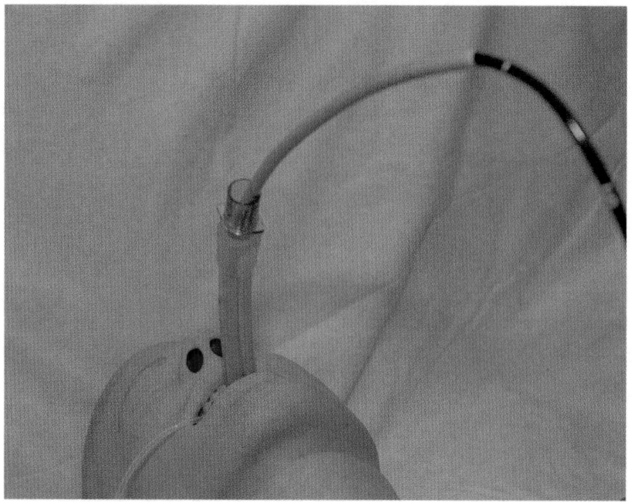

Figure 8.29. An Aintree catheter is passed off the insertion tube, through the LMA, and into the trachea.

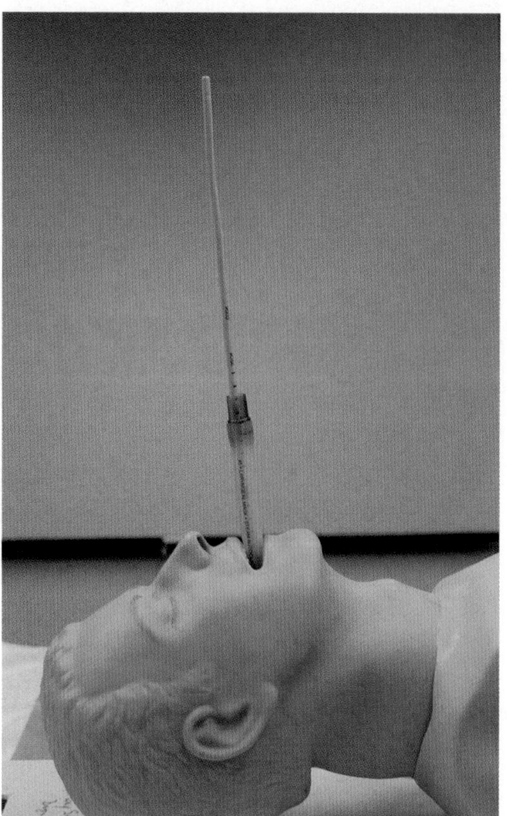

Figure 8.30. The Aintree catheter is left in place in the trachea after the bronchoscope is removed.

The Fastrach device is placed into the airway in the usual fashion (see Chap. 7). Once easy ventilation through the Fastrach has been confirmed, the specialized endotracheal tube is well-lubricated and introduced into the hub of the Fastrach without attaching the adapter to the tube (Figure 8.32). A well-lubricated insertion tube is then run through the endotracheal tube and out the heal of the Fastrach past the epiglottic elevator bar (Figure 8.33). The insertion tube is then steered into the trachea. If the larynx is not

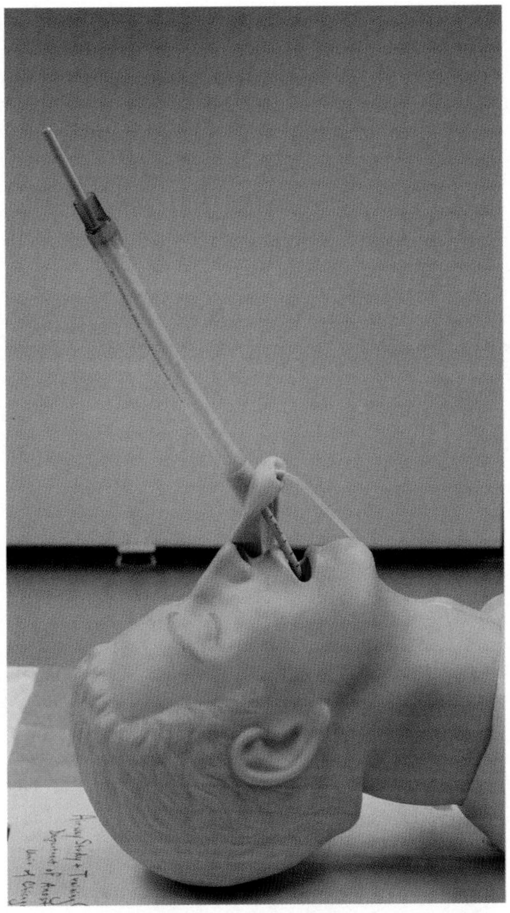

Figure 8.31. The LMA is removed over the Aintree catheter.

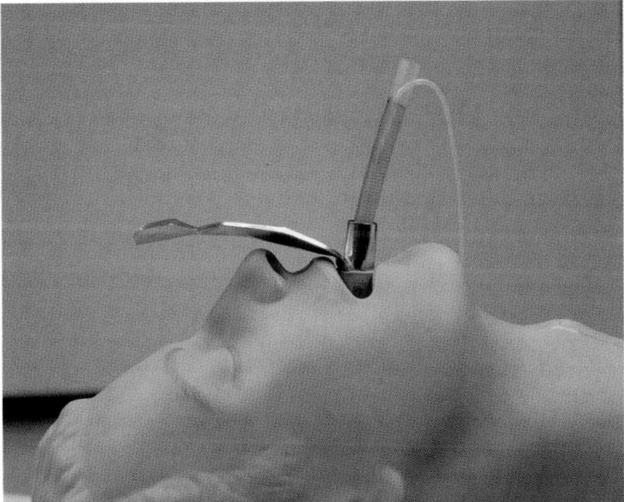

Figure 8.32. A flexible, specialized Fastrach endotracheal tube is inserted into the Fastrach LMA. The adapter hub of the endotracheal tube has been removed to allow the tube's passage through the Fastrach LMA.

visualized upon exiting the Fastrach, posterior rocking of the Fastrach (the Chandy maneuver, see Chap. 7) may align the heel of the Fastrach with the glottic inlet. The endotracheal tube can then be gently advanced over the insertion tube into the trachea and secured in the usual fashion.

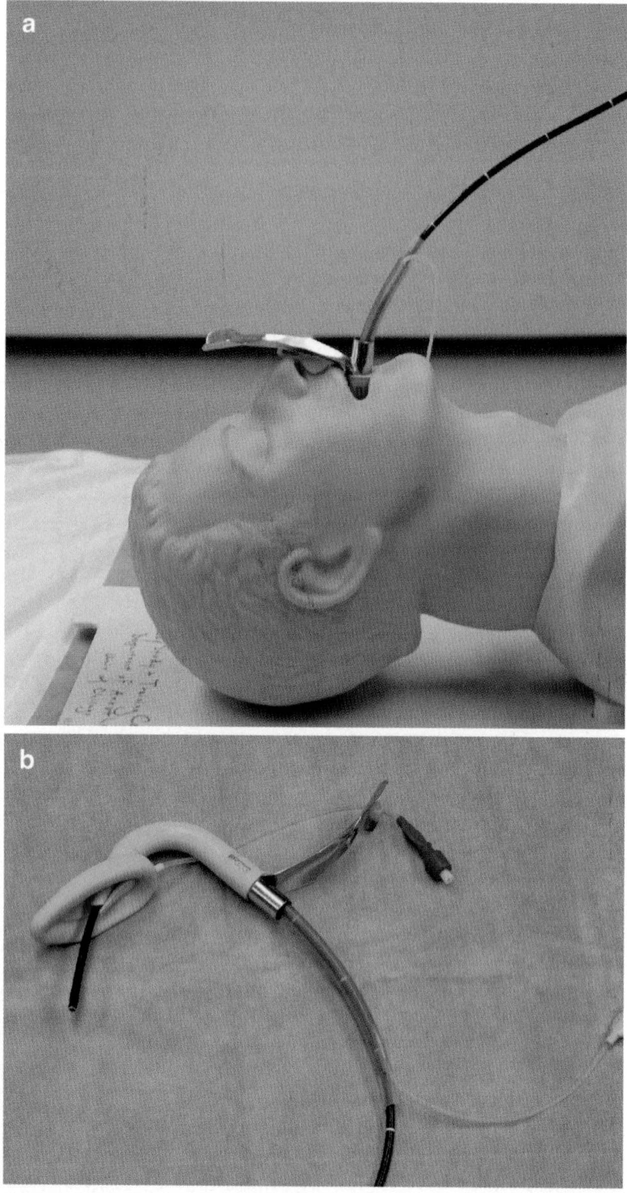

Figure 8.33. (**a**) The bronchoscope is inserted through the endotracheal tube in the Fastrach LMA. (**b**) The bronchoscope's insertion tube tip passes under the Fastrach's epiglottic elevator into the trachea. The endotracheal tube can then be advanced over the insertion tube and into the trachea.

Complications Associated with Fiberoptic Intubations

Because the actual placement of the endotracheal tube is blind (that is, the endotracheal tube is run over the insertion tube and there is no visualization of the endotracheal tube as it passes through the posterior oropharynx or through the cords), it is possible that the endotracheal tube could injure the larynx or that the cuff could end up in the larynx instead of the trachea. Intralaryngeal placement of the cuff can cause recurrent laryngeal nerve injury if the placement is not corrected.

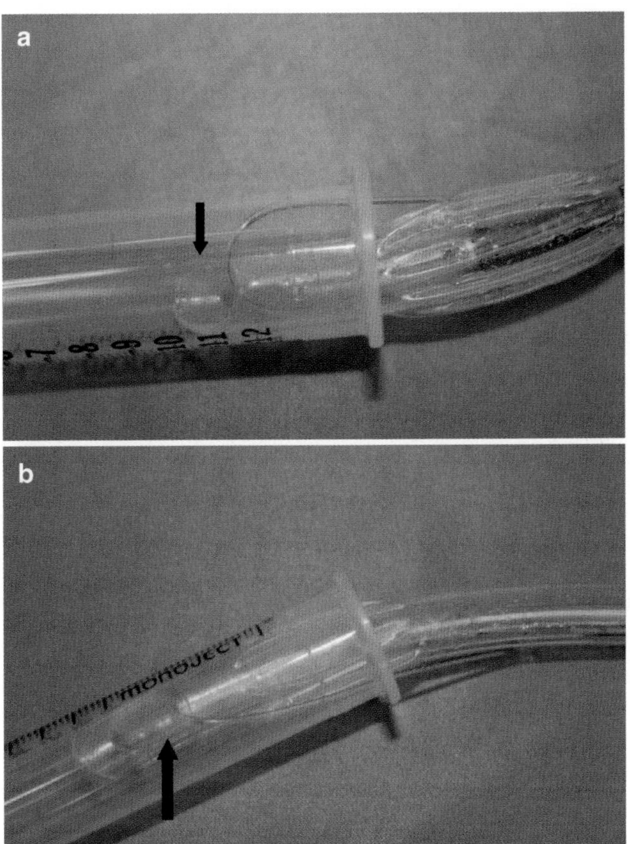

Figure 8.34. (**a**) The epidural catheter is seen extending well beyond the tip of the bronchoscope and emerging at the tip of the endotracheal tube. It then becomes trapped between the outer wall of the endotracheal tube and the surrounding tubular structure (a syringe barrel used to simulate the trachea), making it impossible to withdraw the catheter without pulling the endotracheal tube back. (**b**) The same situation as in (**a**) except the epidural catheter exits the endotracheal tube through the Murphy's eye hole instead of the tip of the endotracheal tube.

In addition, if the insertion tube is too large to fit through the endotracheal tube or it is inadequately lubricated, the outer covering of the insertion tube can be sheered off and obstruct either the endotracheal tube or the airway beyond the tip of the endotracheal tube.

If the bronchoscope is advanced through the Murphy eye of the endotracheal tube (instead of out the tip), it can become stuck. Then the bronchoscope cannot be removed and the endotracheal tube must be removed with the insertion tube in place and the entire procedure started over.

Finally, care must be taken when administering local anesthesia through a catheter inserted through the suction/working port of the bronchoscope. If the tip of the catheter protrudes beyond the tip of the insertion tube, it is possible for it to get drawn down by the tip of the endotracheal tube as it is advanced off of the insertion tube. When this happens, the catheter can become pinched between the tip of the endotracheal tube and the tracheal wall (Figure 8.34) and it becomes difficult or impossible to remove the catheter without manipulating the endotracheal tube[10].

References

1. Ovassapian A, Dykes MHM. The role of fiberoptic endoscopy in airway management. Semin Anesth. 1987;6:93.
2. Heidegger T. Fiberoptic intubation. N Engl J Med. 2011;364:e42.
3. Murphy P. A fibre-optic endoscope used for nasal intubation. Anaesthesia. 1967;22:489–91.
4. Lee SC. Improvement of gas exchange by apneic oxygenation with nasal prong during fiberoptic intubation in fully relaxed patients. J Korean Med Sci. 1998;13:582–6.
5. Davis NJ. A new fiberoptic laryngoscope for nasal intubation. Anesth Analg. 1973;52:807–8.
6. Johnson C, Hunter J, Ho E, Bruff C. Fiberoptic intubation facilitated by a rigid laryngoscope. Anesth Analg. 1991;72:714.
7. Lechman MJ, Donahoo JS, MacVaugh III H. Endotracheal intubation using percutaneous retrograde guidewire insertion followed by antegrade fiberoptic bronchoscopy. Crit Care Med. 1986;14:589–90.
8. Benumof JL. Use of the laryngeal mask airway to facilitate fiberscope-aided tracheal intubation. Anesth Analg. 1992;74:313–5.
9. Chadd GD, Walford AJ, Crane DL. The 3.5/4.5 modification for fiberscope-guided tracheal intubation using the laryngeal mask airway. Anesth Analg. 1992;75:307–8.
10. Prakash PS, Pandia MP. A complication associated with the use of a drug injection catheter through a fiberscope. Anesthesiology. 2008;108:173.

9 The Role of Optical Stylets

Richard Levitan

R. Levitan (✉)
Department of Emergency Medicine, Thomas Jefferson University Hospital,
11th and Walnut Street, 239 Thompson Building, Philadelphia, PA 19107, USA
e-mail: airwaycam@gmail.com

D.B. Glick et al. (eds.), *The Difficult Airway: An Atlas of Tools and Techniques for Clinical Management*,
DOI 10.1007/978-0-387-92849-4_9, © Springer Science+Business Media New York 2013

Introduction

Optical stylets are versatile airway tools now offered in many different designs that are useful for placing endotracheal tubes (ETTs) and confirming location, either used independently, with laryngoscopes, or with supraglottic airways (SGAs). There are wide variations in optical stylet length, malleability, and light sources. Their only common feature is that they provide imaging through an ETT. As they are passed beyond the vocal cords they all permit tracheoscopy.

Maneuverability, a mouth-opening requirement only as wide as the ETT itself, and the capacity for tracheoscopy are distinct advantages of optical stylets over airway imaging devices that are affixed to rigid tongue retractors (such as video and mirror laryngoscopes). Conversely, optical stylets share many of the logistical challenges of flexible fiberscopes, even though their generally shorter length and rigidity provides significantly easier handling. Optical stylets require conforming to the same operating rules of fiberoptics as flexible scopes, namely staying off the mucosa (always following an open channel), recognizing anatomic structures from afar (landmarks are distorted when viewed too closely), knowing your starting position, and proceeding systematically. For practitioners already skilled with flexible fiberoptic devices, optical stylets are quickly adapted and easily used. For those new to fiberoptic anatomy and unfamiliar with the rules of fiberoptics, optical stylets require a methodical and consistent effort to achieve proficiency. Notwithstanding the challenge of achieving skills required for flexible endoscopy, the versatility of optical stylets, especially for facilitating intubation via laryngoscopy or SGAs, can be of great value to practitioners seeking to maximize patient safety in all areas of airway management.

Design Variation

Optical stylets use either fiberoptic rods coupled with a focusing lens or a miniature camera at the distal end of the stylet connected to video imaging screens. Field of view and depth of field both affect performance. With fiberoptic lens-based instruments a wider field of view usually translates into greater fish-eye distortion. This is not the case with newer miniature video chip (CMOS, charged metal oxide sensor) cameras; a wide field of view can be achieved with less noticeable distortion. The depth of field using optical stylets is practically limited by the amount of light projected towards the target. With greater light output landmarks can be recognized from afar, producing less distortion and facilitating directional control. CMOS video generally provides a superior image quality compared with fiberoptics when illumination is reduced. LED illumination is progressively replacing other light sources.

Stylet malleability and length are other features that vary among commercially available optical stylets. The Storz Bonfils Scope (Karl Storz Endoscopy, El Segundo CA) has a fixed shape with a long narrow axis and a 40° distal deflection (Figure 9.1). It provides extraordinary visual clarity (35,000 pixels), and now is also offered in a high-resolution video version. Storz offers both its Bonfils and Brambrink scopes with a DCI (direct coupled interface) connector, a direct, paired connection to an external light source and video monitor.

Clarus Medical's Shikani Stylet (Figure 9.2) and Levitan FPS Stylet (Clarus Medical, Golden Valley MN) are made of malleable steel surrounding fiberoptic bundles (10,000 pixels) (Figure 9.3). The distal end of these devices can be shaped for different applications, including use with and without a laryngoscope, and insertion through an SGA.

All fiberoptic optical stylets (and other fiberoptic scopes) with an eyepiece can be connected to a video camera, using a C-mount coupler. Miniaturization of video cameras and LED illumination now permits direct placement of digital video cameras on the tip of stylets, obviating the need for fiberoptic imaging or lenses. These digital-based imaging systems have integrated, battery-powered video screens, freeing the stylet from external light, power, or video connections. The Video RIFL (Rigid and Flexible Laryngoscope,

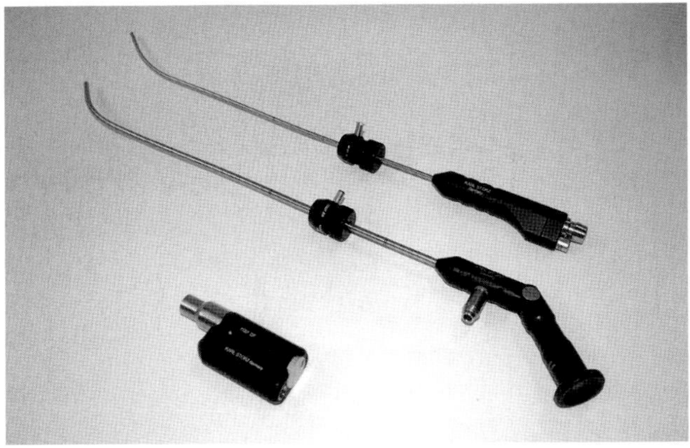

Figure 9.1. Two versions of the Karl Storz Bonfils scope. Top unit has DCI (direct coupled interface) connection which is a paired light guide and video cable connection. Standard model, below, has a pivoting eyepiece. All of Storz's products have a fixed straight shape with a deflection in the distal tip (40°). On both units is an adjustable tube stop. At *bottom left* is a super bright small LED light that attaches to standard model.

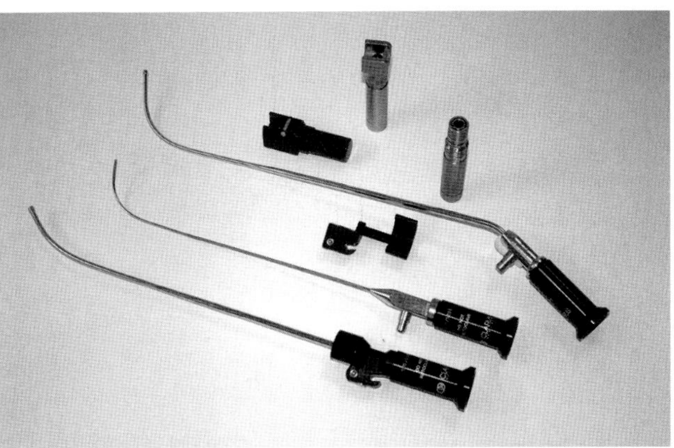

Figure 9.2. Malleable optical stylets produced by Clarus Medical Inc. Shikani (*top*), pediatric version of Shikani stylet (*middle*), and Levitan Stylet (*bottom*). The Shikani has an ACMI light fitting but can be converted to a laryngoscope connection with an adaptor (shown below the Shikani scope). Light sources (*top*) include a custom made, super bright LED light (*top left*), or snap on miniature handles using laryngoscope or ACMI fittings.

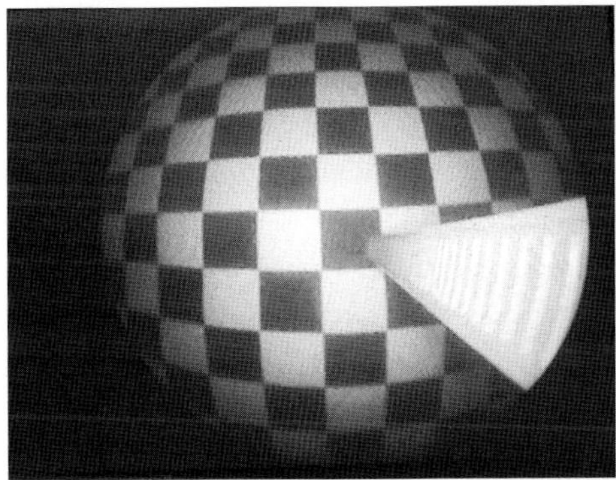

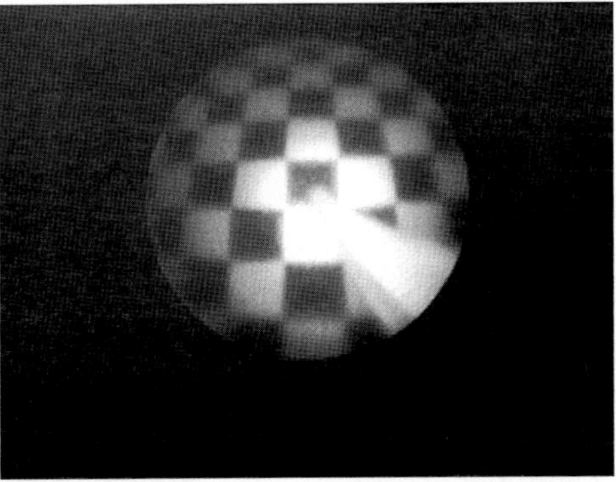

Figure 9.3. Comparisons of images from Storz's 35,000 pixel Bonfils (*left*) and Clarus 10,000 pixel instruments. The Storz product has a greater viewing angle and more peripheral fish-eye distortion. The grid is marked with 1 cm squares. Images were obtained by attaching an endoscopic coupler and video camera and measured from a fixed distance of 5 cm.

AI Medical Devices, Williamston MI) (Figure 9.4) is a novel combination of a rigid scope with an articulating distal tip (0–135°), and an integrated video screen. Clarus Medical has also recently introduced a malleable stylet with an attached video screen (Clarus Video System) (Figure 9.4).

The length of an optical stylet affects its ease of handling and intended use. ETTs from different manufacturers have certain agreed upon industrial standards regarding fittings (such as the 15 mm connectors, etc.), shaping, and markings, but not overall length. Different tube sizes, and even tubes of the same internal diameter (ID) by different manufacturers, have different lengths. This creates the need for some sort of tube stop, or adjustment device, so that different tube lengths can be appropriately positioned over an optical stylet. If the ETT is not positioned correctly, either the scope will be excessively recessed within the ETT or it will protrude beyond the tip of the ETT in an unsafe manner. An excessively recessed scope produces a view that is analogous to looking through a straw—a very narrow optical field making anatomical orientation difficult. A protruding stylet is not protected by the ETT, leaving the distal tip of the stylet exposed to secretions, blood, or other material thereby compromising the image and creating the potential for tissue

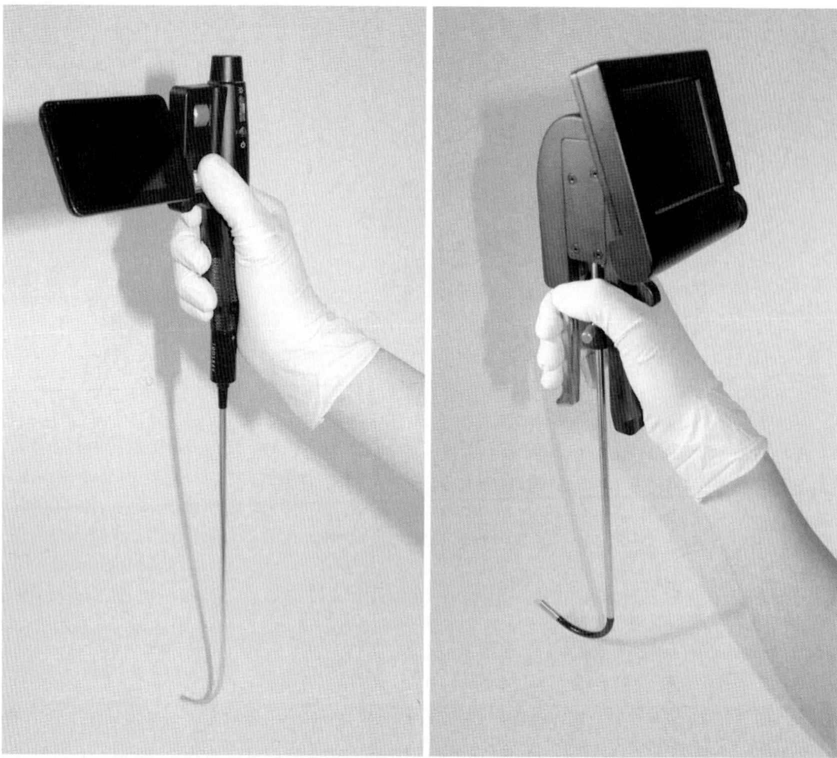

Figure 9.4. Video optical stylets: Clarus model with malleable tip, small lightweight screen (*left*) and AI Medical Video RIFL shown *right*, which has an articulating mechanism and video screen.

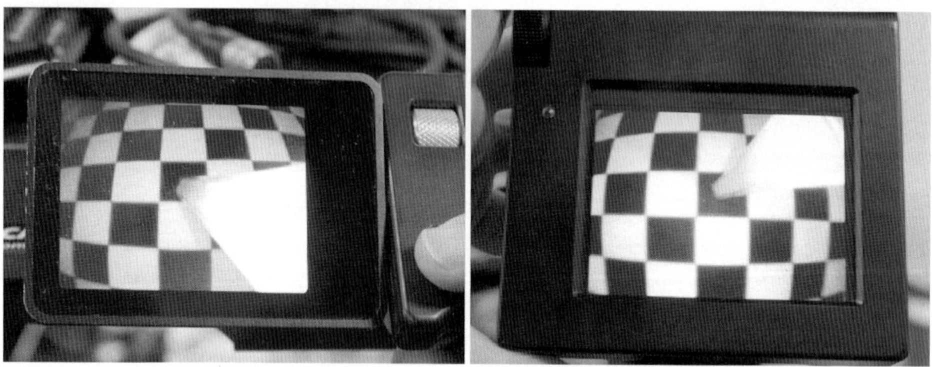

Figure 9.5. Screen shots from Clarus Video Scope and Video RIFL show very similar fields of view on a grid of 1 cm squares (measured 5 cm from target).

injury. The ideal position for an ETT is just overlying (~1 cm) the distal tip of the optical stylet, so the optical element is not exposed, but also not set too far back which would compromise the field of view. Different manufacturers have created a variety of mechanical adjustable tube stop devices that connect with the standard 15 mm plastic hub on an ETT. The Levitan FPS incorporates a fixed tube stop (at its hub) that is not adjustable; the ETT is cut to fit the shortened length of this optical stylet.

Most optical stylets have lengths of approximately 36 cm or longer. This is to accommodate the overlying ETTs and an adjustable tube stop. This distance requires the operator to be somewhat afar in order to bring their eye to the eyepiece. The impact of this length on ease of use is also a function of how the device is to be used. The Storz Bonfils has a fixed, low bend angle (~40°) and was designed for independent use. The operator uses their left hand to distract the jaw, while their right manipulates the scope

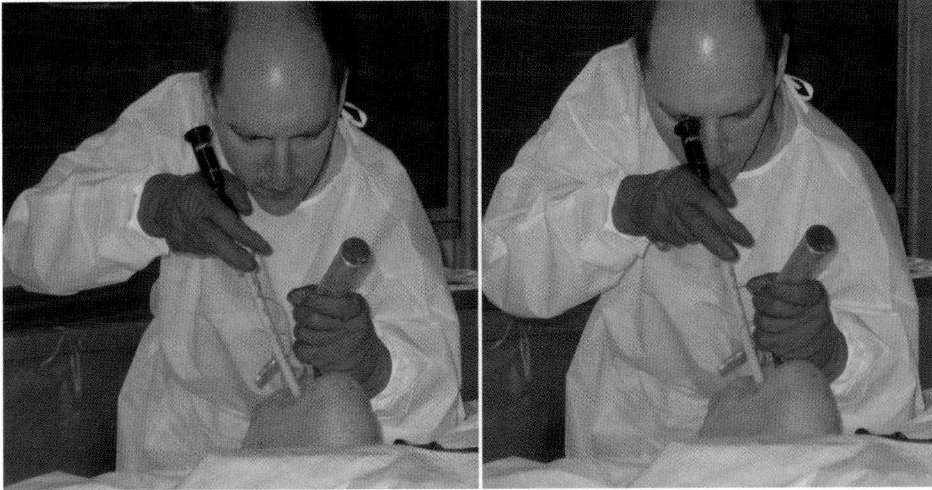

Figure 9.6. The Levitan FPS, showing transition from direct laryngoscopy to using the eyepiece. Note the more vertical orientation of the scope when using the eyepiece.

down the right side of the mouth to the larynx. Depending upon the operator's arm length and their comfort manipulating a relatively long instrument, this may result in a relatively long distance from the operator (and eyepiece) to the patient. There is an articulating eyepiece, however, which can be tilted downward, putting it in a more convenient location. The Shikani Stylet, also designed as an independent device, has a malleable distal section with an intended S-shaped bend approximately 70–90° from the main section. As this is navigated around the curve of the tongue and oropharynx the proximal end of the scope (and eyepiece) will be positioned in a near vertical position, approximately 30 cm above the patient's mouth opening. Depending on the height of the stretcher and the operator this may be ergonomically difficult. It may be helpful to lower the head of the bed or have the operator stand on a stool to gain additional height. Alternatively, standing at the patient's side and facing the patient's head, the operator can roll the device partially into the mouth before moving to a position more directly above the supine patient. In the spontaneously breathing patient, positioning the patient in a semi-sitting or upright position with the operator facing the patient will also address this problem.

The Video RIFL (Figure 9.4) does not have these ergonomic issues, since the operator does not need to use an eyepiece, and the articulating tip can be dynamically changed during the procedure (so there is more freedom of insertion from different positions). Also, the Video RIFL has a video screen that pivots 180°, allowing insertion from above, or facing the patient. The Clarus Video Scope (Figure 9.4) also has a pivoting video screen, though its range is somewhat less than the RIFL (and the tip of the scope does not articulate).

The Levitan FPS is shorter than other optical stylets (29 cm), designed to be used in conjunction with a laryngoscope. It can also be used without a laryngoscope, using a near right angle bend (~70° bend) like the Shikani Stylet, but its overall shorter length eliminates the height problem for most operators (Figure 9.6).

Addressing the ergonomics and manipulation of an optical stylet is important for successful use. Since the device must always move through an open channel, it is critical for the operator to bring their eye to the eyepiece (or observe the video monitor) immediately as the device is inserted. If the tip of a stylet is just pushed into the tongue (or is touching any other mucosa upon insertion) the view is obscured. Specialized oral airways have been developed to assist the manipulation of flexible scopes through the oral route (Ovassapian, Williams, Berman intubating airways) and can be very helpful for providing an open channel to navigate the oropharynx while using optical stylets.

The technical specifications of different optical stylets designs are outlined in Table 9.1. Images of the different products, and differences in optical appearance through the devices, are shown in Figs. 9.1, 9.2, 9.3, 9.4, and 9.5.

Table 9.1. Specifications of fiberoptic and video optical stylets.

Optical stylet	OD (mm)	Length (cm)	Tube (ID)	Pixels/imaging	Comments
Clarus Levitan	5	29	>5.5	10,000	Malleable stylet, fixed eyepiece
Clarus Shikani	5	36.9	>5.5	10,000	Malleable stylet, fixed eyepiece
Clarus Pediatric Shikani	2.4	26.6	3.0–5.0	10,000	Malleable stylet, fixed eyepiece
Storz Bonfils (10331B)	5	40	> 5.5	35,000	40° distal deflection; eyepiece pivots, DCI model (10331BD)
Storz Bonfils (10332B)	3.5	35	4.0–5.5	35,000	40° distal deflection; eyepiece pivots, DCI model (10332BD)
Storz Bambrink (11605C)	2	22	2.5–4.0	35,000	40° distal deflection; eyepiece pivots, DCI model (11605CV)
Clarus Video Scope	5	36.9	>5.5	CMOS video	Malleable stylet, screen ~6 × 4.5 cm; monitor swivels ~120°
AI RIFL	5	36.9	>5.5	CMOS video	Articulating tip 0–135°, screen ~7.5 × 5 cm, monitor swivels 180°

Principles of Optical Stylets and Progressive Visualization

As already noted, there are "rules" when it comes to effectively using optical stylet devices that have a small imaging element and are positioned within an ETT. Laryngoscopes separate and divide tissue and their movement upon insertion is relatively coarse, and the same is true of imaging devices that are connected to tongue retractors (video laryngoscopes, e.g., the GlideScope, McGrath, or optical laryngoscopes, e.g., the Airtraq). With a laryngoscope the operator gets a set-off view of structures (from their dominant eye, a direct line-of-sight view); with video laryngoscopes and optical laryngoscopes the perspective is from within the mouth but above the epiglottis, and there is a panoramic view of the perilaryngeal structures. By contrast, an optical stylet can offer a set-off view of the larynx from afar, or alternatively the tip of the scope may be abutting the mucosa with no identifiable landmarks. With curved blade retractor imaging devices insertion follows the curvature of the tongue and the blade, serving as a retractor, lifts the jaw creating a channel for viewing. With optical stylets, the first "rule" is that the operator must follow the open channel of the airway.

The initial channel to navigate is the oropharynx. In a supine position, the tongue and the epiglottis can collapse backward onto the posterior hypopharynx. This is the reason Ovassapian, Williams, or Berman intubating airways are recommended when using the oral route with flexible scopes in unconscious patients. If not using these airway channels the operator must carefully navigate the tip of the optical stylet to the glottic opening between the anterior tissues (tongue and epiglottis) and the posterior tissues (pharyngeal wall and the posterior larynx). There is a significant curve to the base of the tongue, and also coming forward from beneath the epiglottis into the larynx. The upward distal deflection of all optical stylets assists in this anterior movement. When the tip of an airway instrument needs to be directed anteriorly (under base of tongue and epiglottis) the proximal portion of the instrument will be tilted backward. Depending on the curvature of a device, this sometimes requires using the extreme right corner of the mouth and avoiding the central incisors. Some operators find it is easier to insert a device in the right side of the mouth, and then rotate the tip around the base of tongue (toward midline) as the proximal section of the instrument is brought to a vertical position. The Video RIFL can deal with the curve of the tongue and advancing past the epiglottis by articulating the distal scope anteriorly.

The airway tube of the LMA™, and many other SGAs (see Chap. 7) provides a clear channel around the tongue for optical stylets to move through. Beyond the glottic opening the trachea itself is an open channel.

The second "rule" of optical stylets is to maintain distance from the target. It has already been mentioned that if a landmark is viewed from too close a perspective it is

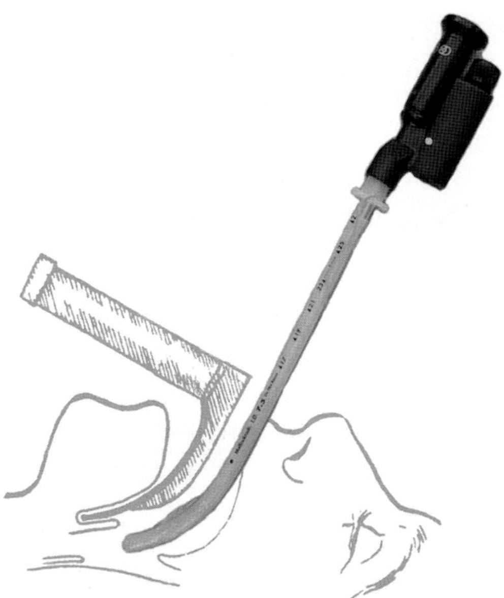

Figure 9.7. Positioning of Levitan FPS in open channel of airway. Notice the laryngoscope is helping to create a channel by lifting tongue and epiglottis (anteriorly).

difficult to recognize. The critical structures that should be recognized from afar are the epiglottis, followed by the posterior (arytenoid) cartilages. Adequate light must be projected down the airway for an operator to see these structures from a distance. When viewed from too close a distance, the epiglottis will be a curvilinear large structure filling the visible field and the posterior cartilages will be large rounded prominences (and not seen as paired structures).

The third and final "rule" of optical stylets is to know your starting position and progress from landmark to landmark. For the purposes of intubation, the "starting position" is the epiglottis. The epiglottis has a fundamentally unique importance in airway anatomy. It is the bridge between the tongue and the glottic opening. It attaches to the base of the tongue at the vallecula and it is the most superior aspect of the laryngeal inlet. It also defines midline, right vs. left. Once the epiglottis is recognized the operator knows the position of the larynx. If the tip of an optical stylet abuts tissue and nothing is identifiable, the operator must *withdraw* and reposition the scope tip into the open channel to locate the epiglottis. This is the exact opposite of laryngoscopy. With a laryngoscope, when no structures are seen the operator *advances* incrementally (down the tongue) until structures become visible. Minor adjustments of an optical stylet may result in a significant change in the resultant view. After the epiglottis is visualized careful movement of the tip is needed to get underneath the epiglottis, and then directing the instrument tip anteriorly (upward) will yield a view of the glottic opening. Depending upon the patient, and the amount of space under the epiglottis, this can be the most challenging aspect of fiberoptic intubation with both flexible scopes and optical stylets. With optical stylets, however, the tip can be used to directly lift the epiglottis as needed. Maneuvers that open the space between the base of tongue–epiglottis and the posterior hypopharyngeal wall can make the difference between success and failure. Options include a jaw thrust, jaw lifting by the operator's left hand, pulling up on the tongue (using a gauze pad to assist with grip), or using a laryngoscope as a tongue retractor (Figure 9.7).

After this step, the next structures that come into view are the posterior cartilages and the interarytenoid notch. The notch may appear as a thin vertical cleft, or a broad flat ridge. The right and left posterior cartilages appear differently. The cuneiform lies more superior than the corniculate on each side, and depending upon the manner in which these two prominences are positioned the operator can distinguish whether they are viewing the right or left posterior cartilages. Above the notch and medial to the posterior cartilages is the glottic opening (with adjacent true and false vocal cords) (Figs. 9.8 and 9.9).

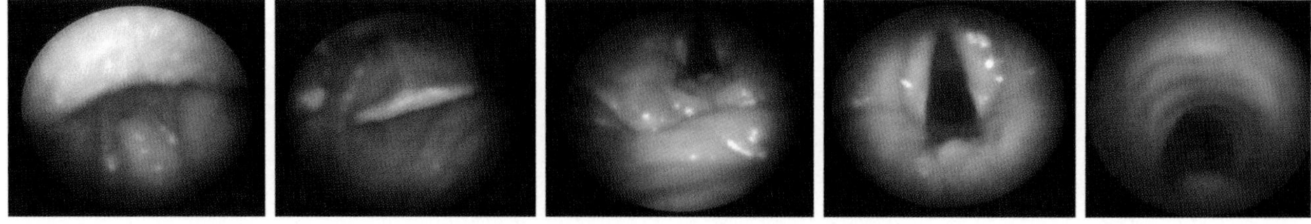

Figure 9.8. Progressive landmarks through an optical stylet: Uvula and base of tongue (*left*), epiglottis, posterior larynx glottic opening, and vocal cords, and tracheal rings (*right*).

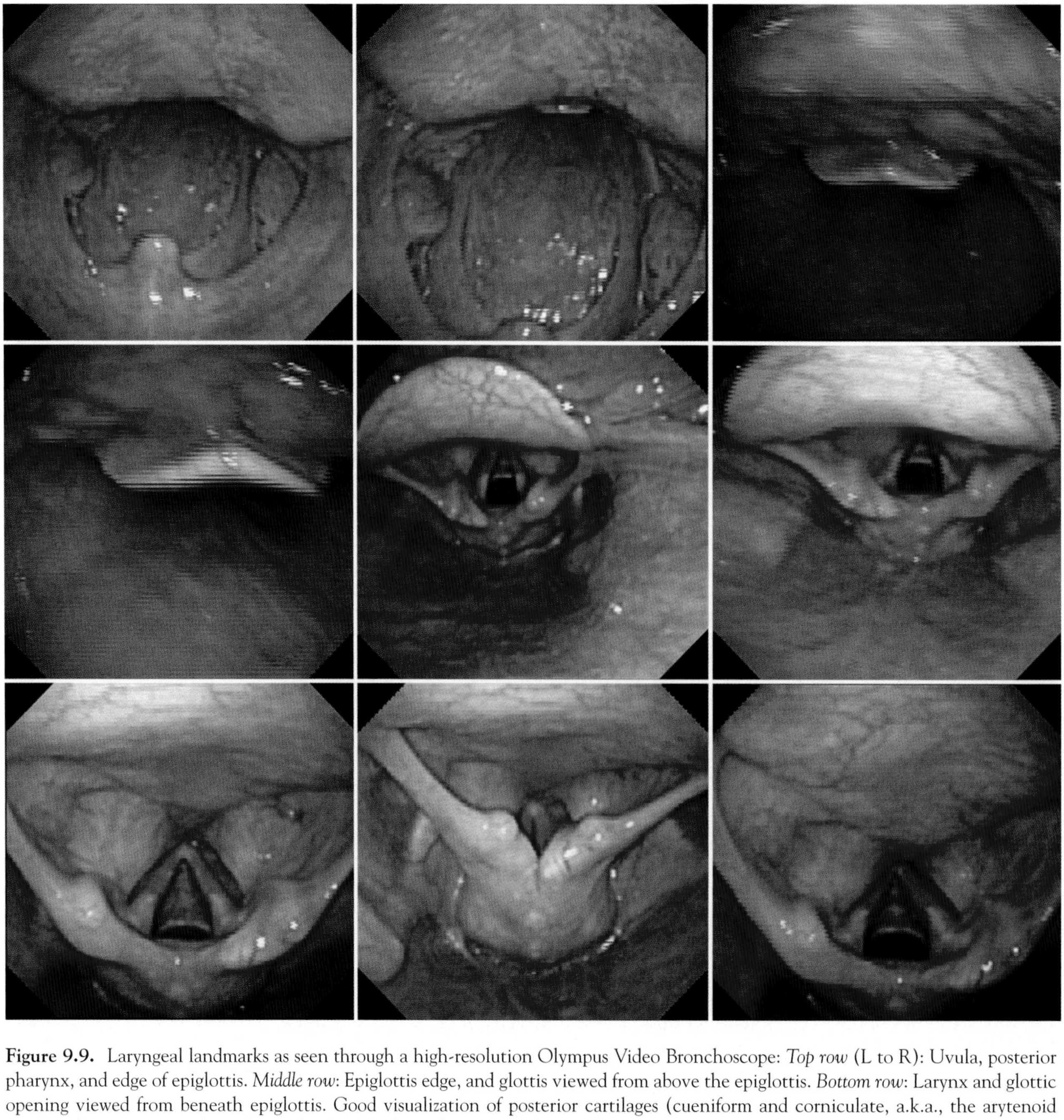

Figure 9.9. Laryngeal landmarks as seen through a high-resolution Olympus Video Bronchoscope: *Top row* (L to R): Uvula, posterior pharynx, and edge of epiglottis. *Middle row*: Epiglottis edge, and glottis viewed from above the epiglottis. *Bottom row*: Larynx and glottic opening viewed from beneath epiglottis. Good visualization of posterior cartilages (cueniform and corniculate, a.k.a., the arytenoid cartilages), interarytenoid notch, epiglottic tubercle, and true and false vocal cords.

Patient Positioning

The importance of patient positioning as it affects the dimensions of the airway at the base of tongue and epiglottis cannot be overstated. A common error is to overextend the head and unknowingly pivot the base of tongue and epiglottis backward, onto the posterior pharyngeal wall. Optimal positioning involves having the patient in ear-to-sternal position and the face plane of the patient should be parallel to the ceiling. Ear-to-sternal notch positioning means aligning the external auditory meatus (the ear) and the sternal notch when viewed from a lateral perspective. In a vertical orientation, this is the position patients naturally assume with respiratory distress (imagine the patient with congestive heart failure, or epiglottitis, for example). It maximizes upper airway patency and in the author's opinion it is the ideal position for mask ventilation, direct laryngoscopy, and all the imaging devices (optical stylets, video and mirror laryngoscopes). Not only does it avoid the problems with overextension, it allows maximal jaw distraction with the least effort. With hyperextension the force vector extending the head is opposing the force vector needed to distract the jaw and tongue making it more difficult to distract the tongue and jaw. With ear-to-sternal notch positioning and a horizontal face plane, the jaw has no mechanical restrictions to forward displacement. A useful way to envision this is to consider the phenomenon of "jaw dropping"—when a person sees something remarkable and their "jaw drops" open. In this position the head comes forward and the face plane is perpendicular to the ground. The jaw has no mechanical restriction and as the person forgets to maintain tension in their masseter muscles, the jaw naturally drops open. Ear-to-sternal notch position and a horizontal face plane recreate this position in a supine person.

The author recommends every patient be placed into optimal position prior to the procedure; however, for some patients dynamic head elevation may be done. While not possible in the morbidly obese, this is easily done in most patients by having an assistant lift the head (from a position aside the patient). This technique can be employed when the epiglottis is viewed but there is not enough space to get underneath it.

Tube Tip Design and Relevance to Optical Stylets

A common feature of all optical stylets is that the tips of these devices are positioned just proximal to the end of an ETT. Accordingly, the shape and design of the overlying ETT affects the view through the stylet. Standard tracheal tubes have a left-facing bevel when viewed down their long axis and an arcuate-shaped curve from proximal to distal. Some designs have a straight cut edge, while others have a "shrouded" tip in which the distal edge of the tube has a rounded edge. Alternatively, the Parker tube (Parker Medical) has a ski tip-shaped symmetric design (Figure 9.10).

If an optical stylet is not inserted close enough to the end of the ETT, the view is like looking through a straw. If the optical stylet projects out from the tube, then it will be susceptible to secretions or other fluids touching the imaging end of the stylet and obscuring the view. Compared to flexible scopes, the slightly retracted position provides a great advantage, protecting the view from secretions.

Depending on how the ETT is secured on an optical stylet, the ETT may rotate in a manner in which the view is straight out the tube tip, or alternatively, the tip and Murphy eye can block the line of sight. With all devices, the operator should optimize the image by adjusting the length and rotation of the ETT prior to use.

The Parker Flex-Tip™ tube (Parker Medical, Highlands Ranch CO) has some mechanical advantages as it advances into the trachea, but for some optical stylets, depending on their field of view, the tip of the ski tip-shaped tube may cover a significant portion of the upper visual field (Figure 9.10).

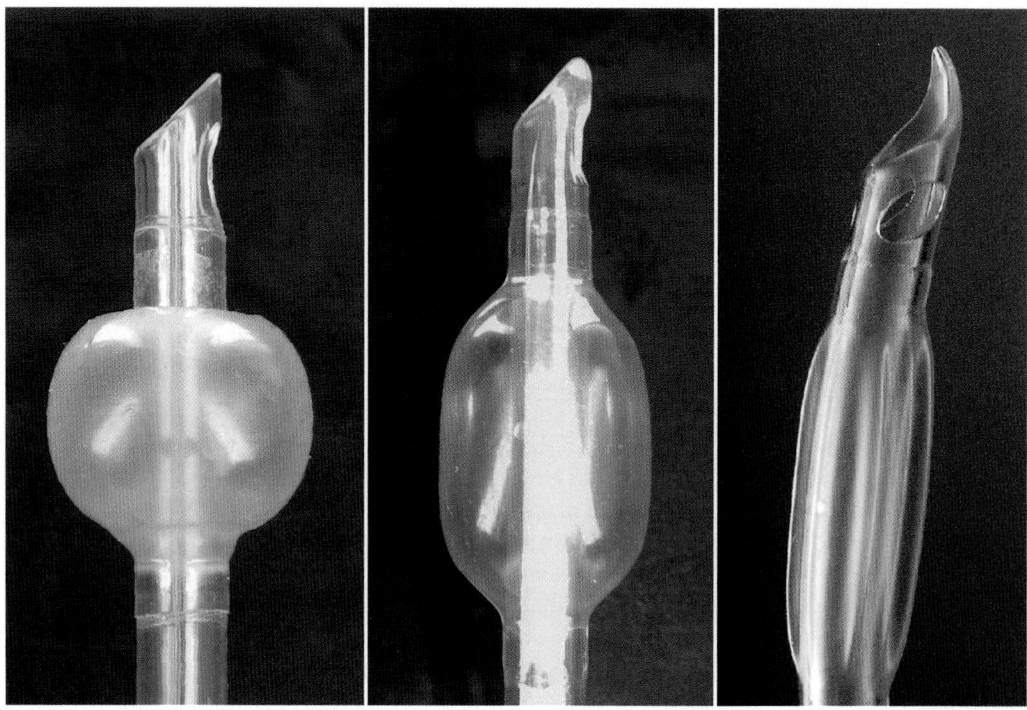

Figure 9.10. Straight cut, left-beveled tube (*left*); shrouded tip left-beveled tube (*middle*); and Parker ski-tip tube (*right*).

Mechanics and Tube Delivery Issues

The mechanics of inserting a rigid instrument through the mouth, and taking advantage of the extreme lateral corner at the right side of the mouth has already been noted.

As tubes are passed from an optical stylet into the trachea, the tube tip may interact with the anterior tracheal rings. This is potentially much more of an issue with optical stylets than standard intubation stylets, because of their rigidity (even the malleable variety) and because operators often use a significant bend angle. When using tracheal tube stylets, a straight-to-cuff bend angle of 35° provides optimal visualization and maneuverability without mechanical problems of tube insertion against the tracheal rings. The original Smiths tracheal introducer (Eschmann gum elastic bougie) has a bend angle of 38°. The author recommends a bend angle of 35° straight-to-cuff when using the Levitan Stylet with a laryngoscope (Figure 9.11). The Bonfils has a fixed bend angle of 40° at the distal tip Whenever bend angles exceed these angles the tip of the tube will interact with the anterior tracheal rings in a manner that can frustrate ETT advancement. This is a common challenge of video and mirror laryngoscopes. It was recognized by Archie Brain in his specially designed ETT for intubation through the Fastrach™ LMA. With optical stylets, this issue is commonly encountered if angled more severely.

One option to lessen the impaction of a left-facing beveled tube on the tracheal rings is to rotate the ETT clockwise as it is advanced off the stylet. This turns the bevel from facing left to facing up, and the leading edge of the tube drops down, disengaging from the tracheal rings. When using an optical stylet in the right hand, the tube is easily advanced with the left hand by encircling the proximal tube with the four fingers of the left hand and turning the wrist clockwise as the tube is pushed down. With all the optical stylets, it is important to advance the ETT rather than withdrawing the stylet to ensure that the ETT is not partially or fully removed from the trachea. Operators should check the depth of tube placement by centimeter markings on the tube prior to device removal.

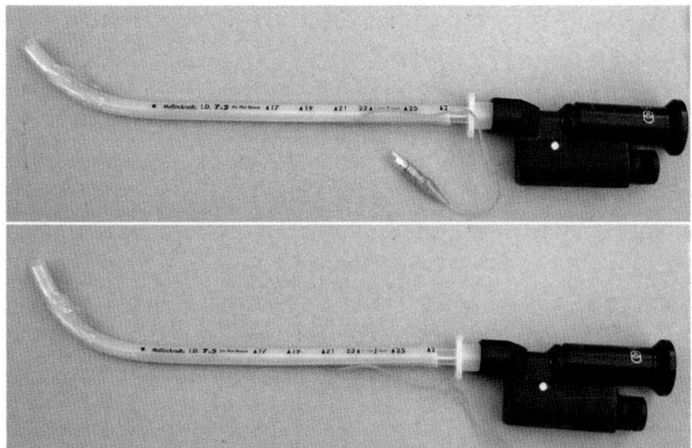

Figure 9.11. The Levitan FPS used with a laryngoscope should have a 35° bend angle (straight to cuff, then bent 35° at the proximal cuff; *top image*). When used without a laryngoscope, the optimal bend angle, rolling the device around the tongue, is 70° (*bottom*).

Oxygen Ports

All of the optical stylets mentioned, except the Video RIFL, have a means of insufflating oxygen through the tube as a means of keeping the distal tip clear of secretions. There is debate about how much this is needed and how much oxygen is safe. The author has used low flow rates 2–4 lpm, but some other users have used as much as 15 lpm. As long as placement is not in the esophagus, and assuming that the time the scope is within the trachea is limited, and that there is a means of air egress, barotrauma risk is minimal.

Cleaning

Optical stylets, like other fiberoptic imaging devices, should not be heat sterilized. A variety of cold cleaning methods (Steris, glutaraldehyde, ethylene oxide, etc.) are recommended by different manufacturers. Since optical stylets do not have working channels (like flexible bronchoscopes) they are significantly easier to clean with less risk of cross contamination between patients.

Combining Optical Stylets with Supraglottic Airways

Depending on the design features of the stylet and the particular SGA, the latter can serve as a conduit for the optical stylet. This may be useful for correctly seating the device, for ventilation or to facilitate placement of an ETT through the SGA.

For this purpose, the best-designed SGA should have a short tube (so an ETT can reach the larynx) with a large bore (to accept an adult-sized tube). It also should have no aperture bars or other mechanical impediments to tube passage. The Cookgas air-Q™ (Mercury Medical, Clearwater FL) has these features, plus a low angle exit from the tube section that also facilitates tube placement. The proximal 15-mm connector can easily be removed and a specially designed stabilizing rod can be inserted in the ETT to enable the removal of the air-Q. An optical stylet (the Air-Vu) for intubation through the air-Q is also available. Another airway that may be particularly useful with optical stylets is the i-gel (Intersurgical Ltd., Wokingham, UK). The tube section is short, the bore large, with an integral bite block and 15-mm connector.

When exiting the tube section of an SGA, the visualized structures are a function of how well placed the device is in relation to the laryngeal inlet. Ideally, only the glottis is seen; occasionally the epiglottis hangs down horizontally across the visual field, and on other occasions only the posterior cartilages are recognizable. If nothing is recognizable, the device may not be in far enough (and the optical stylet is against the base of tongue), or it is too far into the upper esophagus (with the optical stylet contacting the undersurface of the posterior larynx). Alternatively, the epiglottis may be down-folded and the view is that of the vallecula. While holding the optical stylet with the right hand, the operator can perform an "up-down maneuver" (see Chap. 8), withdrawing and reintroducing the SGA to optimize its relation to the laryngeal inlet.

Specific Uses of the Different Instruments, Pediatric Versions

Optical stylets were originally designed as independent devices for intubation. The Bonfils and Shikani are both used in this fashion. The Bonfils was designed for a retromolar, low-angle approach (right side of tongue, paraglossal technique) while the Shikani was intended to be used with a marked bend and rotated around the base of the tongue. Both of these devices could be used in conjunction with a laryngoscope. The Air-Vu (Mercury Medical) is just a fixed curved version of the Shikani designed specifically for passage through an SGA. The Levitan stylet was designed primarily as an adjunct for laryngoscopy, but can be used with a greater bend angle like a Shikani, or passed through an SGA. The Video RIFL was intended as an independent device but can also be used with a laryngoscope or through an SGA.

The Shikani SOS is available in a pediatric version; the Storz Bonfils has a pediatric version called the Brambrinck. These pediatric stylets can be used with ETTs as small as 2.5 cm ID.

Literature Reports of Optical Stylets

Optical stylets are a relatively new addition to the arena of airway management. There have been relatively few large series addressing their efficacy. Most of the reports are anecdotal. The number of citations is related to how long the devices have been produced; the Bonfils has a greater number of reports than the Shikani, which in turn has more reports than the Levitan. There are no published papers yet on the Video RIFL or the video version of the Clarus stylet. Although many clinicians are focused on published papers regarding devices, in the author's opinion, much of the device literature is not truly about the specific device as much as it is about the technical skill of the operator handling the device. Fiberoptic instruments, and optical stylets, are potentially powerful and versatile tools for airway management but they are only as good as the operator using them.

The literature on optical stylets, broken down by device, is listed in the Bibliography.

Disclosure Richard Levitan receives royalties on the FPS Levitan Optical Stylet manufactured and sold by Clarus Medical, Minneapolis, MN.

Bibliography

General or Multi-device Review

1. Gravenstein D, Liem EB, Bjoraker DG. Alternative management techniques for the difficult airway: optical stylets. Curr Opin Anaesthesiol. 2004;17(6):495–8.

Bonfils

2. Powell L, Andrzejowski J, Taylor R, Turnbull D. Comparison of the performance of four laryngoscopes in a high-fidelity simulator using normal and difficult airway. Br J Anaesth. 2009;103(5):755–60.
3. Corbanese U, Possamai C. Awake intubation with the Bonfils fibrescope in patients with difficult airway. Eur J Anaesthesiol. 2009;26(10):837–41.
4. Maeyama A, Kodaka M, Miyao H. [BONFILS retromolar intubation fiberscope VS styletscope for oro-tracheal intubation] [Japanese]. Masui. 2009;58(10):1323–7.
5. Piepho T, Noppens RR, Heid F, Werner C, Thierbach AR. Rigid fibrescope Bonfils: use in simulated difficult airway by novices. Scand J Trauma Resusc Emerg Med. 2009;17(1):33.
6. Corbanese U, Morossi M. The Bonfils intubation fibrescope: clinical evaluation and consideration of the learning curve. Eur J Anaesthesiol. 2009;26(7):622–4.
7. Aucoin S, Vlatten A, Hackmann T. Difficult airway management with the Bonfils fiberscope in a child with Hurler syndrome. Paediatr Anaesth. 2009;19(4):421–2.
8. Baker P, Mahadevan M. The Bonfils fiberscope is not suitable for neonatal intubation. Paediatr Anaesth. 2009;19(4):418.
9. Bhagwat A, Bhadoria P, Wadhawan S, Gupta L. A novel aid for intubation using the bonfils retromolar scope. Acta Anaesthesiol Scand. 2009;53(3):418–9.
10. Xue FS, Luo MP, Liao X, He N. Airway topical anesthesia using the Bonfils fiberscope. J Clin Anesth. 2009;21(2):154–5.
11. Sorbello M, Paratore A, Morello G, Merli G, Belluoccio AA, Petrini F. Bonfils fiberscope: better preoxygenate rather than oxygenate! Anesth Analg. 2009;108(1):386.
12. He N, Xue FS, Xu YC, Liao X, Xu XZ. Awake orotracheal intubation under airway topical anesthesia using the Bonfils in patients with a predicted difficult airway. Can J Anaesth. 2008;55(12):881–2.
13. Bein B, Wortmann F, Meybohm P, Steinfath M, Scholz J, Dörges V. Evaluation of the pediatric Bonfils fiberscope for elective endotracheal intubation. Paediatr Anaesth. 2008;18(11):1040–4.
14. Caruselli M, Zannini R, Giretti R, Rocchi G, Camilletti G, Bechi P, et al. Difficult intubation in a small for gestational age newborn by bonfils fiberscope. Paediatr Anaesth. 2008;18(10):990–1.
15. Liao X, Xue FS, Zhang YM. Tracheal intubation using the Bonfils intubation fibrescope in patients with a difficult airway. Can J Anaesth. 2008;55(9):655–6; author reply 656–7.
16. Mihai R, Blair E, Kay H, Cook TM. A quantitative review and meta-analysis of performance of non-standard laryngoscopes and rigid fibreoptic intubation aids. Anaesthesia. 2008;63(7):745–60; review.
17. Abramson SI, Holmes AA, Hagberg CA. Awake insertion of the bonfils retromolar intubation fiberscope in five patients with anticipated difficult airways. Anesth Analg. 2008;106(4):1215–7, table of contents.
18. Rudolph C, Henn-Beilharz A, Gottschall R, Wallenborn J, Schaffranietz L. The unanticipated difficult intubation: rigid or flexible endoscope? Minerva Anestesiol. 2007;73(11):567–74.
19. Byhahn C, Meininger D, Walcher F, Hofstetter C, Zwissler B. Prehospital emergency endotracheal intubation using the Bonfils intubation fiberscope. Eur J Emerg Med. 2007;14(1):43–6.
20. Buehner U, Oram J, Elliot S, Mallick A, Bodenham A. Bonfils semirigid endoscope for guidance during percutaneous tracheostomy. Anaesthesia. 2006;61(7):665–70.
21. Maeyama A, Kodaka M, Koyama K, Okuyama S, Maruo T, Miyao H. [Newly developed BONFILS retromolar intubation fiberscope for difficult airway]. Masui. 2006;55(4):494–8.

22. Rudolph C, Schneider JP, Wallenborn J, Schaffranietz L. Movement of the upper cervical spine during laryngoscopy: a comparison of the Bonfils intubation fibrescope and the Macintosh laryngoscope. Anaesthesia. 2005;60(7):668–72.
23. Bein B, Caliebe D, Römer T, Scholz J, Dörges V. Using the Bonfils intubation fiberscope with a double-lumen tracheal tube. Anesthesiology. 2005;102(6):1290–1.
24. Maybauer MO, Maier S, Thierbach AR. An unexpected difficult intubation. Bonfils rigid fiberscope. Anaesthesist. 2005;54(1):35–40.
25. Bein B, Yan M, Tonner PH, Scholz J, Steinfath M, Dörges V. Tracheal intubation using the Bonfils intubation fibrescope after failed direct laryngoscopy. Anaesthesia. 2004;59(12):1207–9.
26. Bein B, Worthmann F, Scholz J, Brinkmann F, Tonner PH, Steinfath M, et al. A comparison of the intubating laryngeal mask airway and the Bonfils intubation fibrescope in patients with predicted difficult airways. Anaesthesia. 2004;59(7):668–74.
27. Wong P. Intubation times for using the Bonfils intubation fibrescope. Br J Anaesth. 2003;91(5):757; author reply 757–8.

Levitan

28. Greenland KB, Liu G, Tan H, Edwards M, Irwin MG. Comparison of the Levitan FPS scope and the single-use bougie for simulated difficult intubation in anaesthetised patients. Anaesthesia. 2007;62(5):509–15. Erratum in: Anaesthesia. 2007;62(6):644.
29. Levitan RM, Chudnofsky C, Sapre N. Emergency airway management in a morbidly obese, noncooperative, rapidly deteriorating patient. Am J Emerg Med. 2006;24(7):894–6.
30. Levitan RM. Design rationale and intended use of a short optical stylet for routine fiberoptic augmentation of emergency laryngoscopy. Am J Emerg Med. 2006;24(4):490–5.
31. Paladino L, DuCanto J, Manoach S. Development of a rapid, safe, fiber-optic guided, single-incision cricothyrotomy using a large ovine model: a pilot study. Resuscitation. 2009;80(9):1066–9.
32. Manoach S, Paladino L. Trauma airway salvage using an optical stylet with oxygen insufflation. J Clin Anesth. 2008;20(4):317–8.
33. Kovacs G, Law AJ, Petrie D. Awake fiberoptic intubation using an optical stylet in an anticipated difficult airway. Ann Emerg Med. 2007;49(1):81–3.

Shikani

34. Yao YT, Jia NG, Li CH, Zhang YJ, Yin YQ. Comparison of endotracheal intubation with the Shikani Optical Stylet using the left molar approach and direct laryngoscopy. Chin Med J (Engl). 2008;121(14):1324–7.
35. Stricker P, Fiadjoe JE, McGinnis S. Intubation of an infant with Pierre Robin sequence under dexmedetomidine sedation using the Shikani Optical Stylet. Acta Anaesthesiol Scand. 2008;52(6):866–7.
36. Jansen AH, Johnston G. The Shikani Optical Stylet: a useful adjunct to airway management in a neonate with popliteal pterygium syndrome. Paediatr Anaesth. 2008;18(2):188–90.
37. Young CF, Vadivelu N. Does the use of a laryngoscope facilitate orotracheal intubation with a Shikani Optical Stylet? Br J Anaesth. 2007;99(2):302–3.
38. Young CF, Vadivelu N. Can the Shikani Optical Stylet facilitate intubation in simulated difficult direct laryngoscopy? Conn Med. 2007;71(7):407–8.
39. Turkstra TP, Pelz DM, Shaikh AA, Craen RA. Cervical spine motion: a fluoroscopic comparison of Shikani Optical Stylet vs Macintosh laryngoscope. Can J Anaesth. 2007;54(6):441–7.
40. Evans A, Morris S, Petterson J, Hall JE. A comparison of the Seeing Optical Stylet and the gum elastic bougie in simulated difficult tracheal intubation: a manikin study. Anaesthesia. 2006;61(5):478–81.
41. Duffy MR, Ingham J. The Seeing Optical Stylet for percutaneous tracheostomy. Anaesthesia. 2006;61(3):298–9.
42. Shukry M, Hanson RD, Koveleskie JR, Ramadhyani U. Management of the difficult pediatric airway with Shikani Optical Stylet. Paediatr Anaesth. 2005;15(4):342–5.

Manufacturer's Web Sites

AI MEDICAL: Video RIFL—http://www.aimedicaldevices.com/videorifl.html

CLARUS MEDICAL: Shikani, Levitan, Video Scope—http://www.clarus-medical.com/airway-management/airway_home.htm

STORZ: Bonfils, Brambrinck—http://www.karlstorz.de/cps/rde/xchg/SID-35846978-EB5BAFE8/karlstorz-en/hs.xsl/49.htm

10

The Role of the Lightwand

Ashutosh Wali

Introduction

The lightwand has been used in airway management for more than five decades and was first described to assist direct laryngoscopic orotracheal intubation in 1957[1]. Soon after, in 1959, a study reported the successful use of the lightwand, based on the principle of transillumination of the throat, to facilitate nasotracheal intubation in 29 of 30 patients with severe trismus[2]. The authors noted three concerns that are still valid today: the need for a dark room to appreciate transillumination in the neck, the difficulty in transilluminating patients with thick necks, and the risk of thermal injury[2]. The lightwand was first used as a commercial stylet, later that year[3]. However, the initial interest in the device soon waned, probably because of the difficulty in transillumination of the light through red rubber tracheal tubes that were being used at that time. The lightwand regained popularity

A. Wali (✉)
Baylor College of Medicine, 1709 Dryden, Suite 1700, Houston, TX 77030, USA
e-mail: awali@bcm.edu

D.B. Glick et al. (eds.), *The Difficult Airway: An Atlas of Tools and Techniques for Clinical Management*,
DOI 10.1007/978-0-387-92849-4_10, © Springer Science+Business Media New York 2013

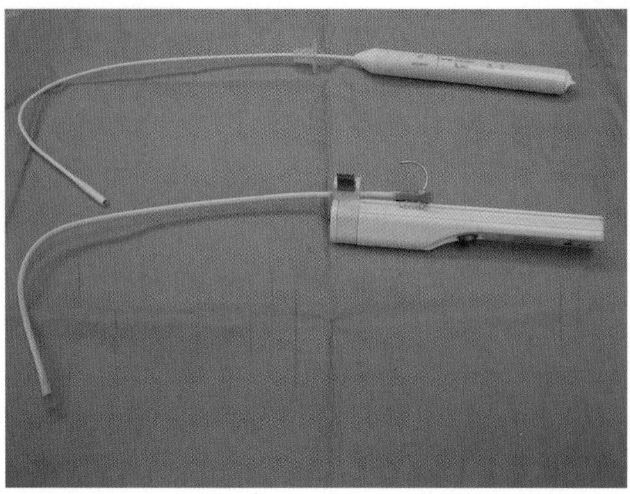

Figure 10.1. The photograph shows two lightwands, the Surch-Lite™ (*top*, Aaron Medical) and the recently discontinued Trachlight™ (*bottom*, Laerdal Medical).

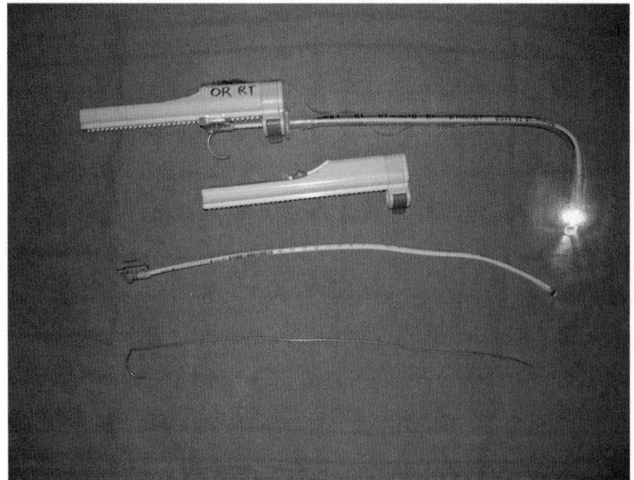

Figure 10.2. The photograph shows an assembled and deconstructed Trachlight™. The three components consist of the handle, the lightwand, and the malleable metal stylet. The tracheal tube is inserted into the 15-mm holder and the green latch is closed, locking it into position. The metal stylet is lubricated and inserted into the flexible light wand until a click is heard indicating that it is secured. The lightwand/stylet is mounted onto the track of the handle by depressing the green tab on its proximal end. The lightwand is advanced within the tracheal tube until the lightwand/stylet is slightly recessed within the distal end. It should be advanced or withdrawn very slightly until a click is heard, indicating that it is locked onto the handle. Turn on the light switch on the back of the handle. The light will flash after 30 s.

with the advent of clear, plastic tracheal tubes in 1985. It was reported to be useful in accurately determining the position of tracheal tubes, with 96 % accuracy, in less than 5 s[4] and was used to facilitate difficult tracheal intubation in adults[5]. Currently, many lightwand devices (e.g., Flexilum™, Concept Corporation, Clearwater FL; Surch Lite™, Aaron Medical, Clearwater FL and Tubestat™, Xomed, Jackonville FL) are available from different manufacturers (Figure 10.1). The Trachlight™ (Laerdal, Wappingers Falls, NY) was the most widely used and studied of these devices (Figure 10.2); however, the manufacturer discontinued this product in 2009 due to declining sales.

Principle

Lightwand-guided tracheal intubation is based on the principle of transillumination of the soft tissues of the neck during the passage of the tracheal tube from the hypopharynx into the larynx and trachea. The thyroid cartilage is the anatomical surface marking for the larynx. A faint midline glow above the thyroid cartilage suggests that the tip of the tracheal tube/lightwand unit is in the vallecula while a bright, well-demarcated light glow in the midline but below the thyroid cartilage suggests upper tracheal entry[6]. It has been claimed that the appearance of the bright glow at the sternal notch indicates that the tip of the tracheal tube/lightwand unit is halfway between the glottic opening and the carina. However, Locker and colleagues have suggested that in adults, the tracheal tube (TT) should be advanced 3 cm beyond the sternal notch to be optimally positioned[7]. Many companies manufacture and market these devices, but the underlying principle remains the same.

Assembly and Positioning

Insert the lightwand into the tracheal tube and attach the lightwand to the tracheal tube with its adaptor. The light bulb at the tip of the lightwand should be within the tracheal tube lumen, a few millimeters above the tip to avoid thermal injury to any soft tissues in the upper or lower airway. A 90° bend of the device assembly is recommended proximal to the cuff (Figure 10.3) to transilluminate the anterior neck and facilitate entry through the laryngeal aperture[8]. Softening of the TT with warm water immersion and lubrication of the lightwand (and inner metal stylet of the Trachlight™) are essential for successful passage of the device assembly.

The intubationist should be at the head of the operating table, and the operating table at a comfortable height, generally lower than that required for direct laryngoscopy. The patient's head should be in maximal extension to allow adequate exposure of the anterior neck and to facilitate lifting the epiglottis away from the posterior pharyngeal wall (Figure 10.4). The sniffing position does not provide an adequate lift to elevate the epiglottis from the posterior pharyngeal wall (Figure 10.5).

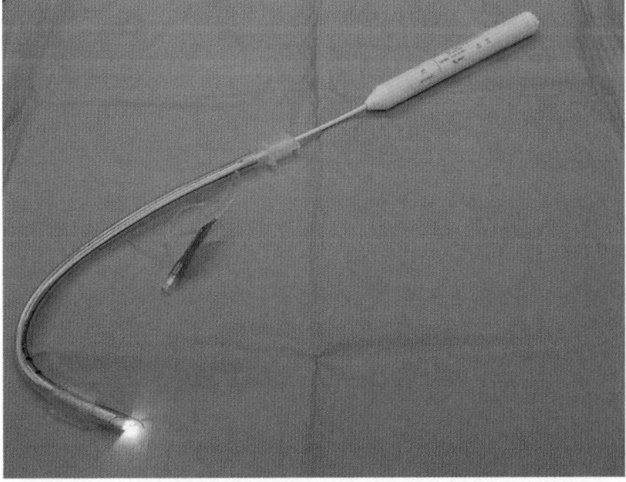

Figure 10.3. A Surch-Lite™ is prepared for use. These are available in 5, 10, and 15-in. lengths. An adjustable tube holder allows the lightwand to be properly positioned with the tracheal tube.

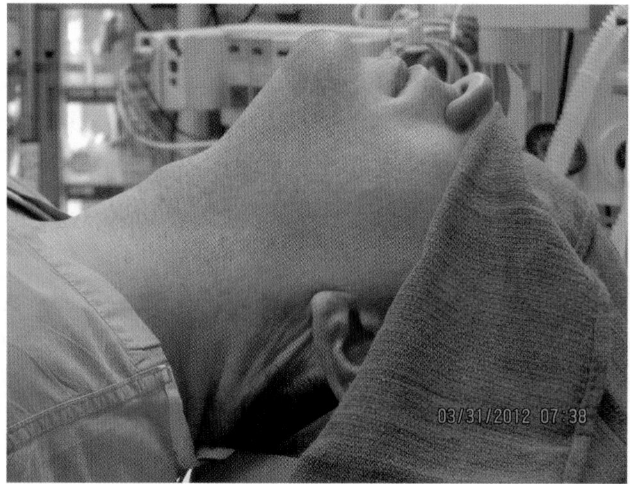

Figure 10.4. The patient is positioned with the head elevated and the neck maximally extended, providing good visibility of the neck.

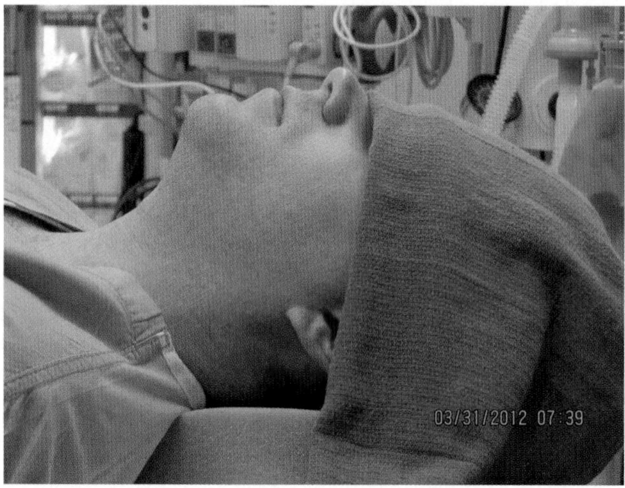

Figure 10.5. The head is elevated on a small pillow, assuming the typical "sniffing position." Some practitioners prefer a neutral position, removing the pillow.

Method

Orotracheal Intubation

Adequate preoxygenation of the patient in the supine position, with maximal head extension, is followed by induction of general anesthesia. The light bulb is switched on. For orotracheal intubation, it is imperative that the intubationist lift the lower jaw with one hand (Figure 10.6) thereby creating space in the hypopharynx and elevating the epiglottis from the posterior pharyngeal wall. Additionally, this maneuver creates an unobstructed path in the midline and facilitates passage of the TT into the upper trachea. Lightwand operation and jaw elevation can be performed with either hand[8,9]. As the lightwand within the TT bypasses the tongue and reaches the vallecula (Figure 10.7), a faint, symmetrical light glow is seen above the thyroid cartilage—suprathyroid glow[10] (Figure 10.8). If the

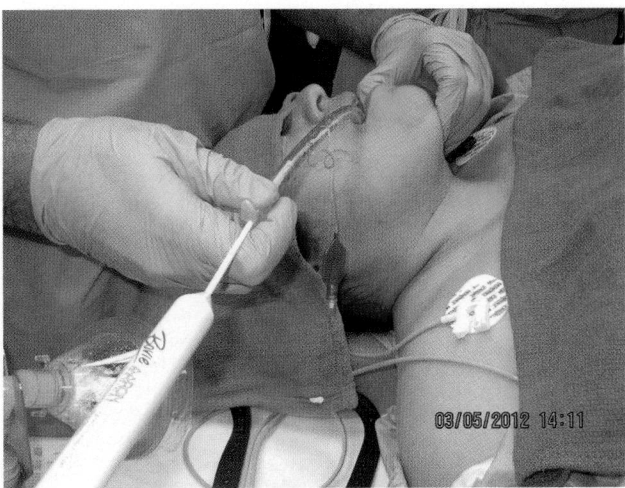

Figure 10.6. Most practitioners hold the lightwand in their dominant hand. The thumb of the other hand is introduced behind the mandibular incisors and a jaw thrust is performed. This elevates the tongue and the epiglottis, creating space to advance the lightwand.

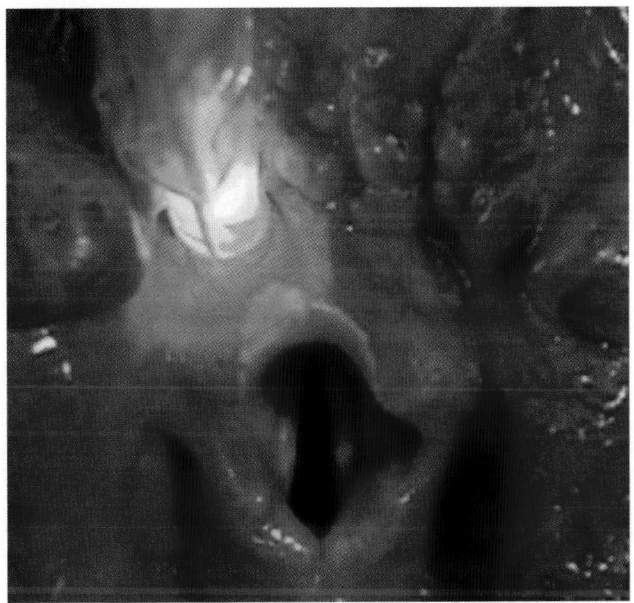

Figure 10.7. The photograph shows a lightwand inserted into the vallecula, slightly to the *left*. (From Agro F, Hung OR, Cataldo R, Carassiti M, Gherardi S. Lightwand intubation using the trachlight: a brief review of current knowledge. Can J Anaesth. 2001;48: 592–9. With kind permission from Springer Science and Business Media).

light glow appears in the lateral part of the neck (Figure 10.9), it suggests that the lightwand assembly is in the piriform fossa[11] (Figure 10.10), and the assembly should be withdrawn slightly and redirected towards the midline. When the lightwand/TT enters the trachea (Figure 10.11), a bright, well-circumscribed glow appears below the thyroid cartilage suggesting entry into the upper trachea[8] (Figure 10.12). If the lightwand/TT assembly is advanced further, the glow is seen in the suprasternal notch, approximating the appropriate depth of insertion[7] (Figure 10.13). If the lightwand/TT assembly enters the esophagus, at best a very dim, diffuse glow is visible in the anterior neck[8] (Figure 10.14). Caution is advised when performing this technique in a very thin patient as esophageal placement may go unappreciated. Confirmatory signs of tracheal placement are always essential.

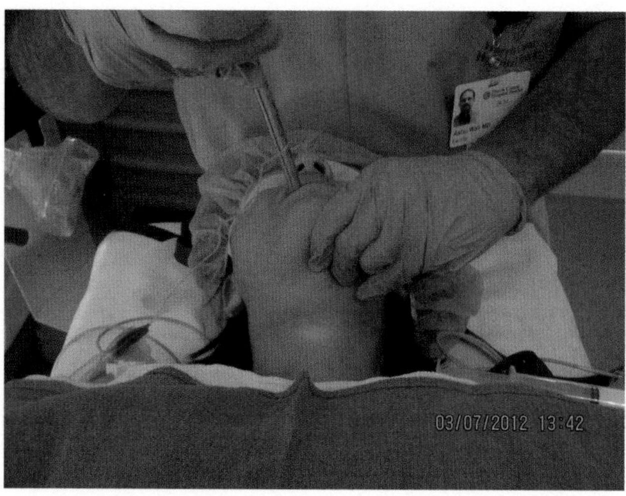

Figure 10.8. This illustrates transillumination of the central neck. The position of the light is midline and cephalad (above the thyroid prominence) indicating that it is likely in the vallecula.

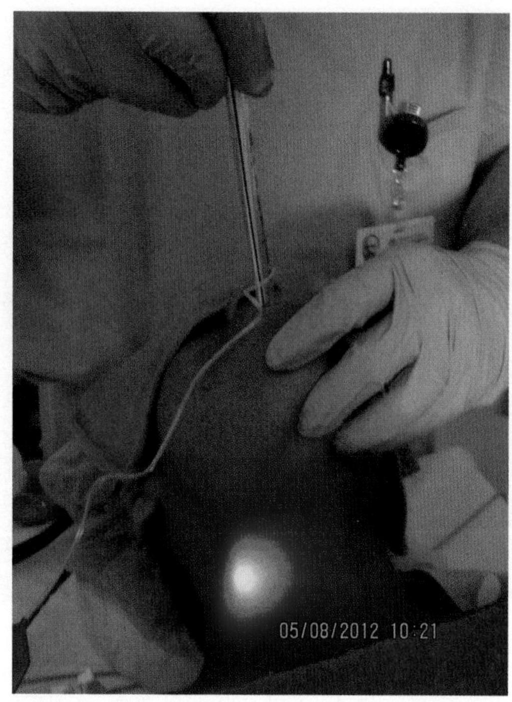

Figure 10.9. The transillumination is well circumscribed but appears slightly to the *right* of the *midline*. The depth suggests that it is either in the vallecula or the right pyriform fossa.

Nasotracheal Intubation

It is important to spray the nasal mucosa with a vasoconstricting nasal spray prior to insertion of the TT/lightwand unit. Additionally, it is important to immerse the tracheal tube in warm, sterile water for softening and to lubricate the nostril, the lightwand, and the TT with a water-soluble lubricant prior to use (Figure 10.15). The remaining steps are essentially similar to orotracheal intubation; however if a Trachlight™ is used, the wire stylet is fully withdrawn prior to use.

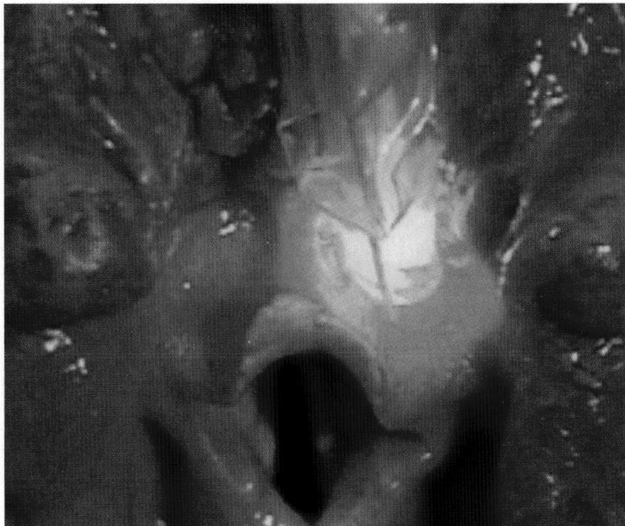

Figure 10.10. The lightwand is positioned on the right side of the vallecula, giving rise to a well-circumscribed light to the *right* of the *midline*, above the thyroid prominence. (From Agro F, Hung OR, Cataldo R, Carassiti M, Gherardi S. Lightwand intubation using the trachlight: a brief review of current knowledge. Can J Anaesth. 2001;48: 592–9. With kind permission from Springer Science and Business Media).

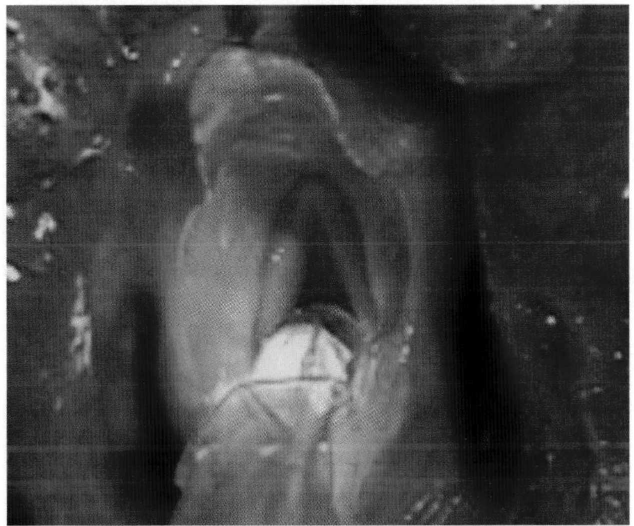

Figure 10.11. This illustrates the lightwand entering the larynx. After passing through the vocal cords, the 90° curvature will produce a bright, well-circumscribed, midline illumination below the thyroid prominence. (From Agro F, Hung OR, Cataldo R, Carassiti M, Gherardi S. Lightwand intubation using the trachlight: a brief review of current knowledge. Can J Anaesth. 2001;48: 592–9. With kind permission from Springer Science and Business Media).

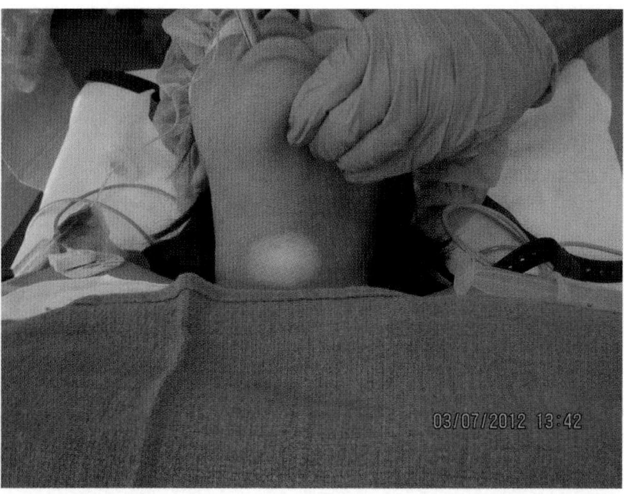

Figure 10.12. A bright *midline*, glow is seen below the thyroid prominence indicating subglottic placement.

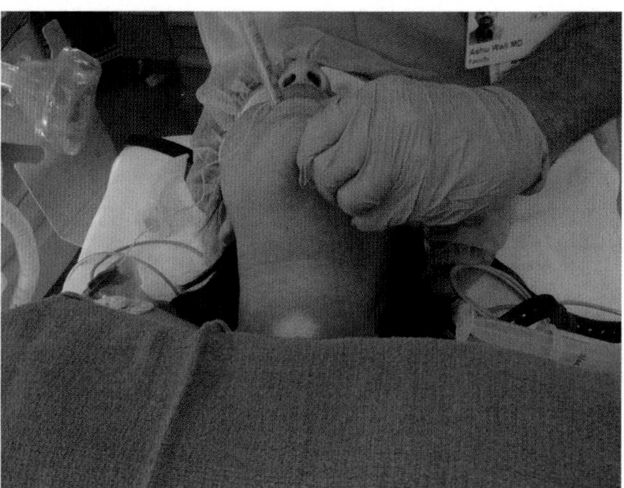

Figure 10.13. The lightwand has been advanced to the sternal notch which generally indicates the appropriate depth, though agreement on this point is not universal (see text for more details).

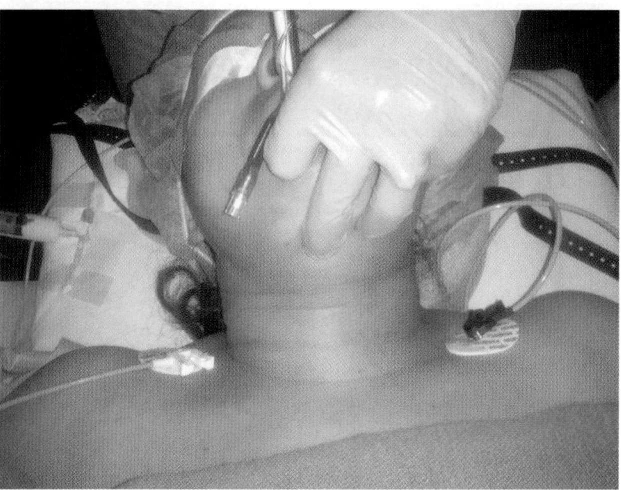

Figure 10.14. When the lightwand is introduced into the esophagus, a diffuse glow or no transillumination is apparent.

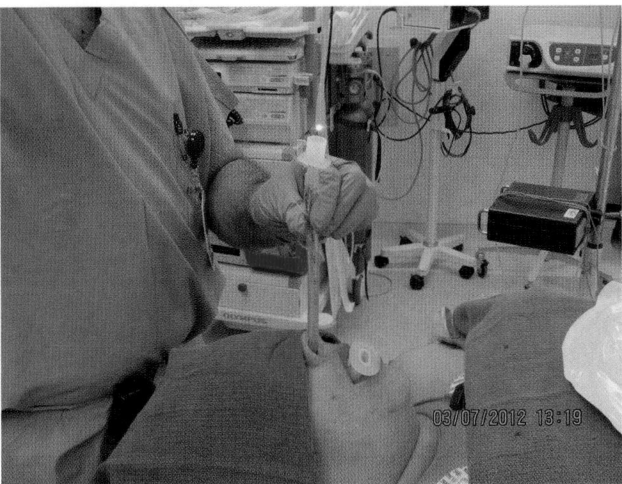

Figure 10.15. The lightwand can also be used in conjunction with nasotracheal intubation. In this circumstance, the light indicates the location of the nasotracheal tube. The nasotracheal tube, the head and neck or the larynx may then be manipulated to facilitate intubation.

Literature Review

Although intubation by transillumination had been described much earlier, Hung and colleagues demonstrated its ease and utility and rekindled interest in the technique[10,12,13]. They conducted a study comparing the use of a lightwand (Trachlight™) with direct laryngoscopy in patients with easy airways. Patients were randomly assigned to one of the two intubation methods: the lightwand was used in 479 patients and direct laryngoscopy in 471 patients. Intubation time was shorter in the lightwand group (15.7 ± 10.8 s vs. 19.6 ± 23.7 s). The incidence of trauma/failure was less in the lightwand group (10/5 vs. 37/13). Similarly, sore throat/hoarseness was less in the lightwand group (82/2 vs. 119/5)[12]. The authors emphasized that at the time of the study, they had used the lightwand device in over 6,000 patients. This level of experience undoubtedly influenced their findings.

A subsequent study looked at lightwand (Trachlight™) in patients with known or suspected difficult airways[13]. The study involved 265 patients, including 206 patients with a previous history of difficult intubation or anticipated difficult airway. Given the option of intubation awake or asleep, 202 patients chose the latter. Oral and nasal intubations were conducted on 183 and 23 patients, respectively. Mean intubation time was 25.7 ± 20.1 s. A single attempt was required in 200 patients; intubation was unsuccessful in two patients. The second cohort consisted of 59 patients in whom the lightwand was used as a rescue device after failed direct laryngoscopy. Lightwand intubation was successful in all cases, requiring 19.7 ± 13.5 s.

Fisher et al. reported on relatively inexperienced anesthesiology residents attempting intubation of 125 children, most under 10 kg using a pediatric Trachlight™. They did not specify the nature of their training or the airway characteristics of the patients. Despite their inexperience, they reported a success rate of 104/125 (83 %). Many of their failures were a consequence of inappropriately large TTs and entrapment within the vallecula, lateral (pyriform fossa) or posterior (esophageal) placement. They recommended the use of a shoulder roll, slight head extension, anterior jaw lift, and careful alignment of the airway axes[14].

Lightwand has been used as an adjunct to other airway devices such as the intubating LMA™ (Figure 10.16), where success rates went up from 76 to 95 % in 172 surgical patients[15], and time to endotracheal intubation was reduced in 100 patients from 38.3 (±10.4) to 26.4 (±9.1) s[16,17]. Addas et al. used the Trachlight™ without its metal stylet to facilitate the performance of a percutaneous tracheostomy in 11 neurosurgical patients[18].

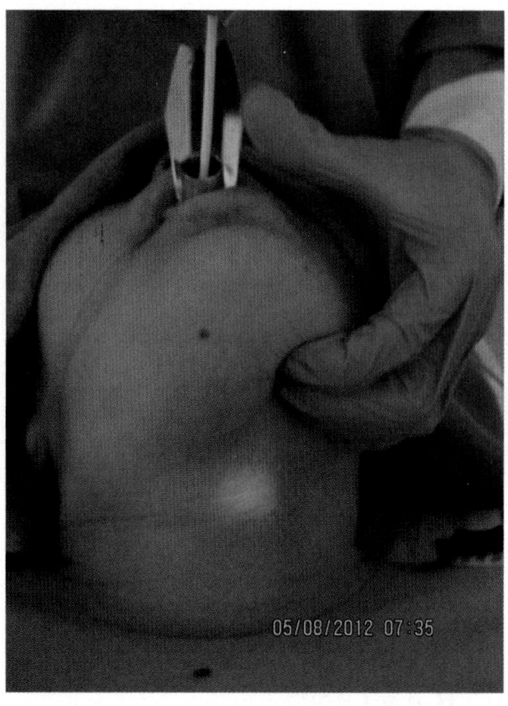

Figure 10.16. Here the lightwand is being used to "visualize" the passage of a tracheal tube through an Intubating LMA™.

Flexible lightwand-guided tracheal intubation via the intubating laryngeal mask, by experienced users, was found to be equally effective in the supine, right lateral, and left lateral position in healthy patients[19].

Hung and coworkers also demonstrated the effectiveness and safety of lightwand-guided retrograde tracheal intubation in 27 patients with cervical spine instability. An epidural catheter was introduced through a cricothyroid puncture and after retrieving it from the mouth, passed through a TT/lightwand. The procedure was accomplished either using general anesthesia or in awake patients with a time to intubation of 205 ± 78 s[20].

A study looked at cervical spine movement during lightwand-guided tracheal intubation and compared it with McCoy laryngoscope-guided tracheal intubation in 20 patients[21]. All patients underwent general anesthesia, including use of muscle relaxants prior to tracheal intubation. Lateral cervical spine X-rays were taken before and after tracheal intubation. Measurements included the distance between the occiput and the first cervical spine δ[C1-O] and the sum of the displacement between the first cervical spine against the third cervical spine and the displacement between the fifth cervical spine against the third cervical spine δ[C1 + C5]. Their results showed that δ[C1-O] was larger and δ[C1 + C5] was smaller. They concluded that lightwand-guided tracheal intubation caused less cervical spine movement than McCoy laryngoscopy and that the lightwand use was easier and safer in patients in whom cervical spine movement is limited or undesirable.

The issue of an optimum technique for safely achieving tracheal intubation in patients with cervical spine injury was also examined in a study of 36 healthy patients participating in a crossover trial. Fluoroscopic cervical spine motion during tracheal intubation with manual in-line stabilization was compared between direct laryngoscopy using a Macintosh 3 blade, GlideScope™ video laryngoscope and a Trachlight™ lightwand. Cervical spine motion was examined at four mobile segments of the cervical spine (Occiput-C1 junction, C1-2 junction, C2-5 segment, and C5-thoracic segment) during bag-mask ventilation, laryngoscopy, and tracheal intubation. The time to tracheal intubation was also noted. Cervical spine motion during bag-mask ventilation was 82 % less at the four motion segments compared to Macintosh laryngoscopy ($p < 0.001$). Cervical spine motion using the lightwand was less than Macintosh laryngoscopy, averaging 57 % less at the four motion segments ($p < 0.03$) with the same time to tracheal intubation. Compared with Macintosh laryngoscopy, cervical spine motion was 50 % less at the C2-5 segment with the GlideScope™ ($p < 0.04$) but there was no significant difference at the other levels. The time to tracheal intubation was 62 % longer with the GlideScope™ compared to direct laryngoscopy with the Macintosh blade ($p < 0.01$). The authors concluded that lightwand-guided tracheal intubation is associated with reduced cervical spine movement compared with the Macintosh laryngoscope[22].

Several studies have compared the hemodynamic changes during lightwand-guided tracheal intubation and direct Macintosh laryngoscopic tracheal intubation. A study of 40 patients, randomized equally between the two groups, found no difference in changes in mean arterial pressure and heart rate between the two groups[23]. Another study of 40 patients concluded that the lightwand significantly attenuated the hemodynamic response to tracheal intubation (compared to direct laryngoscopy) in normotensive patients, but not in hypertensive patients[24] and a third study of 88 patients, over the age of 60 years, concluded that the lightwand significantly attenuated the hemodynamic changes to tracheal intubation (compared to fiberoptic bronchoscopy) in normotensive patients, but not in hypertensive patients[25]. Finally, among patients with coronary artery disease, undergoing elective coronary artery bypass grafting, lightwand-guided intubation did not significantly modify the hemodynamic responses to tracheal intubation as compared with direct laryngoscopy[26].

Casati and colleagues compared the effects of direct laryngoscopy and lightwand-guided tracheal intubation in 50 patients. They found no differences in the changes in intraocular pressure, mean arterial pressure, and heart rate with laryngoscopy or tracheal intubation[27].

A study from Japan used the Trachlight™ in a very different manner, allowing it to protrude various distance beyond the tip of the TT. In their hands, extrusion of 1–2 cm beyond the tracheal tube tip, at an angle bend of 40–60° (rather than 90° recommended by the manufacturer and most other investigators) was optimal. Difficult tracheal intubation was defined as two or more attempts required to achieve tracheal intubation. Patients in the "obese" cohort (mean body weight 73 ± 9 kg) were more likely to be difficult. Unfortunately, the authors did not indicate the experience level of the operators[28]. The authors had previously demonstrated the thermal safety of a protruding lightwand in cats[29] but it cannot be assumed that a device stiffened with a metal stylet will behave like a flexible bougie.

A study on 60 female patients, undergoing abdominal hysterectomy, showed that application of cricoid pressure significantly prolonged the time to tracheal intubation using the Surch-Lite™ (48.5 vs. 28 s) and the number of patients requiring more than one attempt (4 vs. 0). There was one failure and that occurred in the cricoid pressure group[30].

Another study compared the lightwand with direct laryngoscopy during awake, tracheal intubation for emergency surgery in 60 ASA-I patients. Time to tracheal intubation was shorter, the number of intubation attempts fewer, the incidence of sore throat was less, and changes in mean arterial pressure were less in the lightwand group[31].

Favaro and coworkers modified the Trachlight technique for nasotracheal intubations by leaving the metal stylet in place, but creating a 90° bend at a point equal to the distance from the mental symphysis to the angle of the mandible. They attempted nasotracheal intubation on 123 patients, 76 of whom had no features predictive of difficulty and 47 with limited mouth opening. The latter group was sedated but spontaneous ventilation was maintained. Success rates were similar in both groups (98.4 vs. 92.6 %), with most patients being intubated on the first attempt[32].

An interesting paper looked at varying the location of the 90° bend of the lightwand tip, in accordance with the thyro-*mandibular* (TMD) length. Patients with shorter TMD lengths benefitted from shorter distal lengths of the Trachlight (6.5 vs. 8.5 cm) resulting in reduced "search times" and a higher success rate. In patients with TMD greater than

5.5 cm, no statistical differences were found. Of interest, this study was conducted in Taiwan where TMDs may be shorter than among occidentals[33].

The effectiveness and safety of lightwand-guided tracheal intubation, by novice users, was studied in 150 ASA I or II patients undergoing elective surgery. The overall intubation success rate was 92 % (87.68 % after first attempt). Minor trauma, such as mucosal bleeding or laceration, was noted in 5.33 % of the patients. The authors concluded that lightwand-guided tracheal intubation was effective and safe even in inexperienced hands[34].

Some patients need tracheal intubation in the lateral decubitus position. This issue was studied in 120 patients, randomly allocated to the supine, right lateral, or left lateral position. Time to tracheal intubation was similar between groups with a comparable incidence of successful first attempt tracheal intubation, hoarseness, sore throat, mucosal injury, and dysrhythmias. However, there was a trend toward more esophageal intubations among those intubated in the lateral position. The authors concluded that lightwand-guided tracheal intubation can be performed easily using a technique similar to the supine position[35].

Indications

The above studies suggest the following clinical indications for the lightwand: patients with restricted cervical spine movement or in whom limited cervical movement is desirable, limited mouth opening, poor dentition, expensive dental work, coronary artery disease/hypertension where tachycardia and hypertension may be detrimental, and facial trauma. Needless to say, prior proficiency with the technique is required to realize the potential benefits.

Problems

Some reported complications include light bulb disconnection[36], thermal injury from prolonged use, and subluxation of the arytenoid cartilage. Some limitations include the need (with some devices) to reduce the ambient light in the room, inadequate transillumination of the neck in the obese individual, an uncooperative awake patient, patients with an upper airway mass, and patients where cricoid pressure may be required during rapid sequence induction of anesthesia. It is important to bear in mind that both success and complication rates will vary with devices and operator experience.

Conclusion

The lightwand is a part of the American Society of Anesthesiologists Difficult Airway Algorithm (ASA-DAA)[11], published in 2003, as a means to provide an alternative to tracheal intubation in the nonemergency pathway. Over the last 50 years, it has been used successfully in patients with easy and known difficult airways, in the unanticipated difficult airway, in awake and anesthetized patients, and by the oral or nasal route. It has been used as an adjunct to intubation through a supraglottic airway, retrograde intubation, and percutaneous tracheotomy. While interest in this technique has waned with the availability of indirect methods of viewing the larynx such as fiberoptic and video stylets and laryngoscopes, there are many who regret the retreat of these low-cost, low-tech devices for reasons that may reflect an insufficient revenue stream for their manufacturers.

References

1. Macintosh R, Richards H. Illuminated introducer for endotracheal tubes. Anaesthesia. 1957;12(2):223–5.
2. Evans T. Device for Blind Nasal Intubation. 1959;20(2):221.
3. Berman RA. Lighted stylet. Anesthesiology. 1959;20(3):382–3.
4. Stewart RD, LaRosee A, Kaplan RM, Ilkhanipour K. Correct positioning of an endotracheal tube using a flexible lighted stylet. Crit Care Med. 1990;18(1):97–9.
5. Olson KW, Culling DC. An alternative use for a nasotracheal tube. Can J Anaesth. 1989;36(2):252–3.
6. Hung OR, Stewart RD. Intubating stylets. In: Hagberg CA, editor. Benumof's airway management principles and practice. Philadelphia, PA: Mosby Elsevier; 2007. p. 463.
7. Locker GJ, Staudinger T, Knapp S, Burgmann H, Laczika KF, Zimmerl M, et al. Assessment of the proper depth of endotracheal tube placement with the trachlight. J Clin Anesth. 1998;10(5):389–93.
8. Hung OR, Stewart RD. Illuminating stylet (lightwand). In: Benumof JL, editor. Airway management principles and practice. St. Louis, Missouri: Mosby-Year Books, Inc.; 1996. p. 342.
9. Kuo YW, Yen MK, Cheng KI, Tang CS, Chau SW, Hou MF, et al. Lightwand-guided endotracheal intubation performed by the nondominant hand is feasible. Kaohsiung J Med Sci. 2007;23(10):504–10.
10. Hung OR, Stewart RD. Lightwand intubation: I–a new lightwand device. Can JAnaesth. 1995;42(9):820–5.
11. Practice guidelines for management of the difficult airway: an updated report by the American Society of Anesthesiologists Task Force on Management of the Difficult Airway. Anesthesiology. 2003;98(5):1269–77.
12. Hung OR, Pytka S, Morris I, Murphy M, Launcelott G, Stevens S, et al. Clinical trial of a new lightwand device (trachlight) to intubate the trachea. Anesthesiology. 1995;83(3):509–14.
13. Hung OR, Pytka S, Morris I, Murphy M, Stewart RD. Lightwand intubation: II–clinical trial of a new lightwand for tracheal intubation in patients with difficult airways. Can J Anaesth. 1995;42(9):826–30.
14. Fisher QA, Tunkel DE. Lightwand intubation of infants and children. J Clin Anesth. 1997;9(4):275–9.
15. Fan KH, Hung OR, Agro F. A comparative study of tracheal intubation using an intubating laryngeal mask (fastrach) alone or together with a lightwand (trachlight). J Clin Anesth. 2000;12(8):581–5.
16. Chan PL, Lee TW, Lam KK, Chan WS. Intubation through intubating laryngeal mask with and without a lightwand: a randomized comparison. Anaesth Intensive Care. 2001;29(3):255–9.
17. Dimitriou V, Voyagis GS, Brimacombe J. Flexible lightwand-guided intubation through the ILM. Acta Anaesthesiol Scand. 2001;45(2):263–4.
18. Addas BM, Howes WJ, Hung OR. Light-guided tracheal puncture for percutaneous tracheostomy. Can J Anaesth. 2000;47(9):919–22.
19. Dimitriou V, Voyagis GS, Iatrou C, Brimacombe J. Flexible lightwand-guided intubation using the intubating laryngeal mask airway in the supine, right, and left lateral positions in healthy patients by experienced users. Anesth Analg. 2003;96(3):896–8.
20. Hung OR, al-Qatari M. Light-guided retrograde intubation. Can J Anaesth. 1997;44(8):877–82.
21. Konishi A, Kikuchi K, Sasui M. Cervival spine movement during light-guided orotracheal intubation with lightwand stylet (trachlight). Masui. 1998;47(1):94–7.
22. Turkstra TP, Craen RA, Pelz DM, Gelb AW. Cervical spine motion: a fluoroscopic comparison during intubation with lighted stylet, GlideScope, and Macintosh laryngoscope. Anesth Analg. 2005;101(3):910–5.
23. Hirabayashi Y, Hiruta M, Kawakami T, Inoue S, Fukuda H, Saitoh K, et al. Effects of lightwand (Trachlight) compared with direct laryngoscopy on circulatory responses to tracheal intubation. Br J Anaesth. 1998;81(2):253–5. Epub 1998/11/14.
24. Nishikawa K, Omote K, Kawana S, Namiki A. A comparison of hemodynamic changes after endotracheal intubation by using the lightwand device and the laryngoscope in normotensive and hypertensive patients. Anesth Analg. 2000;90(5):1203–7.

25. Nishikawa K, Kawamata M, Namiki A. Lightwand intubation is associated with less hemodynamic changes than fibreoptic intubation in normotensive, but not in hypertensive patients over the age of 60. Can J Anaesth. 2001;48(11):1148–54.
26. Montes FR, Giraldo JC, Betancur LA, Rincon JD, Rincon IE, Vanegas MV, et al. Endotracheal intubation with a lightwand or a laryngoscope results in similar hemodynamic variations in patients with coronary artery disease. Can J Anaesth. 2003;50(8):824–8.
27. Casati A, Aldegheri G, Fanelli G, Gioia L, Colnaghi E, Magistris L, et al. Lightwand intubation does not reduce the increase in intraocular pressure associated with tracheal intubation. J Clin Anesth. 1999;11(3):216–9.
28. Nishiyama T, Matsukawa T, Hanaoka K. Optimal length and angle of a new lightwand device (trachlight). J Clin Anesth. 1999;11(4):332–5.
29. Nishiyama T, Matsukawa T, Hanaoka K. Safety of a new lightwand device (trachlight): temperature and histopathological study. Anesth Analg. 1998;87(3):717–8.
30. Hodgson RE, Gopalan PD, Burrows RC, Zuma K. Effect of cricoid pressure on the success of endotracheal intubation with a lightwand. Anesthesiology. 2001;94(2):259–62.
31. Nishikawa K, Kawana S, Namiki A. Comparison of the lightwand technique with direct laryngoscopy for awake endotracheal intubation in emergency cases. J Clin Anesth. 2001;13(4): 259–63.
32. Favaro R, Tordiglione P, Di Lascio F, Colagiovanni D, Esposito G, Quaranta S, et al. Effective nasotracheal intubation using a modified transillumination technique. Can J Anaesth. 2002;49(1):91–5.
33. Chen TH, Tsai SK, Lin CJ, Lu CW, Tsai TP, Sun WZ. Does the suggested lightwand bent length fit every patient? The relation between bent length and patient's thyroid prominence-to-mandibular angle distance. Anesthesiology. 2003;98(5):1070–6.
34. Amornyotin S, Sanansilp V, Amorntien V, Tirawat P. Effectiveness of lightwand (trachlight) intubation by 1st year anesthesia residents. J Med Assoc Thai. 2002;85 Suppl 3:S963–8. Journal Article.
35. Cheng KI, Chu KS, Chau SW, Ying SL, Hsu HT, Chang YL, et al. Lightwand-assisted intubation of patients in the lateral decubitus position. Anesth Analg. 2004;99(1):279–83.
36. Stone DJ, Stirt JA, Kaplan MJ, McLean WC. A complication of lightwand-guided nasotracheal intubation. Anesthesiology. 1984;61(6):780–1.

11 Role of Retrograde Intubation

Martin Dauber

Introduction

When the view into the upper airway is obscured by tumor, blood, or other visual obstructions of the upper airway, it can be helpful to introduce a guide from below the glottis directed cephalad to the mouth or nose, and use this to direct an endotracheal tube (ETT) into the trachea. Although the ETT is passed through the glottis in an antegrade direction, this technique is referred to as retrograde intubation. Retrograde intubation of the trachea was first described in 1960 by Butler and Cirillo[1]. The technique involves introduction of a wire through the cricothyroid membrane or the membranous space between the cricoid cartilage and the first tracheal ring into the airway. The wire is then directed cephalad and is used to help guide an ETT into the trachea. Although infrequently used, retrograde intubation can be an extremely useful tool in the anesthesiologist's armamentarium for managing difficult airways, and it has been used successfully in many clinical situations. Common indications for the procedure include failure of other airway techniques, anatomical abnormalities, and the presence of blood or secretions in the proximal airway that obscure the glottic structures. Specialized kits are available that include all the necessary equipment for retrograde intubations (e.g., the Cook Retrograde

M. Dauber (✉)
Department of Anesthesia & Critical Care, The University of Chicago,
Chicago, IL 60637, USA
e-mail: mdauber@dacc.uchicago.edu

D.B. Glick et al. (eds.), *The Difficult Airway: An Atlas of Tools and Techniques for Clinical Management*,
DOI 10.1007/978-0-387-92849-4_11, © Springer Science+Business Media New York 2013

Intubation Set, Cook Incorporated, Bloomington, IN), but the necessary supplies—consisting of a long guide wire approximately .038″ caliber, a needle or large-bore intravenous catheter able to accommodate the guide wire, a hemostat, and a tube exchange catheter—are usually available without one of these kits.

Historical Development

The retrograde intubation technique was first described in a patient with a large carcinoma of the extrinsic larynx who presented for resection. Prior experience had demonstrated that difficulties encountered during laryngoscopy of patients with bulky laryngeal tumors resulted in pre-laryngectomy tracheostomies in 40% of cases. As laryngectomies became more commonly performed in the late 1950s retrograde tracheal intubation was often used as the preferred method to intubate these patients, as it enjoyed a high success rate and relatively few complications. The initial technique described was an "open" one, as the wire was passed through a tracheostomy or a surgical incision in the neck. An orotracheal tube was then passed along the wire into the trachea and used for the duration of the laryngectomy[2].

Subsequent modifications of the technique eliminated the neck incision, instead a large-bore needle was inserted through the cricothyroid membrane and an epidural catheter (and later, a guide wire) was passed through the needle. The catheter was then directed cephalad through the larynx and the tip of the catheter was recovered from the mouth. The catheter or wire was then used to guide an ETT into the trachea. Bourke and Levesque noted a problem when passing the ETT toward the trachea. When the wire was released from its insertion site in the neck, to allow the tip of the ETT to pass into the trachea, the tip of the guide wire could flip out of the larynx resulting in the ETT being introduced into the esophagus. To avoid this problem they proposed a modified approach whereby the catheter guide was passed through the side hole (i.e., Murphy's eye) instead of through the tip of the ETT and then passed up through the ETT (Figure 11.1). This way, when the ETT was run down the catheter the beveled distal end of the ETT would be 2 cm caudad to the catheter insertion site at the cricothyroid membrane (Figure 11.2). This made it less likely that the ETT would flip into the esophagus when the catheter was released[3]. Another way to keep the ETT from flipping into the esophagus when the guide is removed is to enter the airway with the needle lower in the neck (e.g., between the cricoid ring and the first tracheal ring or between the first and second tracheal rings) instead of through the cricothyroid cartilage (Figure 11.3).

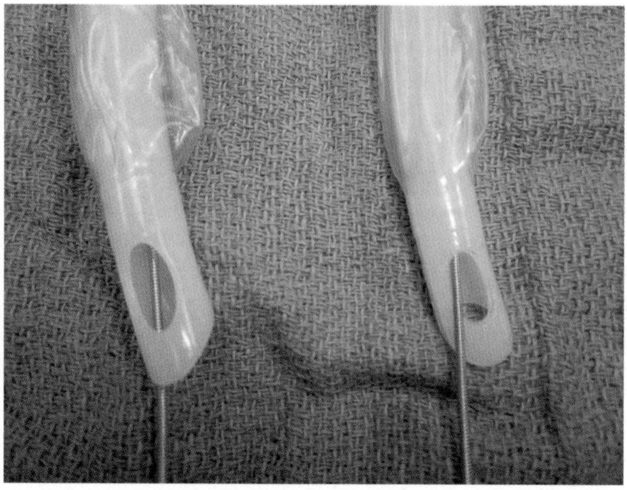

Figure 11.1. Wire threaded via lumen (*left*) and via Murphy's eye (*right*).

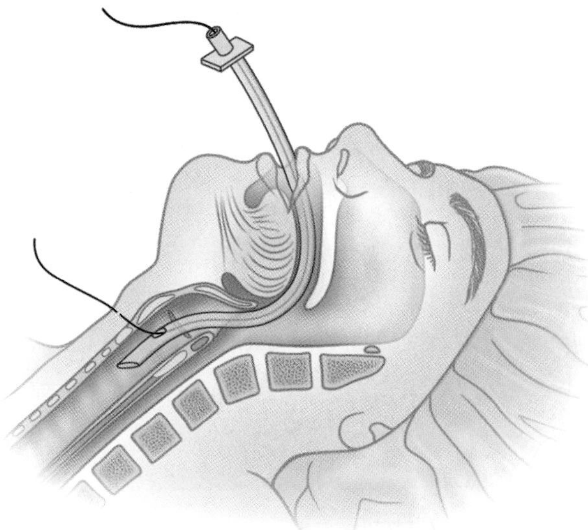

Figure 11.2. Endotracheal tube in place. Note the tip placement 2 cm. inferior to cricothyroid membrane.

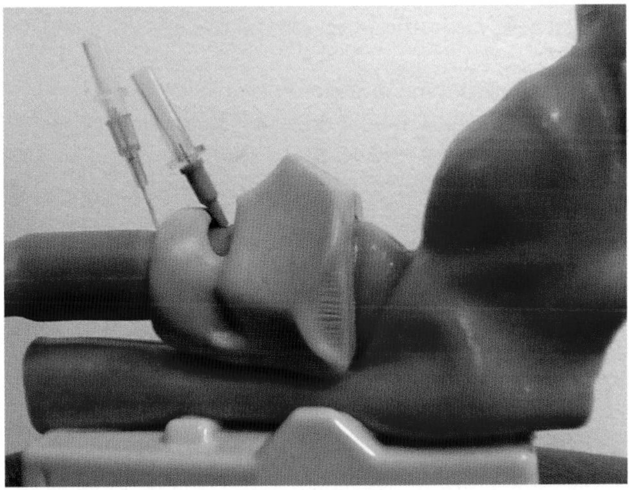

Figure 11.3. *Blue* needle via cricothyroid membrane. *Pink* needle via space between coid cartilage and first tracheal ring.

Techniques

Retrograde intubation involves placing an ETT over a guiding catheter or wire that has been directed into the mouth or nose from its initial placement into the airway at the level of the cricoid cartilage. It is often a final or rescue maneuver in a difficult airway experience or algorithm[4]. Depending upon the particular circumstances, and the preparation time available, one may use a variety of procedures and equipment. *Elective* retrograde intubation, employed either as a teaching/learning experience or as a planned approach for a known difficult airway, can be performed under ideal conditions with all necessary and supplemental equipment readily available. It can be performed using local anesthesia with or without sedation, or under general anesthesia with or without spontaneous ventilation, depending upon the patient, operator, and situation.

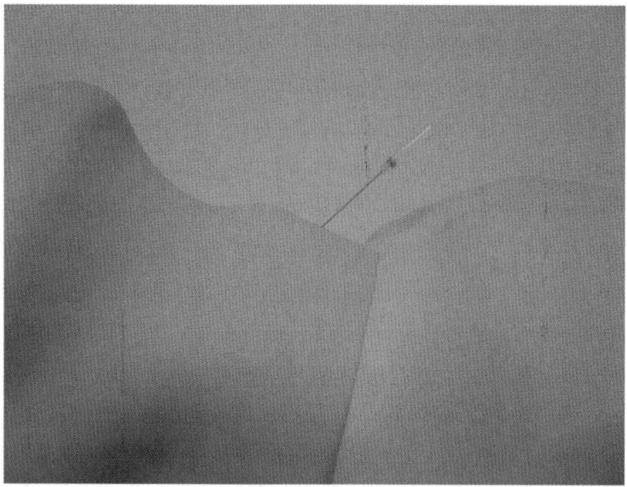

Figure 11.4. Needle angled at 30° to horizontal to facilitate cephalad course of wire.

Alternatively, in an emergency, it may be necessary to expediently use equipment at hand.

For an elective retrograde intubation, the following equipment is recommended:

1. Emergency/resuscitative medications, an oxygen source, and equipment for bag-mask ventilation
2. Iodine, alcohol, or chlorhexidine skin preparation solution
3. Local anesthetic (such as 1 or 2% lidocaine) in a 3-cc syringe, 25-ga needle
4. Midsize syringe (10–12 cc) half-filled with 0.9% NS
5. 16 ga or 18 ga thin-walled intravenous catheter or needle
6. Fifty centimeter (or longer) wire of approximately 0.035″ caliber—ensure that the wire passes easily through the needle or intravenous catheter before puncturing the cricothyroid membrane
7. Hemostat
8. Airway exchange catheter (e.g., Aintree)
9. Optional: flexible bronchoscope with a suction channel through which the wire will easily pass. If a bronchoscope is to be used, a longer wire (usually 110 cm) will be necessary

As noted previously, Cook Critical (Bloomington, IN) sells both adult and pediatric-sized kits that contain all the necessary items. Familiarity with the contents, prior to opening the trays, is advised.

The procedure is best performed by one individual while a second monitors the patient and maintains oxygenation, ventilation, and sedation levels as appropriate. A shoulder roll should be placed transversely to provide neck extension and facilitate identification of and access to the cricothyroid membrane. If the cricothyroid membrane is not accessible, then the membranous spaces above the first or second tracheal rings may be used instead. The overlying skin is prepped in a sterile fashion. Unless the patient is under general anesthesia, local anesthetic is then injected over the membrane with a 25-ga needle.

Puncture of the cricothyroid membrane perpendicular to the skin is performed with a 16-ga or 18-ga intravenous catheter or needle connected to a 10 to 12-cc syringe, half-filled with saline. Unequivocal aspiration of air and bubbling confirms entry into the airway. The tip of the needle should then be angled approximately 15–30° cephalad to facilitate passage of the wire toward the glottis (Figure 11.4). The wire should pass easily through the needle. If it does not thread easily, it is likely that the needle is not in the airway, and it should be replaced. After the wire is in the airway, the needle or intravenous catheter is removed, and a hemostat is tightly applied to the end of the wire protruding

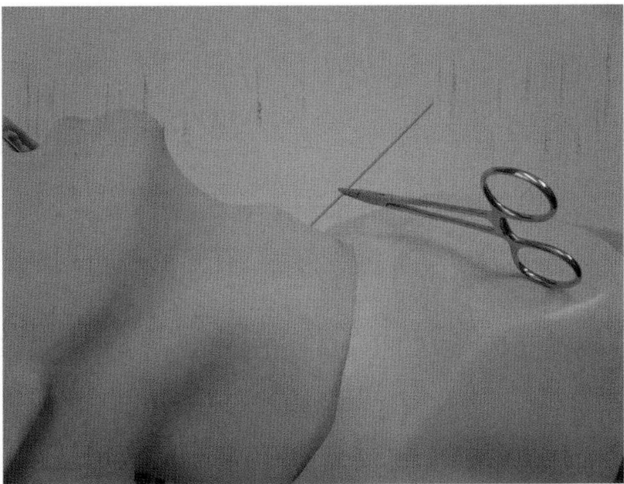

Figure 11.5. Hemostat applied to neck end of wire to prevent loss of wire.

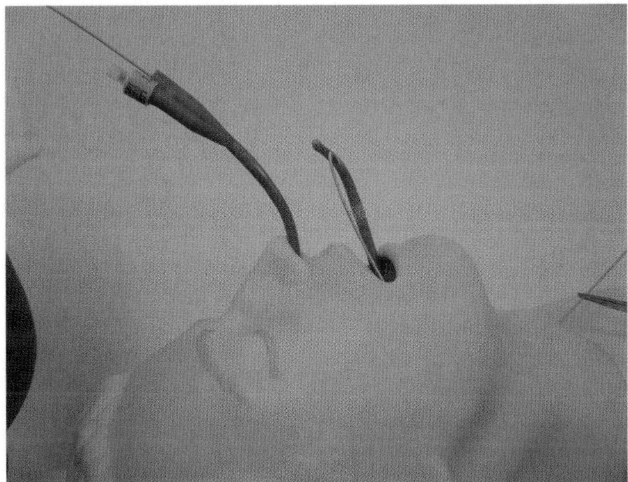

Figure 11.6. *Red* rubber catheter inserted via nose through mouth to allow easy passage of the wire into the nare for nasal intubation.

from the neck (Figure 11.5). This prevents the end of the wire from being pulled into the trachea even when traction is applied.

Once the wire is in place several alternative maneuvers can be performed. Most often, the wire finds its way out of the mouth as it is directed cephalad from the insertion site. If the wire comes out through the nose, and orotracheal intubation is desired, a finger sweep of the oropharynx or Magill forceps can be used to retrieve the wire from the mouth. If a nasal intubation is desired and the wire exits the mouth, a red rubber catheter can be passed through one of the nares into the mouth and the wire can be passed up through the red rubber catheter and out the nostril (Figure 11.6).

Once the wire is appropriately placed, an ETT can be threaded over the wire by one of three methods, each with its advocates (Figure 11.7):

1. Pass the wire though the lumen of the tube[5]
2. Pass the wire through the lumen, and out the Murphy's eye (this author's preference)
3. Pass the wire through the Murphy's eye into the lumen of the tube[4]

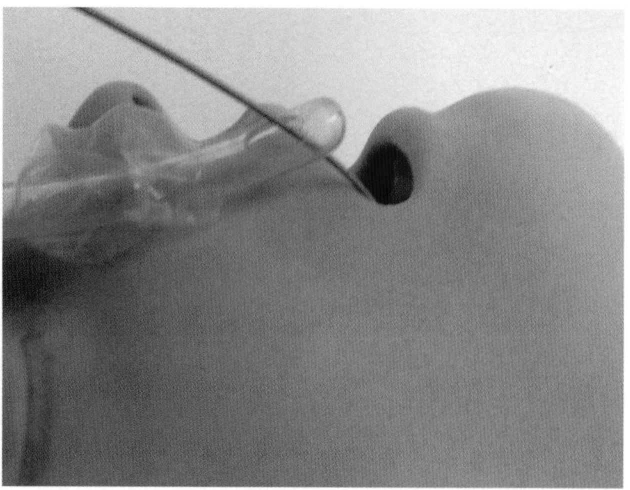

Figure 11.7. Wire passed through lumen and out Murphy's eye.

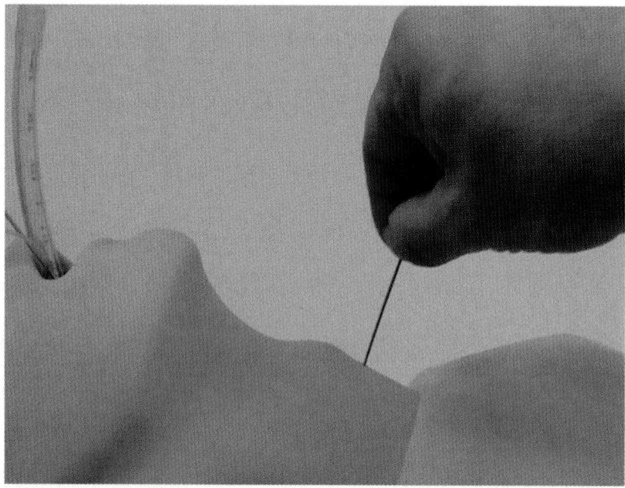

Figure 11.8. Wire being gently pulled and withdrawn.

Tension should be applied to the wire from above as the tube is gently advanced towards the trachea. When the tip of the ETT reaches the wire insertion point in the trachea and hemostat that is securing the neck end of the wire gets snug, gentle pressure is exerted on the ETT as it enters the trachea. The wire is then withdrawn through the neck (Figure 11.8). Confirmation of correct endotracheal placement should then be carried out as usual.

Several variations on the above technique have been described. After the wire exits the mouth or nose, an airway exchange catheter (e.g., Aintree) can be threaded over the wire. The exchange catheter is advanced in a manner similar to the above-described method for the ETT. Once the tip of the tube exchange catheter has reached the level of the wire insertion site in the neck, the wire can be withdrawn and an ETT is passed into the trachea over the exchange catheter. The ETT is then advanced and confirmed to be correctly placed[6]. In another variation, an ETT is loaded over a fiberoptic bronchoscope. The wire, that is exiting the mouth or nose, is inserted through the suction lumen of the distal end of the scope (Figure 11.9) with the suction port adapter on the bronchoscope body removed to allow the exit of the wire. The bronchoscope is then run down along the wire to the level of the wire insertion. The wire is then pulled out either through the neck or through the suction port on the handle of the bronchoscope. The view from the tip of

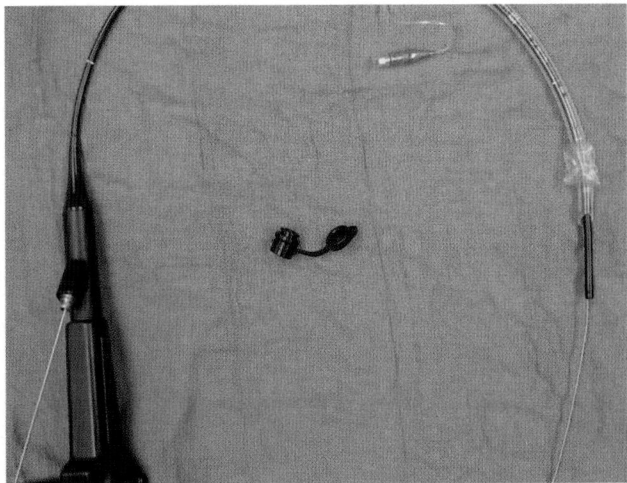

Figure 11.9. Wire placed in suction lumen of fiberoptic bronchoscope with an endotracheal tube loaded on the scope's insertion tube.

the scope should be looking directly into the trachea, so the bronchoscope can be advanced to the mid-trachea under visual control. Finally, the ETT is passed over the bronchoscope into the trachea (just as is done with a standard bronchoscopic intubation)[7]. It is important to verify that the wire is small enough to pass through the suction channel before placing the wire through the needle in the neck if a bronchoscope is to be used.

Contraindications to Retrograde Intubation

There are circumstances when retrograde intubation is relatively contraindicated. If it is not possible to identify the cricothyroid membrane or membranous spaces above the first or second tracheal rings then it may not be possible to safely introduce the needle into the trachea. The inability to identify the membranous spaces can result from the presence of a thyroid goiter (or other pretracheal mass), from morbid obesity, or from severe cervical flexion. An abscess overlying the cervical puncture site would also be a contraindication to retrograde intubation. Coagulopathy is a relative contraindication to the cervical puncture. The risk of bleeding is greater if the needle is inserted below the level of the cricoid ring. While more caudal entrance to the airway presents a higher risk of bleeding, particularly in the coagulopathic patient, more cephalad entry poses a greater risk of laryngeal injury.

Applications for this Technique

The literature is replete with case reports, proposed uses and indications, and comparisons of retrograde intubation techniques. Also, as this is an uncommonly performed procedure, the benefits and practicality of several training models have been studied. The American Society of Anesthesiologists has published its practice guidelines for management of the difficult airway, and these include recommendations for using retrograde intubation. In addition to proposing retrograde intubation for management of the difficult airway, the guidelines also recommend retrograde equipment be part of the contents of the difficult

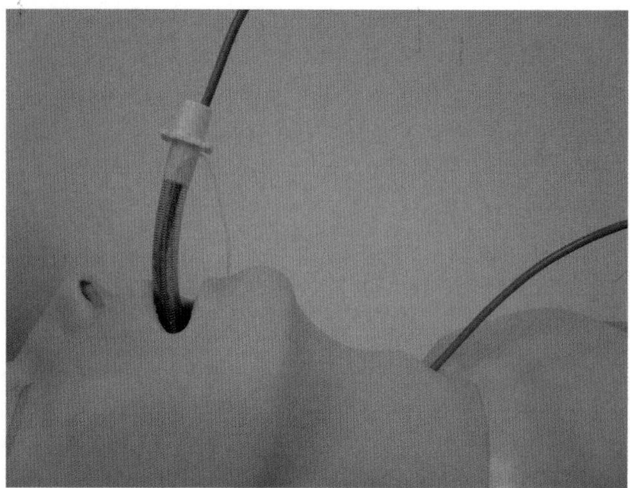

Figure 11.10. Exchange catheter used in place of bougie to facilitate threading of endotracheal tube.

airway cart[8]. A Canadian national survey demonstrated greater comfort and use of this technique among older anesthesiologists, though overall the usage rate was still very low[9].

One advantage of the retrograde technique is that unlike most intubation techniques it can be accomplished without requiring visible airway landmarks. Like the unguided intubating LMA technique, intubation can be performed "blindly" when the retrograde wire is in place to guide the ETT into the trachea. One case demonstrating this advantage of retrograde intubation detailed multiple failed attempts at rigid and flexible laryngoscopy in a patient with severe rheumatoid arthritis, constrictive pericarditis, and copious oropharyngeal bleeding in whom retrograde intubation was successfully accomplished[10]. The ability to use retrograde intubation when other more expensive techniques/devices are unavailable was demonstrated in a neurologically intact patient who had sustained a traumatic fracture of the C2 transverse process and presented in a halo traction device. A flexible bronchoscope was unavailable, and retrograde nasotracheal intubation was successfully performed[11]. A variation of retrograde intubation involving the retrograde passage of a gum elastic bougie through a failed cricothyroidotomy incision into the oropharynx has also been described. Once the bougie was in place an ETT was threaded over it into the trachea[12] (Figure 11.10). This approach is similar to the originally described method that used an open surgical insertion and an epidural catheter as a guide[1].

As retrograde intubation techniques are rarely used, teaching trainees how to perform retrograde intubations can pose challenges. Recently several articles recommending different educational pathways for the technique have appeared. Some have proposed using fresh cadavers to teach the infraglottic procedures, showing that the passage of a tube exchange catheter through the ETT prior to advancement into the trachea leads to higher rates of success[13]. A group of residents was instructed on the technique on preserved cadavers using the Cook® retrograde kit. After a single demonstration of the process there was a significant increase in the number of residents who believed they could perform the procedure correctly[14]. Although airway training manikins can be used to teach retrograde intubation skills, they are expensive and wear out quickly when used for invasive procedures[15]. This author's preference for teaching colleagues and residents has been to use patients coming for laryngectomy who are candidates for fiberoptic intubation. After transcricothyroid instillation of local anesthetic, rather than removing the intravenous catheter, a wire is placed as per the above technique. The trainee can then attempt retrograde intubation with or without flexible bronchoscopic guidance. One advantage of this educational technique is that the risk of damage to the larynx is mitigated by the fact that the larynx is surgically removed before the end of the case.

Conclusion

Retrograde intubation of the trachea is one more technique that has its place in the airway management armamentarium. Those already skilled with airway procedures can learn and employ the technique as part of a rescue sequence for the difficult intubation. With commonly available equipment or specialized commercially available kits, it can be smoothly and safely applied to a wide range of clinical situations to facilitate endotracheal intubation.

References

1. Butler FS, Cirillo AA. Retrograde tracheal intubation. Anesth Analg. 1960;39:333–8.
2. Powell WF, Ozdill T. A translaryngeal guide for tracheal intubation. Anesth Analg. 1967;6:231–4.
3. Bourke D, Levesque PR. Modification of retrograde guide for endotracheal intubation. Anesth Analg. 1974;53:1013–4.
4. Shantha TR. Retrograde intubation using the subcricoid region. Br J Anaesth. 1992;68:109.
5. Dhara SS. Retrograde intubation: a facilitated approach. Br J Anaesth. 1992;69:631.
6. Parmet JL, Metz S. Retrograde endotracheal intubation: an underutilized tool for management of the difficult airway. Contemp Surg. 1996;49:300–6.
7. Bissinger U, Guggenberger H, Lenz G. Retrograde-guided fiberoptic intubation in patients with laryngeal carcinoma. Anesth Analg. 1995;81:408–10.
8. Practice guidelines for management of the difficult airway; an updated report by the ASA task force on management of the difficult airway. Anesthesiology.2003; 98:1269–77.
9. Wong DT, Lai K, Chung FF, Ho RY. Cannot intubate-cannot ventilate and difficult intubation strategies: results of a Canadian national survey. Anesth Analg. 2005;100:1439–46.
10. Lechman MJ, Donahoo JS, Macvaugh H. Endotracheal intubation using percutaneous retrograde guidewire insertion followed by antegrade fiberoptic bronchoscopy. Crit Care Med. 1986;14:589–90.
11. Bhardwaj N, Yaddanapudi S, Makkar S. Retrograde tracheal intubation in a patient with a halo traction device; Letter to editor. Anesth Analg. 2006;103:1628–9.
12. Marciniak D, Smith CE. Emergent retrograde tracheal intubation with a gum-elastic bougie in a trauma patient. Anesth Analg. 2007;105:1720–1.
13. Lenfant F, Benkhadra M, Trouilloud P, Freysz M. Comparison of two techniques for retrograde tracheal intubation in human fresh cadavers. Anesthesiology. 2006;104(1):48–51.
14. Hatton KW, Price S, Craig L, Grider JS. Educating anesthesiology residents to perform percutaneous cricothyroidotomy, retrograde intubation, and fiberoptic bronchoscopy using preserved cadavers. Anesth Analg. 2006;103:1205–8.
15. Salah N, Mhuircheartaigh RN, Hayes N, McCaul C. A comparison of four techniques of emergency transcricoid oxygenation in a manikin. Anesth Analg. 2010;110(4):1083–5.

12

The Role of the Combitube and Laryngeal Tube

Michael Woo and Michael F. O'Connor

M. Woo (✉) • M.F. O'Connoer
Department of Anesthesia & Critical Care, The University of Chicago,
5841 South Maryland Avenue, MC 4028, Chicago, IL 60637, USA
e-mail: mwoo@dacc.uchicago.edu

D.B. Glick et al. (eds.), *The Difficult Airway: An Atlas of Tools and Techniques for Clinical Management*,
DOI 10.1007/978-0-387-92849-4_12, © Springer Science+Business Media New York 2013

Introduction

First described in 1987[1], the Combitube combines the lumen of an endotracheal tube with an esophageal obturator airway. The dual lumen design facilitates airway management for the skilled or novice operator. Like a conventional endotracheal tube, it can be inserted into the trachea blindly or using direct laryngoscopy. Like an esophageal obturator or LMA, it can also be introduced blindly. If the Combitube resides in the esophagus, the obturator (blue) lumen can be used to ventilate the patient. The number of attempts to successful placement should be minimized since ventilation is possible whether the device is placed in the esophagus or trachea. The structural features of the esophageal-tracheal Combitube (ETC) are detailed in Figure 12.1.

Complications associated with its use and the high cost of this single-use product have precluded the Combitube from elective in-hospital use. Newer airway devices have supplanted its place in the management of difficult airways. Nevertheless, it remains more widely available than most of its alternatives, and training rescuers to use it is substantially easier[2–4].

Indications

The Combitube has been successfully used in multiple settings, including emergent pre-hospital settings, in-hospital emergencies, in-hospital airway rescue, and elective in-hospital surgery.

The Combitube is endorsed (Class IIa) by the American Heart Association for the support of ventilation and oxygenation during resuscitation and the peri-arrest period. In randomized trials, ventilation via a Combitube compared favorably to an endotracheal tube[5].

The American Society of Anesthesiologists describes the Combitube as a commonly cited technique to manage difficult ventilation[6]. Many case reports describe successful airway rescue in "cannot intubate-cannot ventilate" situations. These situations include not only CPR and resuscitation, but obstetrics, ICU, and airway rescue in the operating room[7,8].

Elective airway management has faded as a realm for the Combitube due to complications ranging from minor (tongue engorgement, sore throat), to severe (subcutaneous emphysema, pyriform sinus rupture), and life threatening (esophageal tear, pneumopericardium)[9–11]. While these complications can be serious, they are preferable to severe hypoxia and its consequences, which is why the Combitube remains available as a rescue device. Keys to minimizing minor and severe trauma include use of a rigid laryngoscope to facilitate Combitube placement and using a smaller device (see Table 12.1)[12].

Placement of the Esophageal Combitube

Placement of the ETC may be divided into two phases: a placement phase during which the device is placed in the airway, and a ventilation phase during which one or both cuffs are inflated; then ventilation is attempted and confirmed. The placement phase may be blind or blind and aided with a laryngoscope. Laryngoscopy may reveal a view of the glottis which permits endotracheal intubation with the ETC.

The ventilation phase consists of cuff inflation(s) and selection of lumens to attempt ventilation. The sequence of cuff and lumen selections is dependent on the clinical scenario. In emergencies, time to ventilation is minimized by fully inflating the pharyngeal and distal cuffs, and testing ventilation via the blue lumen (labeled "1"). Statistically, blind placement typically results in the ETC in the esophageal position, thus ventilation is more probable via the blue lumen. Figure 12.2 reflects the phases of routine ETC placement.

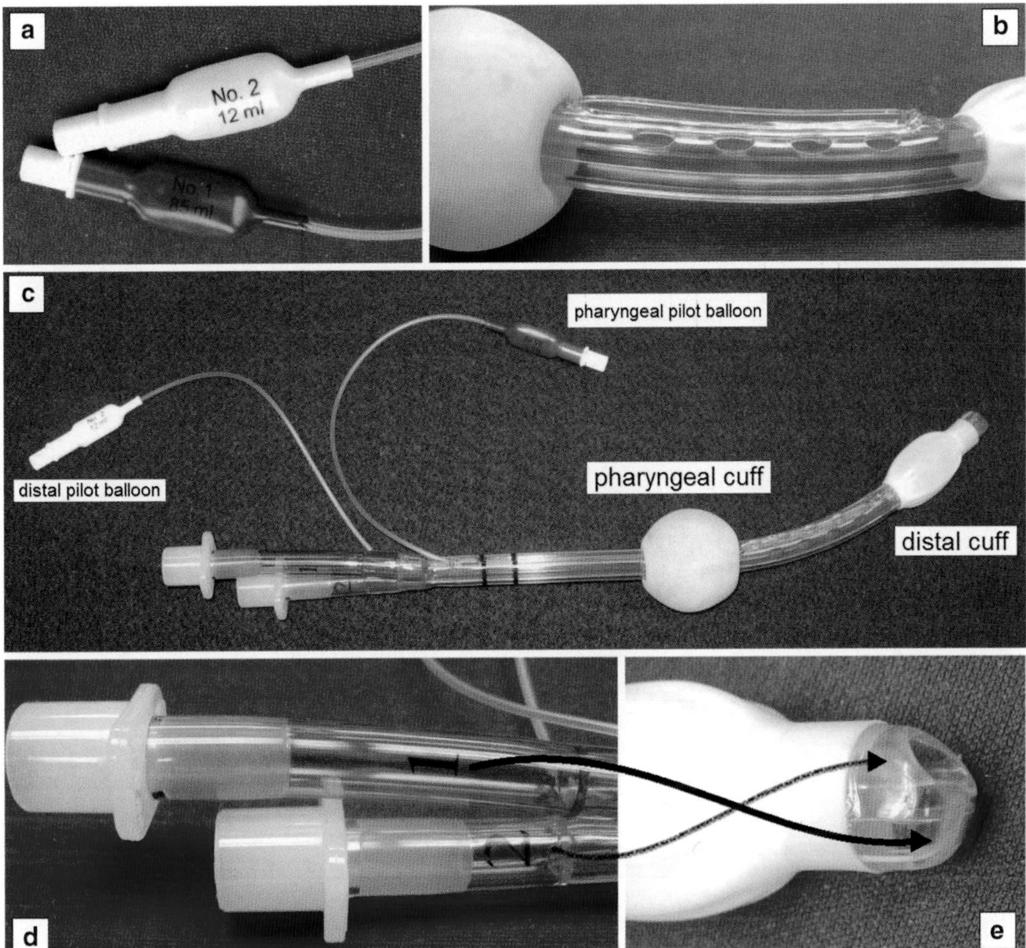

Figure 12.1. Anatomy of a Combitube. (**a**) Each cuff inflates separately. The *blue* (No. 1) pilot balloon connects to the proximal (pharyngeal) cuff. The cuff capacity is 85 mL for the Combitube SA (small adult). The *white* (No. 2) pilot balloon connects to the distal cuff. Cuff capacity is12 mL. (**b**) Eight side ports of the *blue*-topped lumen (labeled "1") open between the proximal (pharyngeal) and distal cuffs. In the likely event of esophageal intubation, ventilation occurs via these holes. Air is forced into the glottis because of the seals of the *yellow* pharyngeal cuff (*blue* pilot balloon) and the *white* esophageal cuff (*white* pilot balloon). (**c**) The Combitube is a double lumen device designed to permit ventilation whether placed in the trachea or esophagus. If tracheally placed, the device seals the trachea via the distal cuff (*white* pilot balloon) and ventilates via the distally opening lumen (labeled "2"). If esophageally placed, the device creates two seals: proximally in the pharynx with the pharyngeal cuff (*blue* pilot balloon) and distally in the esophagus with the distal cuff (*white* pilot balloon). Ventilation occurs via the side ports of the *blue*-topped lumen (labeled "1"). If placed in the esophagus, the *open* lumen can be used to decompress the stomach. (**d**) Blow *blue* first. The *blue* lumen (labeled "1") opens via side ports located between cuffs. This lumen extends to the end of the device where it ends blindly (*solid line*, Box **D-E**). Blind placement results in esophageal placement 95 % of the time; thus conventional wisdom advises to ventilate via the blue lumen first to confirm esophageal placement. The clear lumen (labeled "2) also extends to the end of the device but ends in an open orifice (*shaded line*, Box **D-E**). (**e**). The end of the device reveals one open orifice (from the clear lumen, labeled "2"), and one "dead-end" orifice (from the *blue* lumen, labeled "1").

Table 12.1. Size selection of ETC.

	Distal cuff recommended volume (mL)	Pharyngeal cuff recommended volume (mL)	For use in patients (height recommendation)
37 F SA (small adult)	10–12	85	Under 5 ft
41 F	10–15	100	Over 5 ft

Many reports suggest the 37 F SA ETC is effective in patients up to 6 ft in height[24]

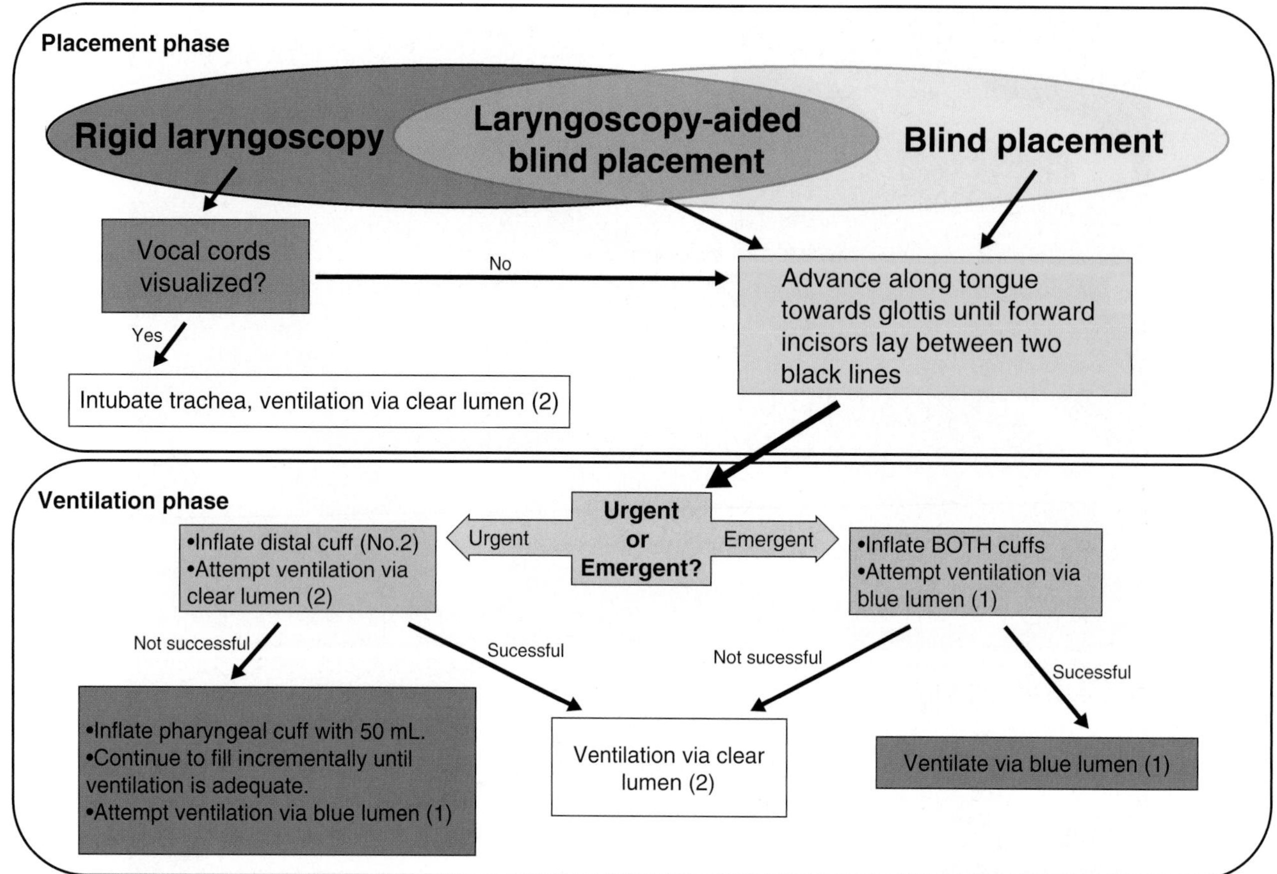

Figure 12.2. For routine ETC use, the placement phase starts with one of three situations: laryngoscope with glottic view, laryngoscope-aided blind, and blind unassisted. The algorithm for the ventilation phase is dependent on the urgency of the clinical scenario. When possible, a minimal inflation technique is preferable to minimize the risk of pharyngeal trauma.

Placement Phase

Placement with Laryngoscope, Vocal Cords Visualized

The ETC may be placed endotracheally akin to a conventional endotracheal tube. The distal cuff should be inflated (labeled white, No. 2), and ventilation should be initiated via the distal lumen (clear, labeled "2"). The pharyngeal cuff need not be inflated.

Blind Placement, with Laryngoscope, Blind Placement, without Laryngoscope

In this situation, the laryngoscope serves to mobilize the tongue, but the glottis is not visualized. The ETC is placed blindly until the patient's teeth rest between the two black lines (Figure 12.1, Box C). The ETC is inserted along the tongue in the direction of the glottis. If a laryngoscope is not available, the mandible and tongue are grasped and lifted and extended. Once the forward incisors rest between the black lines, one can proceed to the ventilation phase.

The head may remain in neutral position. Care should be taken to avoid contact with the posterior pharyngeal wall. The modified Lipp maneuver (described below) may decrease posterior pharyngeal trauma[13]. Esophageal placement is more likely.

Modified Lipp Maneuver

This maneuver consists of a concerted bend of the ETC in the area between the pharyngeal and distal cuffs. The induced curve should help avoid trauma along the posterior pharynx. The modified Lipp maneuver is shown in Figure 12.3.

Ventilation Phase

Emergent

In emergent situations the priority is minimal time to ventilation and oxygen delivery. Both cuffs are inflated to recommended volumes. The circuit should be attached initially to the blue lumen, labeled "1." Ventilation should be confirmed via conventional techniques. If ventilation is not possible via the blue lumen, the circuit should be attached to the clear lumen, labeled "2," and ventilation should be confirmed via conventional techniques.

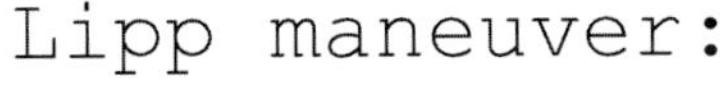

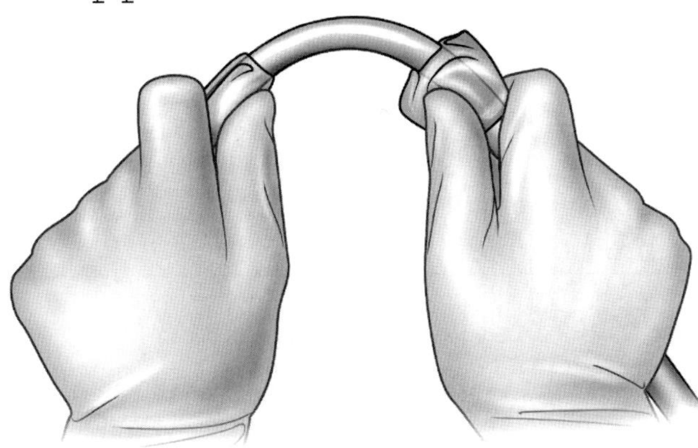

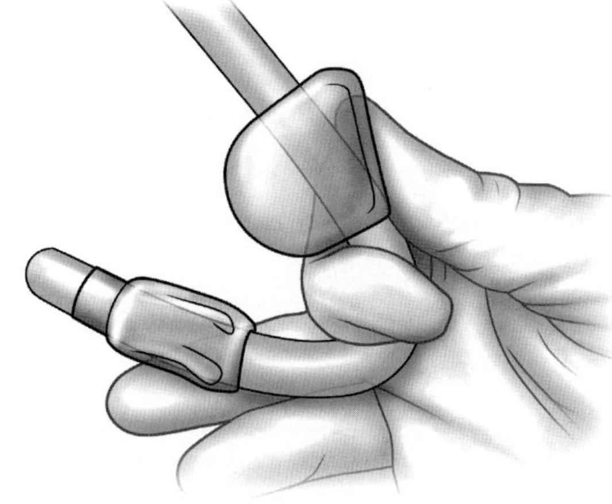

Figure 12.3. Figure of modified Lipp maneuver.

Non-emergent

If the clinical scenario allows for time, pharyngeal complications may be avoided using a minimal inflation technique. In this sequence, the pharyngeal cuff is inflated to less than the manufacturer's recommended volume. A volume of 50 mL is frequently clinically effective[14]. Lumen selection may start with the clear lumen (labeled "2"), but should quickly progress to the blue lumen if necessary. Ventilation should continue with the least amount of volume in the pharyngeal cuff to ensure adequate tidal volumes.

Lateral Placement to Avoid Tongue Engorgement

Tongue engorgement may be lessened by placement of the device lateral to the tongue. In this technique, the tongue is displaced with the same hand that opens the mouth. The device is placed at the opposite corner of the mouth, and eventually lies at the angle of the mouth as its final position.

In elective surgeries using this lateral placement technique, tongue engorgement was decreased in incidence and duration. Device effectiveness appears unaffected by lateral placement, as cuff leaks did not occur[15].

Minimal Leakage Technique to Avoid Tongue Engorgement

The minimal leakage technique has been recommended to decrease compression of lingual veins and thus tongue engorgement[16]. The technique is described for the oropharyngeal cuff of the Combitube SA which is rated for 85 mL.

The proximal (blue) cuff is inflated with 50 mL of air, then inflated in 10 ml increments until the air leak is extinguished. Air leaks are identified by auscultation at the neck or comparison of exhaled tidal volumes. Typical cuff volumes ranged from 40 to 85 mL[17].

Complications Associated with Combitube Use

Ninth and Twelfth Cranial Nerve Dysfunction

Zamora et al. report a patient who awoke with sore throat, dysphagia, tongue deviation, and posterior tongue numbness following Combitube placement for a Caesarean section. Symptoms resolved completely after 3 months[18].

Esophageal Perforation

Esophageal perforation has been reported in many arenas including the operating room[19] and out-of-hospital rescue. Presenting symptoms include subcutaneous emphysema, pneumomediastinum, and pneumopericardium. The key to improved outcome is early diagnosis and treatment.

The mechanism of injury appears more than mechanical, as esophageal tears occur beyond the end of the device[20].

Pyriform Sinus Perforation

Pyriform sinus perforation following Combitube placement was reported in a case of angioedema and respiratory arrest. The patient presented with massive subcutaneous emphysema, pneumomedistinum, and pneumopericardium[21].

Endotracheal Intubation After Combitube Placement

There might be occasions when a Combitube is used for emergency rescue, but an ETT is required for prolonged ventilation of the patient. The technique using the flexible bronchoscope to facilitate the conversion from Combitube ventilation to endotracheal intubation with a standard ETT is shown in Figure 12.4.

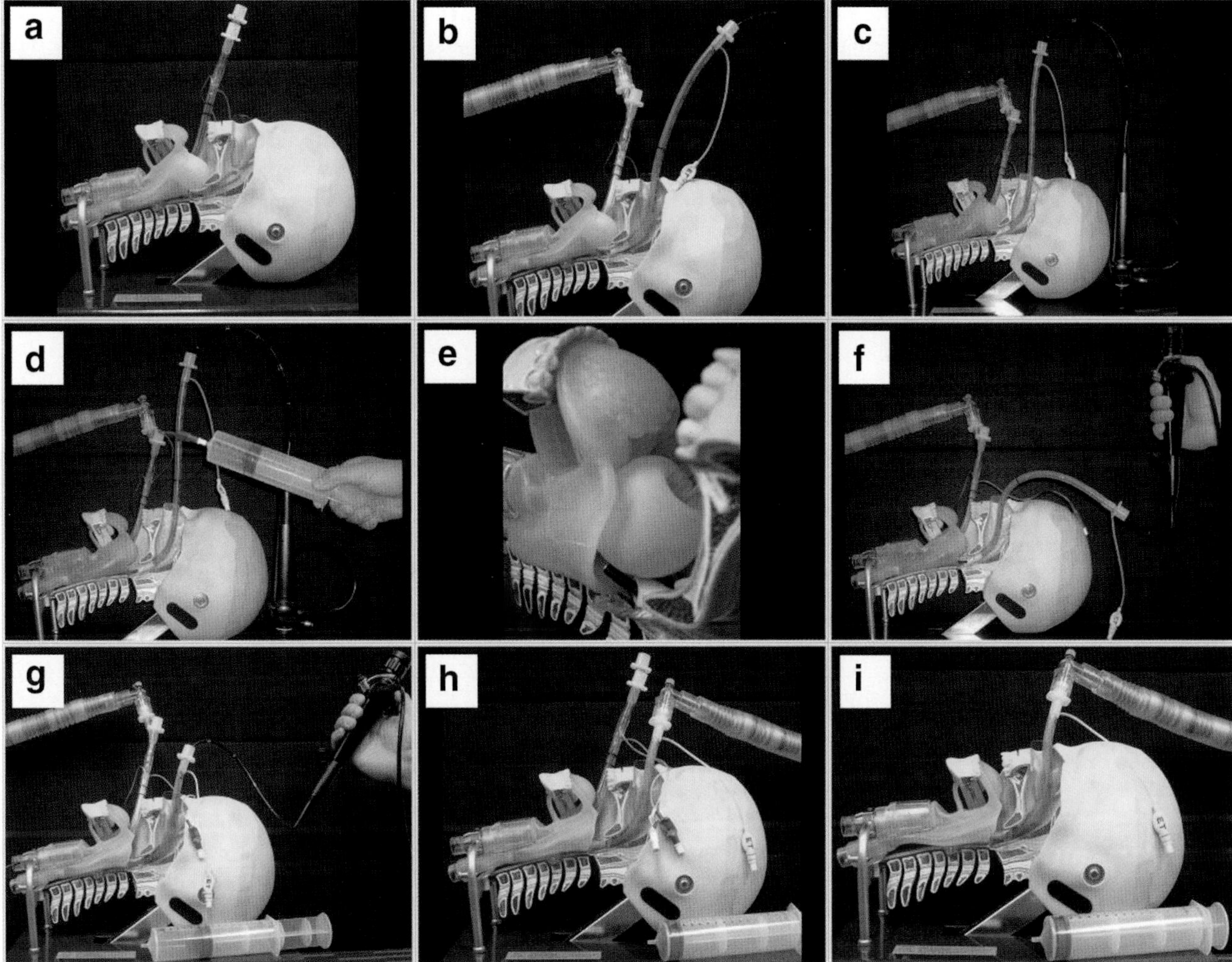

Figure 12.4. Conversion of Combitube to endotracheal tube facilitated by use of a flexible bronchoscope. (**a**) Combitube placed in the esophageal position. While ventilation continues via the blue lumen (labeled "1"), the stomach may be decompressed via gentle suction to the clear lumen (labeled "2"). (**b**). Reinforced endotracheal tube placed nasally while mechanical ventilation continues. (**c**) Flexible bronchoscope is introduced through the endotracheal tube, visualizing the pharyngeal cuff of the Combitube. (**d**) The pharyngeal cuff is partially or completely deflated to allow the bronchoscope to pass through to the glottis. (**e**) The endotracheal tube may be advanced alongside the cuff of the Combitube. This will allow for reinflation of the pharyngeal cuff, and thus positive pressure ventilation can continue during bronchoscopy. (**f**) The bronchoscope is guided into the trachea. (**g**) The pharyngeal cuff of the Combitube is sufficiently deflated to permit advancement of the endotracheal tube into the trachea. (**h**) Endotracheal placement of the endotracheal tube is confirmed, ventilation continues via the endotracheal tube. (**i**) The distal (esophageal) cuff of the Combitube is deflated, and the Combitube is removed.

Next Generation Devices

EasyTube

In many respects, the EasyTube represents the next generation ETC. Structural similarities include dual lumens, dual cuffs, and two inflation ports. Modifications include a larger ventilation port distal to the pharyngeal cuff that accommodates a flexible bronchoscope. Below the distal cuff, the EasyTube is smaller than the ETC as it contains a single lumen. The ETC contains two lumens, of which one ends in a dead end[22].

King LT, LT-D, LTS-D

The King LT (laryngeal tube) series of airways are smaller, simplified versions of the ETC. Similarities to the ETC include dual cuffs and ventilation ports between the cuffs. The two cuffs are connected, thus it is possible to inflate both via a single inflation point. The original King LT is a single lumen device which ends at the distal cuff. The LTS has a second lumen which extends to the tip of the device. It is designed for suction of the esophagus. The proximal opening of the suction lumen does not allow for connection to a breathing circuit. The advantage in these devices is their simplicity. One inflation port and one ventilation lumen dispense with the need for inflation or ventilation algorithms. One disadvantage is the inability to ventilate the patient if the device should happen to reside in the trachea. The "D" signifies the disposable version of the device[23].

Conclusion

Because of its unrivaled ease of placement, the Combitube remains an important and potentially life-saving tool in the hands of both first responders and in-hospital care providers. Unfortunately, the large size and relative stiffness of the Combitube has led to a range of potentially severe complications and so other devices are generally preferred where possible.

References

1. Frass M, Frenzer R, Zdrahal F, et al. The esophageal tracheal combitube preliminary results with a new airway for CPR. Ann Emerg Med. 1987;16:768–72.
2. Rumball CJ, MacDonald D. The PTL, combitube, laryngeal mask, and oral airway: a randomized prehospital comparative study of ventilatory device effectiveness and cost effectiveness in 470 cases of cardiorespiratory arrest. Prehosp Emerg Care. 1997;1:1–10.
3. Tanigawa K, Shigematsu A. Choice of airway devices for 12,020 cases of nontraumatic cardiac arrest in Japan. Prehosp Emerg Care. 1998;2:96–100.
4. Russi Christopher S, Lonny M, Hartley MJ. A Comparison of the King-LT to endotracheal intubation and combitube in a simulated difficult airway. Prehosp Emerg Care. 2008;12(1):35–41.
5. American Heart Association Guidelines for Cardiopulmonary Resuscitation and Emergency Cardiovascular Care: Part 7.1: Adjuncts for Airway Control and Ventilation Circulation, Dec 2005; 112: IV-51 - IV-57.
6. http://www.asahq.org/For-Members/Practice-Management/Practice-Parameters.aspx#airway. Practice Guidelines for Management of the Difficult Airway. Anesthesiology 2003; 98:1269–77.
7. Zamora JE, Saha TK. Combitube rescue for Cesarean delivery followed by ninth and twelfth cranial nerve dysfunction. Can J Anaesth. 2008;55(11):779–84.
8. Frass M, Frenzer R, Mayer G, Popovic R, Leithner C. Mechanical ventilation with the esophageal tracheal combitube (ETC) in the intensive care unit. Emerg Med J. 1987;4:219–25.

9. Richards C. Piriform sinus perforation during esophageal-tracheal combitube placement. J Emerg Med. 1998;16(1):37–9.
10. Gaitini Luis A, Vaida Sonia J, Somri M, et al. The combitube in elective surgery: a report of 200 cases. Anesthesiology. 2001;94:79–82.
11. Vézina D, Lessard MR, Bussières J, Topping C, Trépanier CA. Complications associated with the use of the esophageal-tracheal combitube. Can J Anaesth. 1998;45(1):76–80.
12. Mercer MH, Gabbott DA. The influence of neck position on ventilation using the combitube airway. Anaesthesia. 1998;53:146–50.
13. Urtubia RM, Frass M, Staudinger T, Krafft P. Modification of the Lipp maneuver for blind insertion of the Esophageal-Tracheal Combitube. Can J Anaesth. 2005;52(2):216–7.
14. Gaitini LA, et al. Minimal inflation volume for combitube oropharyngeal balloon. J Med Ar. 2010;8(3):27–32.
15. Ahmed SM, Rizvi KA, Khan RM, Zafar MU, Nadeem A. Less tongue engorgement with lateral placement of the Esophageal Tracheal Combitube. Acta Anaesthesiol Scand. 2008;52(6):834–7. Epub 2008 May 19.
16. Rabitisch W, Kolster WJ, Burgmann H, et al. Recommendation of the minimal volume technique to avoid tongue engorgement with prolonged use of the Esophageal-Tracheal Combitube. Ann Emerg Med. 2005;45(5):565–6. author reply.
17. Urtubia RM, Aguila CM, Cumsille MA. Combitube®: a study for proper use. Anesth Analg. 2000;90:958–62.
18. Zamora JE, Saha TK. Combitube rescue for Cesarean delivery followed by ninth and twelfth cranial nerve dysfunction. Can J Anaesth. 2008;55(11):779–84.
19. Bagheri SC, Stockmaster N, Delgado G, Kademani D, Carter TG, Ramzy A, et al. Esophageal rupture with the use of the Combitube: report of a case and review of the literature. J Oral Maxillofac Surg. 2008;66(5):1041–4.
20. Klein H, Williamson M, Sue-Ling HM, et al. Esophageal rupture associated with the use of the Combitube™. Anesth Analg. 1997;85:937–9.
21. Richards C. Piriform sinus perforation during esophageal-tracheal combitube placement. J Emerg Med. 1998;16(1):37–9.
22. Gaitini LA, Yanovsky B, Somri M, Tome R, Mora PC, Frass M, et al. Prospective randomized comparison of the easytube and the esophageal-tracheal Combitube airway devices during general anesthesia with mechanical ventilation. J Clin Anesth. 2011;23(6):475–81.
23. http://www.kingsystems.com/medical-devices-supplies-products/airway-management/supraglottic-airways/
24. Roland W, Shawn D, Bernhard P. Is the Combitube® a useful emergency airway device for anesthesiologists? Anesth Analg. 1999;88(1):233.

13

The Role of Transtracheal Jet Ventilation

Julio Cortiñas-Díaz and Seth Manoach

J. Cortiñas-Díaz (✉)
Department of Surgery, Service of Anesthesiology, University of Santiago de Compostela School of Medicine, Hospital Clinico Universitario, Santiago de Compostela, 15703, Spain
e-mail: jcortinas@mundo-r.com

S. Manoach
Department of Anesthesiology and Emergency Medicine, Division of Critical Care Medicine, SUNY Downstate Medical Center, Kings County Hospital, Brooklyn, NY 11203, USA

D.B. Glick et al. (eds.), *The Difficult Airway: An Atlas of Tools and Techniques for Clinical Management*, DOI 10.1007/978-0-387-92849-4_13, © Springer Science+Business Media New York 2013

Introduction

Transcutaneous transtracheal jet ventilation (TTJV) is a minimally invasive ventilatory modality that uses a catheter to insufflate oxygen or air at high pressure (0.5–4.0 bar, or 8–60 psi) into the tracheal lumen. To perform TTJV, one can use an automatic jet ventilator or a manual trigger-activated device.

The use of a transtracheal catheter to provide oxygenation was first reported in the mid-twentieth century by Reed and Jacoby[1,2]. In 1971, Spoerel et al.[3] employed a jet to provide transtracheal ventilation at rates less than 40 breaths/min (LFJV or low-frequency jet ventilation), and in 1977 Klain and Smith[4] described high-frequency jet ventilation (HFJV), which employs rates greater than 1 Hz (60 breaths/min). This chapter will focus on LFJV, as that is most commonly employed when TTJV is used to facilitate difficult airway management or rescue a patient who cannot be intubated or ventilated using other means.

Indications for TTJV

Accessing the tracheal lumen transcutaneously through the cricothyroid membrane, or between the tracheal rings if cricothyroid puncture is impossible, is the *rescue* ventilation technique of choice for apneic patients in *extremis* in whom it is not feasible to establish an airway using less invasive means, such as, mask ventilation, direct or indirect laryngoscopy, or supra and extraglottic devices (see Figure 13.1). When a patient's life is threatened by hypoxia, airway managers must act without delay. In such situations, the only absolute contraindications to the trans-cricothyroid membrane approach are traumatic fracture of the larynx and tracheal transection with retraction of the distal portion toward the mediastinum. Every airway management algorithm and clinical guide includes TTJV in the approach to the "cannot intubate–cannot ventilate" scenario[5,6]. This scenario can arise in both pre-hospital and in-hospital situations, and is particularly likely to occur in the emergency department, operating room, or critical care unit.

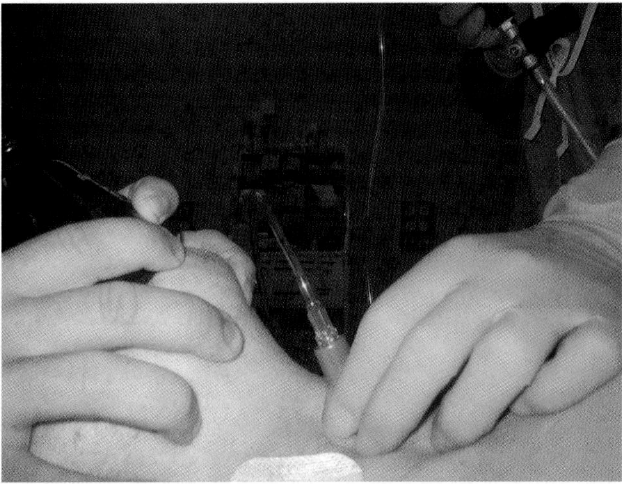

Figure 13.1. In this case the TTJV was used to salvage a patient who could not be intubated and who could barely be ventilated by face mask. Emergency transtracheal ventilation is being performed while the catheter is hand-secured by the anesthesiologist.

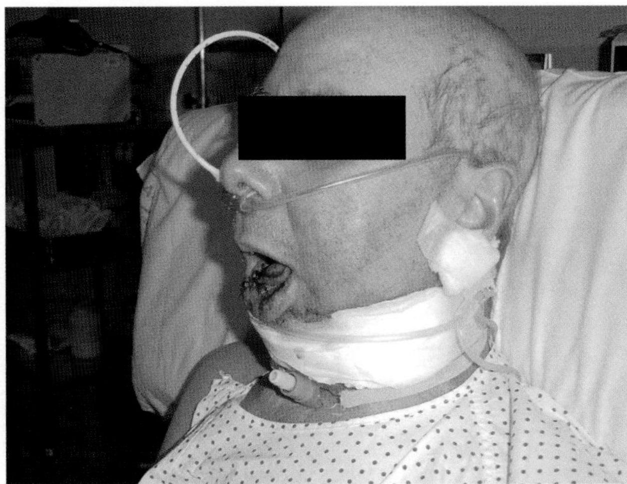

Figure 13.2. A transtracheal catheter can be left in place postoperatively in case a patient with a difficult airway needs to be emergently ventilated. This patient had surgery for a lingual tumor (photo courtesy of Dr. Pablo Otero).

In the field of Anesthesiology, "cannot intubate–cannot ventilate" situations had an estimated rate of 0.01–2: 10,000 cases during the pre-supraglottic device era[7]. Of course "cannot intubate–cannot ventilate" situations are much more likely to occur in patients presenting with airway pathology. Airway management personnel who do not have surgical training must be able to perform either cricothyroidotomy or TTJV when faced with an airway emergency that cannot be rescued otherwise. Tracheostomy is slower, more difficult, and more likely to cause iatrogenic injury[8]. TTJV is a trusted alternative to surgical cricothyroidotomy because it is proven to provide both oxygenation and ventilation[9] and because it is technically easier to perform, as it is similar to peripheral venous cannulation.

In cases in which there is time, and in which a difficult airway is anticipated, some authors introduce a catheter into the tracheal lumen to *prevent* hypoxia and loss of airway control during the process of intubation using other techniques. In fact, ventilation through a transcricoid catheter can facilitate fiberoptic bronchoscopy or direct laryngoscopy because retrograde escape of air through the cords and up toward the pharynx can lead the laryngoscopist to the glottis[10–12]. Prophylactic use of a transtracheal catheter can be extended to the immediate postoperative period in patients with difficult airways (see Figure 13.2). As in other situations, the catheter will allow rapid airway control and ventilation of patients known to be extremely difficult to intubate or ventilate using other means[13].

A third possibility for the use of TTJV is *elective*, for example, in ENT cases, tracheal surgery, and other procedures which are performed upon an airway open to the atmosphere, or in which it is desirable to have an immobile surgical field that is free of endotracheal tubes or other airway devices (Figure 13.3). The use of TTJV in such cases can facilitate the operative intervention while avoiding the need for tracheostomy at the outset of the procedure[14]. The most common use of TTJV is elective, although it is not used at all centers that perform ENT surgery.

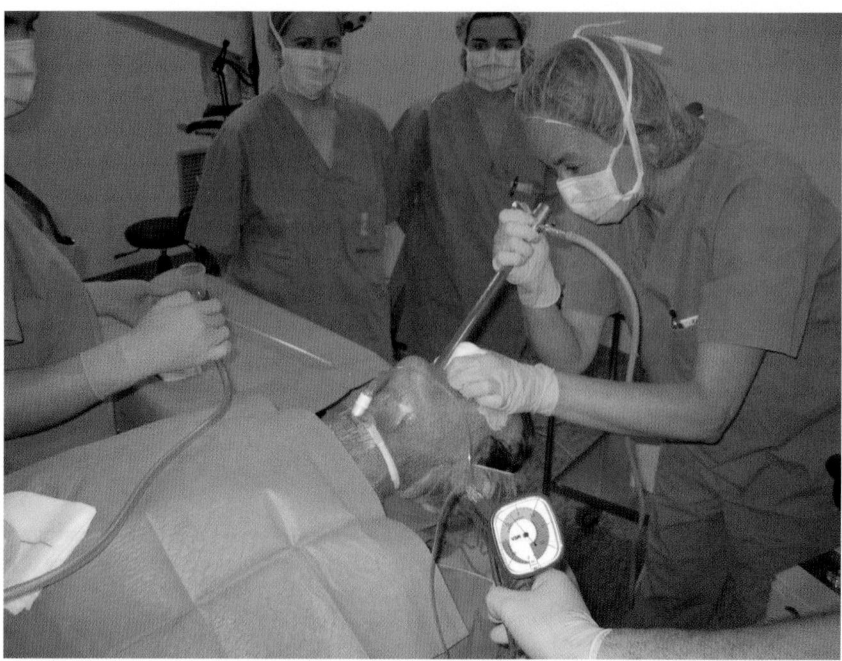

Figure 13.3. Exploration of the aerodigestive tract under general anesthesia with TTJV.

Contraindications

Contraindications include severe coagulopathy, local infection, local infiltration with tumor, complete effacement of anatomic landmarks of the anterior neck (secondary to extreme fixed cervical flexion, radiotherapy, morbid obesity, etc.), complete expiratory obstruction, unavailability of necessary equipment, and severe intrathoracic airway obstruction. As above, the only absolute contraindications to the procedure are tracheal transection, and for transcricoid TTJV, laryngeal fracture.

Equipment

In the majority of cases, oxygen is the gas used during TTJV. One should have access to a high-pressure oxygen source in order to assure the necessary tidal volume for oxygenation and ventilation. The driving pressure is determined by the gas source, the regulator controlling gas flow from the source, the tubing conveying that flow to the jet injector or ventilator, and the tubing and catheter used with the jet equipment. The ventilatory rate is controlled by the operator using either an automatic ventilator or, as is more common when using TTJV specifically for difficult airways, a manual injector.

During the last 25 years, there have been numerous publications describing "homemade" jet ventilation devices. Such devices are often ineffective, incapable of providing adequate driving pressure for transtracheal catheter ventilation in adults. Examples include catheters coupled with standard resuscitation bags or conventional anesthesia circuits[15,16]. As a result, critiques of these designs have also been published. These critiques have reviewed the fundamental physics of TTJV as this relates to the flow generated in the catheter, the pressure that this flow creates, and resistance to the movement of gas[17–20].

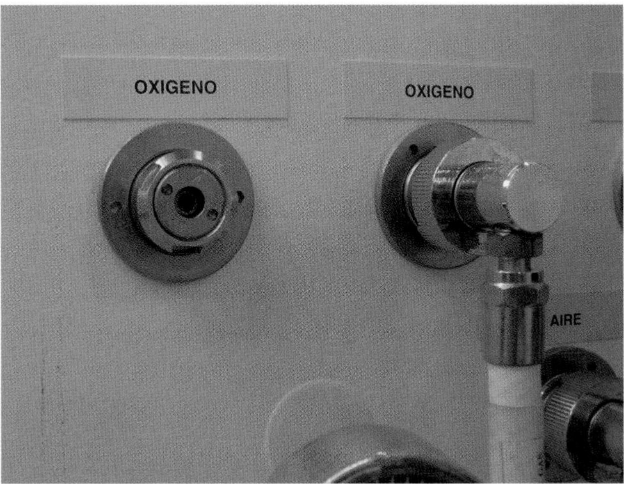

Figure 13.4. Three-tooth wall outlet specifically for oxygen in the operating room. Note the air connector below and to the right of the oxygen connections.

Gas Source

The sources typically available to administer oxygen are:

- Oxygen supplied to the various hospital units and delivered to the bedside via pipes that are fed by a centralized oxygen source.
- Portable oxygen tanks.
- Anesthesia machines.

Centralized Oxygen

Centralized oxygen is the best source for consistent high pressure (greater than 40 psi). Oxygen is obtained from the centralized or "wall" oxygen source via specific connections that are often color-coded to distinguish the various wall feeds (see Figures 13.4 and 13.5). In the US, oxygen sources have green connectors, air connectors are yellow, and wall suction is white. Low compliance tubing connects from the green oxygen port to the jet ventilator. The manual trigger mechanism and the pressure regulator on the jet ventilator in turn control the amount of oxygen administered to the patient.

Oxygen Tanks

Oxygen is delivered from medical tanks using low- or high-flow flowmeters. The pressure inside the tank can be as much as 200 bar (3,000 psi). High-flow regulators can maintain a steady state pressure of approximately 100 psi, with flows as high as 320 L/m, which exceeds the requirements for providing TTJV. In the US, oxygen in large tanks is maintained at a pressure of 2,000 psi and the standard regulators maintain a steady state pressure of 50 psi.

Low-flow regulators are often found on small, easily transportable oxygen tanks (see Figure 13.6). When maximally opened and before gas is allowed to flow, these tanks and regulators can reach a pressure of 120 psi but, once gas flow occurs, pressure falls off and then stabilizes between 0 and 5 psi. This pressure guarantees a steady flow of up to 15 L/min. In order to assure sufficient tidal volume when employing TTJV with a small tank and low-flow regulator, some authors have recommended that the flowmeter be opened completely (15 L/m), and that an I:E ratio of 1:1 be used with a rate of 30 breaths/min[21]. Other authors[22] have shown that with 40 psi (from a wall source or tank) and a low flow

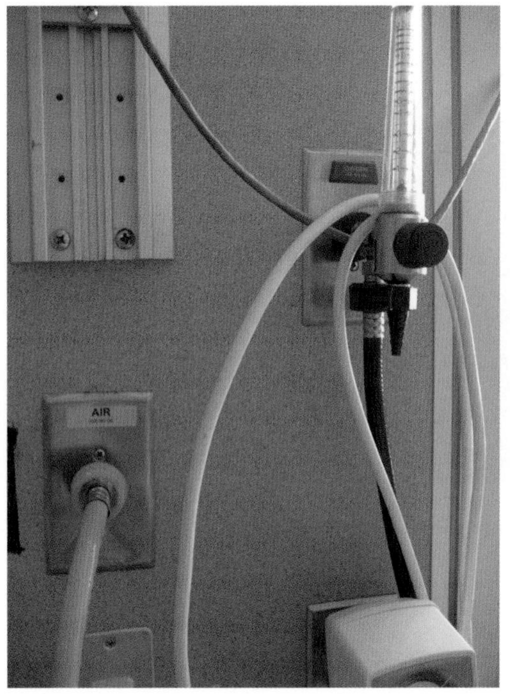

Figure 13.5. Centralized oxygen source via specific connections are often distinguished by different colors and signs.

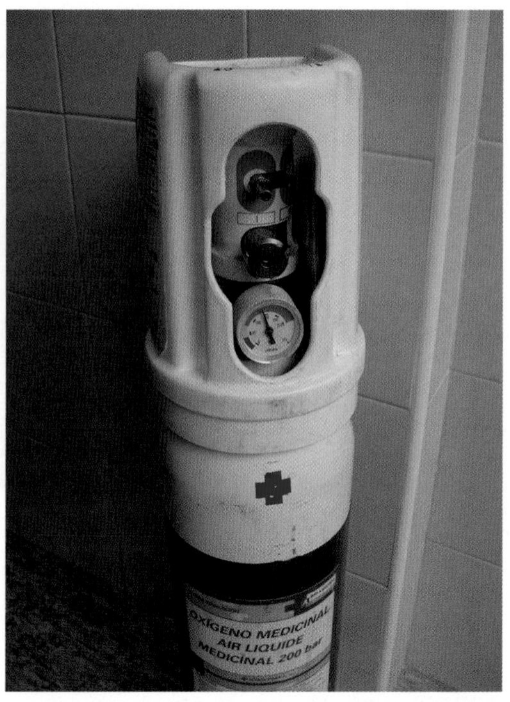

Figure 13.6. Small transportable oxygen tank with protected low-flow regulator. The oxygen inside this tank is pressurized to 200 bar but its outlet is regulated to no more than 3 bar.

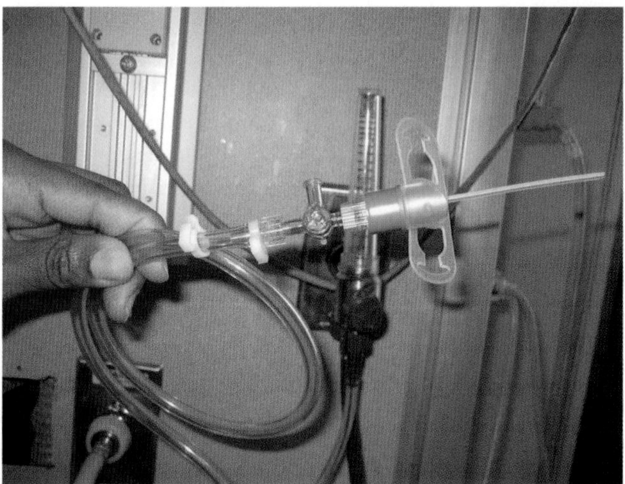

Figure 13.7. Self-assembled device made with a three-way stopcock connected to a high pressure oxygen source by noncompliant tubing, as described by Bould et al.

meter opened to 15 L/m, one can reach pressures and flows similar to those achieved with a variable pressure injector (Manujet™ VBM Medizintechnik, Sulz, Germany), set to100–150 kPa (15–22 psi). If the flowmeter is opened even further, surpassing 15 L/m, one can reach pressures and flows similar to that provided by the Manujet with 400 kPa (60 psi). Both groups suggest that low-flow regulators could be used in this way in pre-hospital or in-hospital settings where a centralized oxygen source is not available (see Figure 13.7).

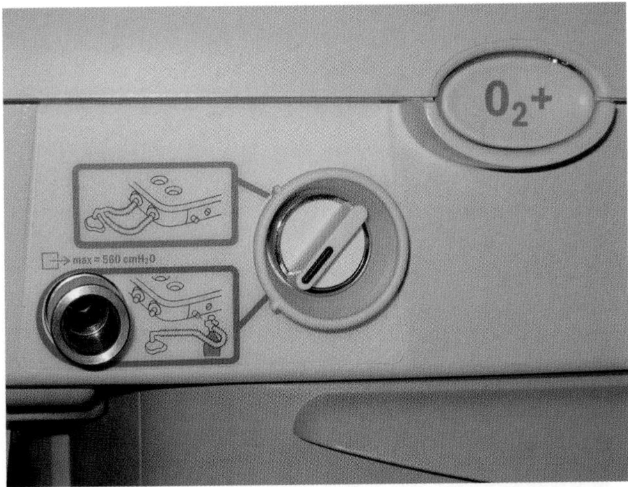

Figure 13.8. Anesthesia-machine flush valve of the Datex-Ohmeda S/5 Avance. Note that the maximum pressure is less than 1 atm.

Anesthesia-Machine Flush Valve

Unless an anesthesia machine has a high-pressure connection specifically tailored for jet ventilation, the common gas outlets are not at present adequate oxygen sources to provide jet ventilation (see Figure 13.8). This is because they do not provide enough driving pressure or because they have relief valves that limit the pressure. That said, some can provide partial and temporary ventilatory support[23]. We recommend consulting the technical specifications for the anesthesia machine used in one's practice, keeping these specifications in a place where they are readily available, and identifying an adequate TTJV gas source in one's usual place of work. These measures will assure that TTJV can be administered in an emergency, should it become necessary to do so.

Pressure-Flow Regulators

There are two ways in which jet ventilation can be administered; by an electrically controlled jet ventilator (see Figure 13.9) or a hand-triggered jet injector. Of the two, the manual unit is more widely used. Injectors used in clinical practice should be authorized for medical use, and should have a pressure regulator (see Figure 13.10a, b), be easy to use, not require any assembly, and have demonstrated efficacy (see Figures 13.11 and 13.12). The devices should permit the use of working pressures between 0 and 50 psi (see Figure 13.13), and allow careful control over the volume. There are several such injectors on the market (see Figures 13.11 and 13.12). Those in common use include the BE 183-SUR (Instrumentation Industries, Bethel Park PA, USA) and the Manujet (Medizintechnik GmbH, Sulz, Germany). Both devices allow gas flow to be regulated on the injector itself so the operator does not have to adjust the wall- or tank-mounted regulator. Both also have easy-to-read pressure gauges. The trigger on the BE-183-SUR is thumb activated, while the Manujet features a handgrip trigger. Both devices have been used extensively in clinical and research settings.

Other effective instruments with the possibility to ventilate have been proposed for TTJV in emergency situations, particularly when special equipment is not immediately available. These include self-assembled devices consisting of a three-way stopcock, connected by a noncompliant tubing to a high-pressure oxygen source (see Figure 13.7), or the commercialized Enk Oxygen Flow Modulator (Cook, Bloomington, IN) that permits flow and pressure release through its side ports (see Figure 13.14).

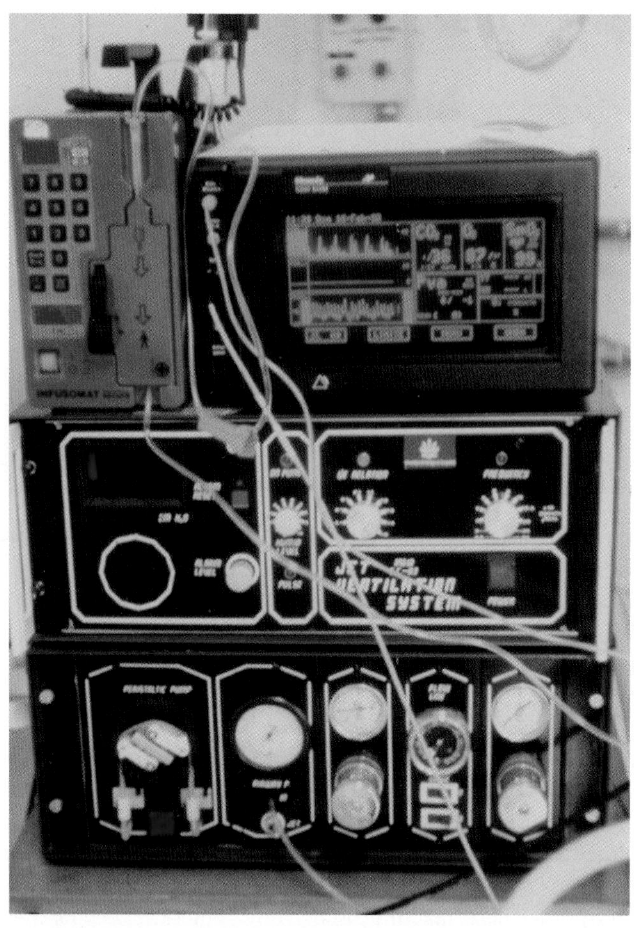

Figure 13.9. The "Santiago II" respirator for high-frequency jet ventilation, developed by Dr. Vicente Ginesta. Note the pump used for humidifying the insufflated gas as well as the respiratory gas monitors.

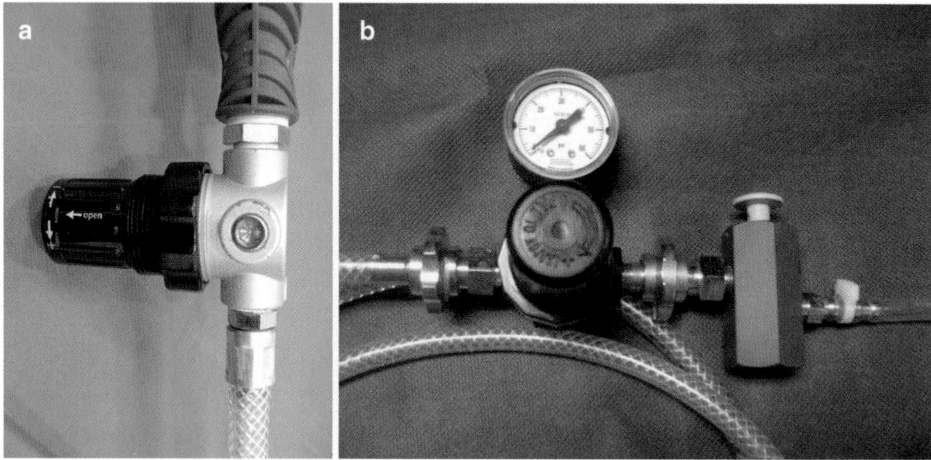

Figure 13.10. (**a**) Manujet pressure regulator. A spring and membrane mechanism allow the operator to change driving pressure. (**b**) Trigger, pressure regulator, and gauge of the BE 183-SUR.

Both could provide sufficient flow and pressure to ventilate and oxygenate but it should be kept in mind that neither assures precise control of the driving pressure. As a result insufficient ventilation can ensue or, in the case of severe upper airway obstruction, these devices could cause the lower airways to reach dangerous pressure levels[24–26].

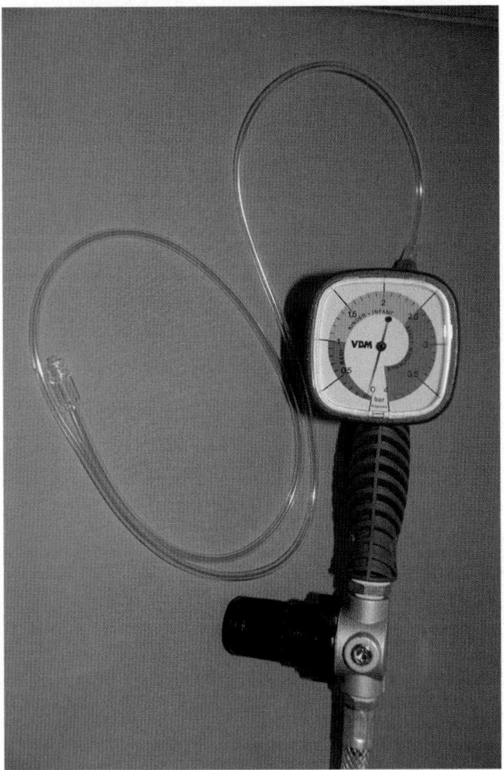

Figure 13.11. Manujet injector. Large-bore tubing for conducting gas from the source to the injector, pressure regulator, handle with trigger and manometer, and small-bore tubing for conducting gas from the injector to the catheter.

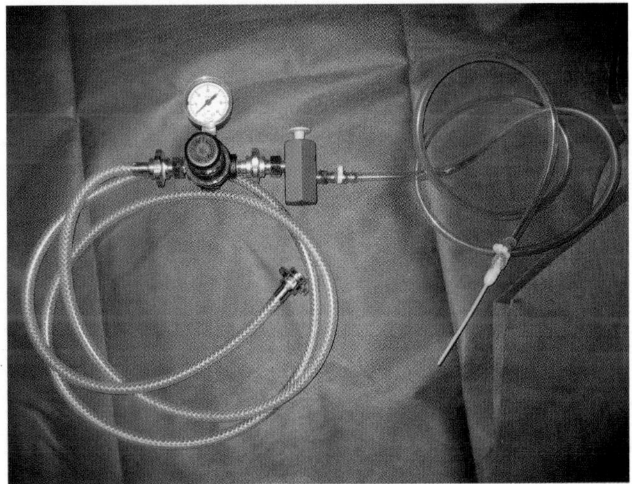

Figure 13.12. BE 183-SUR. Large-bore tubing for conducting gas from the source to the injector, pressure regulator, handle with trigger and manometer; and small-bore tubing for conducting gas from the injector to the catheter (a Cook catheter is deployed here).

Gas Conduits

The tubing used with a jet injector should be noncompliant and of greater caliber than the transtracheal catheter so as to permit flow without dampening pressure. The connections to the proximal and distal end of the tubing between the ventilator and the catheter must be secure and resistant to inadvertent loosening. An example of such an attachment is the Luer-Lok. In general, the proximal connector is female and the distal one is male (see Figure 13.15).

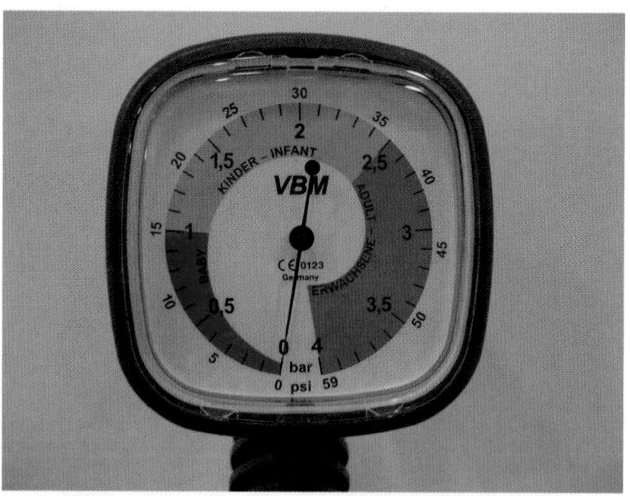

Figure 13.13. Manometer with different recommended driving pressures that can be set according to the age or size of the patient.

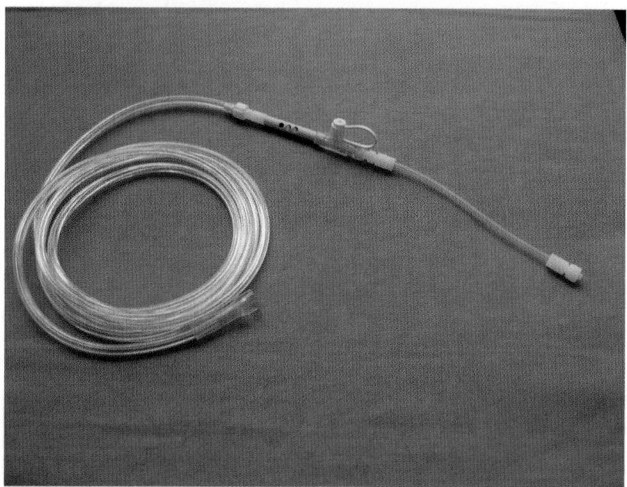

Figure 13.14. Enk oxygen flow modulator. The holes are manually covered and uncovered to alternate between inspiration and expiration.

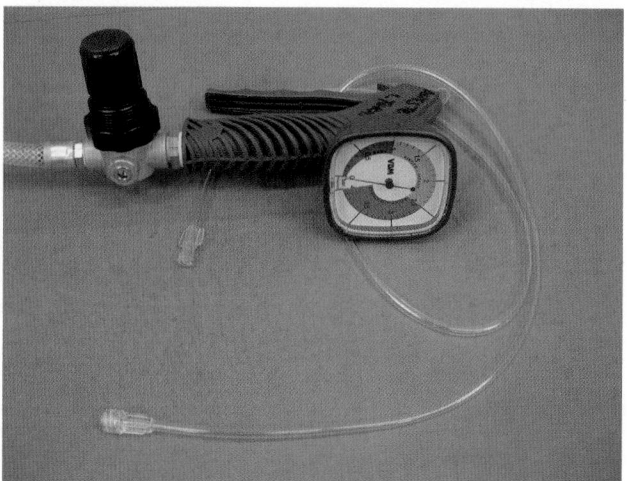

Figure 13.15. Noncompliant tubing and injector. The connections to the proximal and distal end of the tubing must be secure and resistant to inadvertent loosening. Note the female connector for the trigger and the male connector on the catheter side.

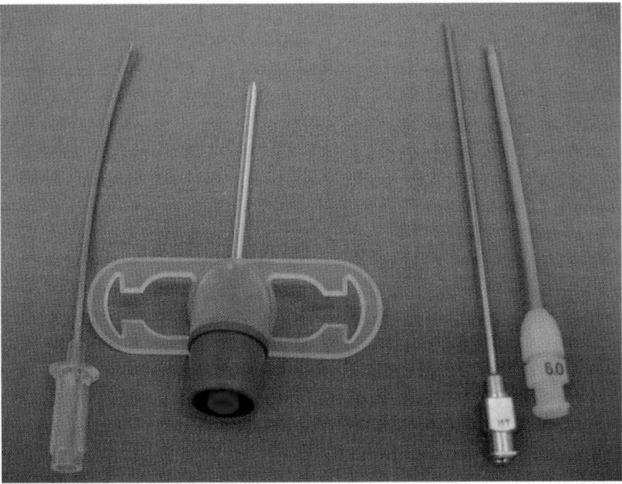

Figure 13.16. Catheters and needles shown, VBM TM 13G and Cook TM 6 Fr. Note the curved Ravussin (VBM) needle vs. the straight Cook one.

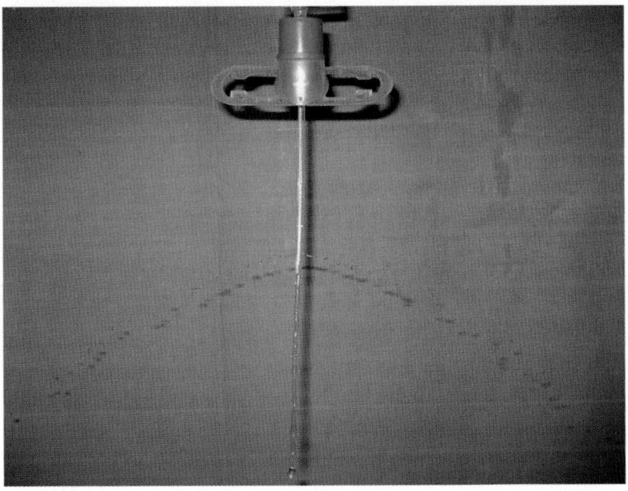

Figure 13.17. Spurts of IV fluid simulating the exit of gas from a Ravussin catheter. The two lateral openings were designed to diminish the Venturi effect.

Types of Catheter (See Figure 13.16)

Specifically for TTJV:

1. The Ravussin Jet Ventilation Catheter (VBM Medizintechnik Gmbh, Sulz, Germany) is 70 mm long, made of teflon (not flammable), and mounted on a steel needle. The catheter is anatomically curved, and has two distal lateral holes that are 0.8 mm in diameter (see Figure 13.17). This design is intended to keep the catheter far from the tracheal wall and reduce gas entrainment caused by the venturi effect. It is marketed in sizes 13G for adults, 14G for children, and 16G for infants. Two lateral attachments permit adjustment to the nearest millimeter to allow fixation around the neck with a Velcro band (see Figure 13.18)[27].
2. The Cook catheter is a straight catheter that is coil-reinforced to prevent kinking (see Figure 13.19). It is marketed as a 2 mm internal diameter catheter in 5.0 and 7.5 cm lengths. The shorter length will cause the less resistance to flow, but may be too short

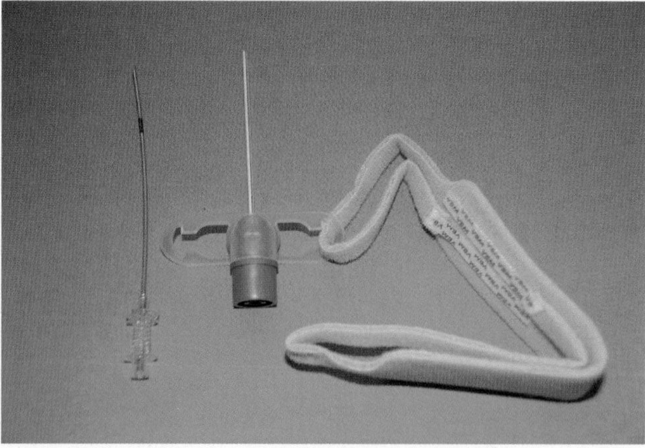

Figure 13.18. Ravussin 13G catheter with needle and neck band for securing the device.

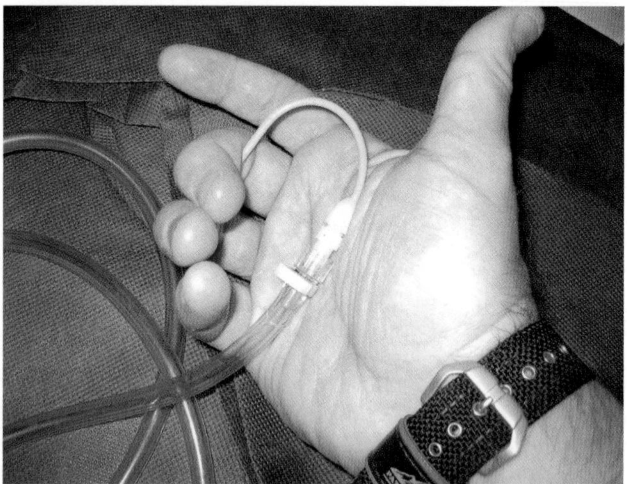

Figure 13.19. The Cook catheter has a reinforcing coil that resists kinking.

for very obese patients. Anecdotally, we have found that the coils make this catheter less likely to kink or shear off the needle during placement. We have experienced shearing of the catheter when the needle has abutted the edge of the cricoid or thyroid cartilages. In those cases, the needle has on occasion continued through the membrane, while the catheter itself has sheared off or "unpeeled" against the lip of the cartilage. This is probably more likely to occur in patients who are obese or otherwise have obstructed anatomic landmarks, because it is more difficult to control the trajectory of the catheter.

Other catheters that have been used for TTJV:

Authors have described the use of intravenous catheters, either single or multiple lumen (to permit monitoring of airway pressure and CO_2), as well as arterial, epidural, and other catheters (see Figure 13.20). Longer, more flexible catheters are more likely to whip around and impact the tracheal wall[28]. Standard intravenous catheters have thin walls and kink more easily compared to those specifically designed for TTJV. If such catheters are used, recommended sizes for TTJV are 16G, 14G, or 12G, depending on patient age. More rigid non-TTJV catheters and needles (e.g., 16G epidural needles) carry a higher risk of injuring the posterior tracheal wall[29–31]. We advise strongly against using intravenous and other non-TTJV catheters if it is at all possible to use a catheter designed for TTJV. Non-TTJV catheters cannot be relied upon, but may serve as a bridge in an emergency.

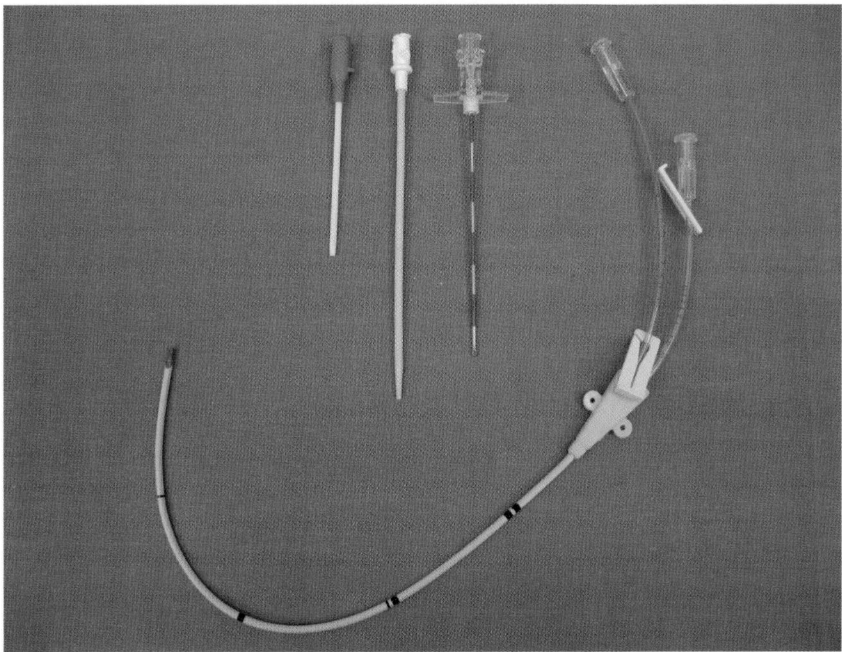

Figure 13.20. Catheters that have been used for TTJV: A double lumen central venous catheter allows ventilation through one lumen and capnography through the other one. The length and small diameter of multi-lumen central venous catheters result in high resistance to flow. As a result, these catheters are unlikely to provide successful ventilation. In addition, they may whip around the trachea and this may result in trauma. Also shown is a 13G intravenous catheter, a 18G vessel dilator, and an epidural needle. Intravenous catheters are more likely to kink. The straight, rigid, and sharp epidural needle is more likely to perforate the posterior wall of the trachea.

Anatomy

The cricothyroid space is found on the anterior surface of the neck, between the inferior border of the thyroid cartilage and the superior border of the cricoid cartilage. The cricothyroid membrane sits in this space. The membrane is the most superficial portion of the subglottic airway and at times the space can be easily appreciated on visual inspection as a depression between the thyroid and cricoid cartilages. In other cases this landmark can only be recognized by palpating the laryngeal cartilages approximately one and a half fingerbreadths below the thyroid prominence or "Adam's apple" (see Figures 13.21 and 13.22).

Occasionally, clinicians will need to make use of larger anatomic landmarks that are less precise than those described above. These reference points will be apparent even in patients who are obese or have other conditions that may efface the finer anatomic features of the neck. They include the crease at the border of the chin and neck and the suprasternal notch. From the suprasternal notch, the membrane can often be found using the index finger. To do this, one places the patient in neutral position, puts the right ring finger in the notch, and allows the index and middle fingers to fall superiorly along the midline of the neck.

The dimensions of the cricothyroid membrane are approximately 1 cm in height and 3 cm in width. In some adults, the membrane may be as small as 0.5 cm in height[32]. The membrane is separated from the skin by the anterior cervical fascia and by fatty subcutaneous tissue. The membrane is practically avascular, although very fine branches of the superior thyroid artery anastomose along the lateral portions of the superior third. In the center of the membrane there is only ligament, which is fatty in its medial aspect. The small cricothyroid muscles are located laterally along this ligament.

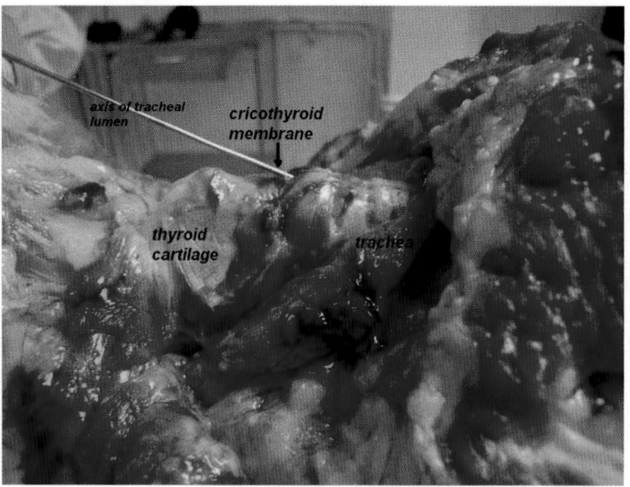

Figure 13.21. Dissection of the anterior region of the neck showing the laryngeal anatomy. The metal guide inserted through the cricothyroid membrane shows the longitudinal axis of the trachea.

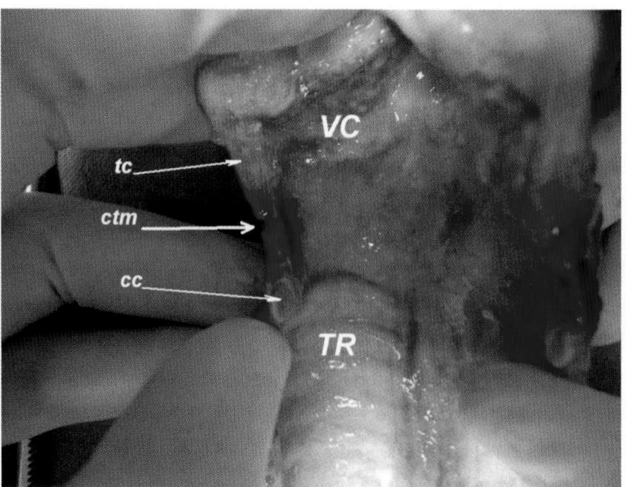

Figure 13.22. Larynx open in the sagittal plane. One can appreciate the cricothyroid membrane, with a too high puncture (sectioned, along the cut edge), and above that, the right vocal cord and false vocal cord. (*VC* vocal cords; *tc* thyroid cartilage; *ctm* cricothyroid membrane; *cc* cricoid cartilage; *TR* trachea).

Upon crossing the cricothyroid membrane, one enters the tracheal lumen. The vocal cords are located more than a centimeter superiorly, which, if the landmarks are clearly identified, makes injury unlikely during transcricoid catheter placement. The thyroid gland is usually located sufficiently remote from the cricothyroid membrane that it should not be injured, although the distance between the two structures depends on the size of the gland. In some cases, for example, in a patient with a goiter, the gland can cross the membrane. The great vessels of the neck, the carotid arteries and jugular veins, sit on either side of the airway, and for this reason, clinicians should be very careful to stay close to the midline. The membranous trachea, which is not protected by cartilaginous rings, is located posteriorly. Behind the membranous trachea is the esophagus. Although the posterior tracheal wall is somewhat protected by the circumference of the cricoid ring at the level of the membrane itself, the catheter must be pointed both posteriorly and caudally during insertion.

While placing the catheter, one must be vigilant about not penetrating the membranous trachea and entering the esophagus. As the trachea runs toward the base of the neck, it runs progressively deeper and therefore becomes more difficult to access. It is critical that airway managers do not confuse the cricothyroid and thyrohyoid membrane. The latter sits between the superior border of the thyroid cartilage and the hyoid bone. This mistake occurs more often in patients with short, fat necks. It is a grave error, as a puncture of the thyrohyoid cartilage leads into the supraglottic airway, and not the tracheal lumen.

In infants and small children, the larynx is very small, and below the cords it is shaped like an inverted funnel, very narrow at the level of the cricoid, and with somewhat firm tissue between the cartilages. These features make the transcricoid approach more difficult, and make surgical cricothyroidotomy particularly problematic in children less than 10 years of age[33]; transcricoid jet ventilation is the only emergent subglottic rescue technique that is recommended in this age group[34] for all but very experienced surgical subspecialists.

Technique for Performing Cricothyroid Puncture and Tracheal Catheterization

Although patients should be anesthetized or, if conscious, have received local anesthesia, it may be necessary to proceed directly to cricothyroid puncture in emergencies. When cricothyroid puncture is contraindicated or impossible, one may perform TTJV between the tracheal rings, although this may carry a greater risk of complications[30].

Procedure (see sequence of Figures 13.23, 13.24 and 13.25)

1. *Extend* the neck as much as possible. The chin can significantly interfere with the orientation of the catheter during placement. This, in turn, can lead to a greater risk of

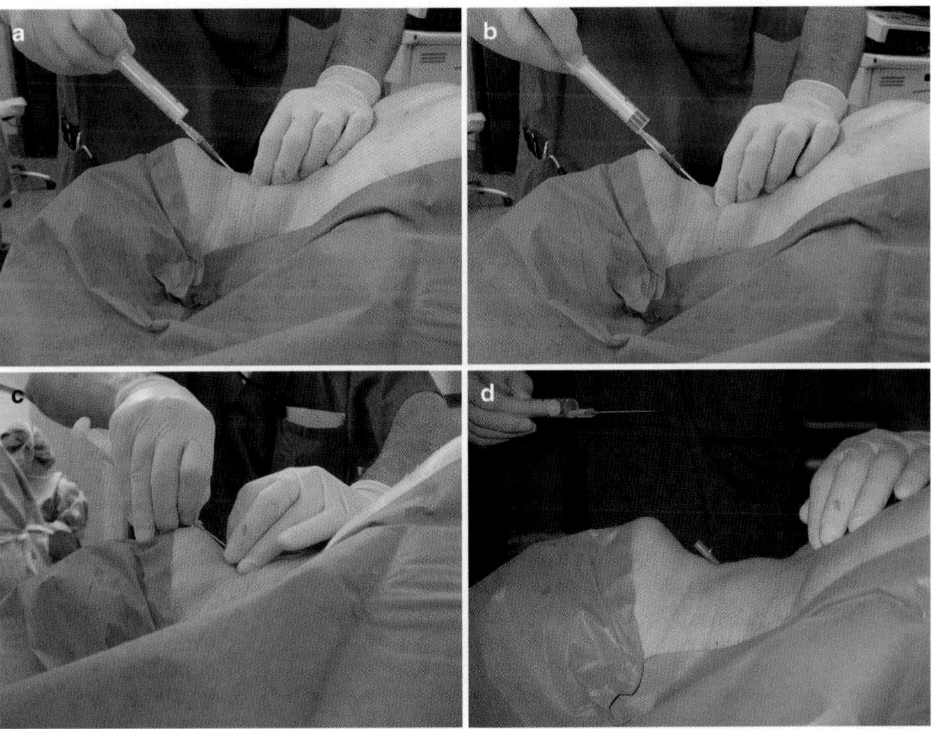

Figure 13.23. (**a, b**) Aspirating while puncturing with a 14G venous catheter; (**c**) Firmly holding the needle, one slides the catheter into the tracheal lumen. (**d**) Catheter placed in the tracheal lumen through the cricothyroid membrane.

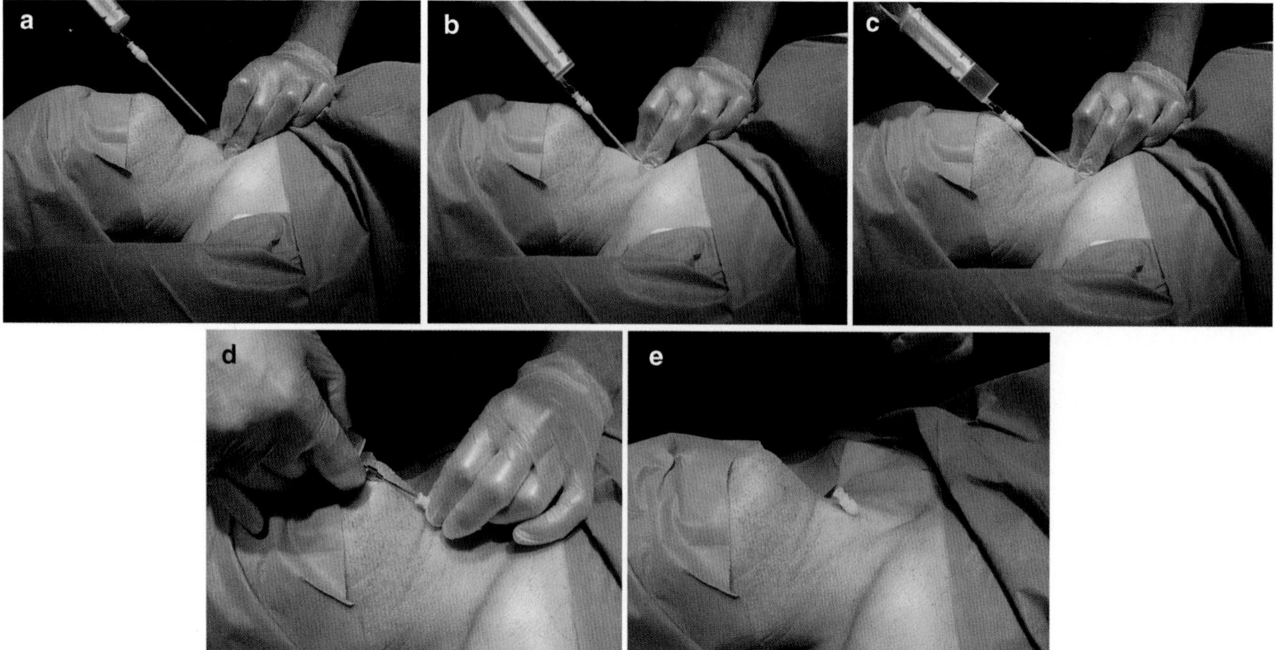

Figure 13.24. (a) Initiating puncture with the Cook catheter. The operator's nondominant hand firmly secures the larynx in the midline, marking the location of the cricothyroid membrane and avoiding any displacement during cannulation. (b) One advances the needle while stabilizing the larynx and continuously aspirating, so that entry into the trachea can be detected. (c) Loss of resistance to aspiration as the needle is advanced marks entry into the tracheal lumen. (d) Holding the needle firmly, one slides the catheter off the needle and further into the trachea. (e) Final placement of the catheter in the trachea, prior to being held in place by hand or by suturing the hub to the skin.

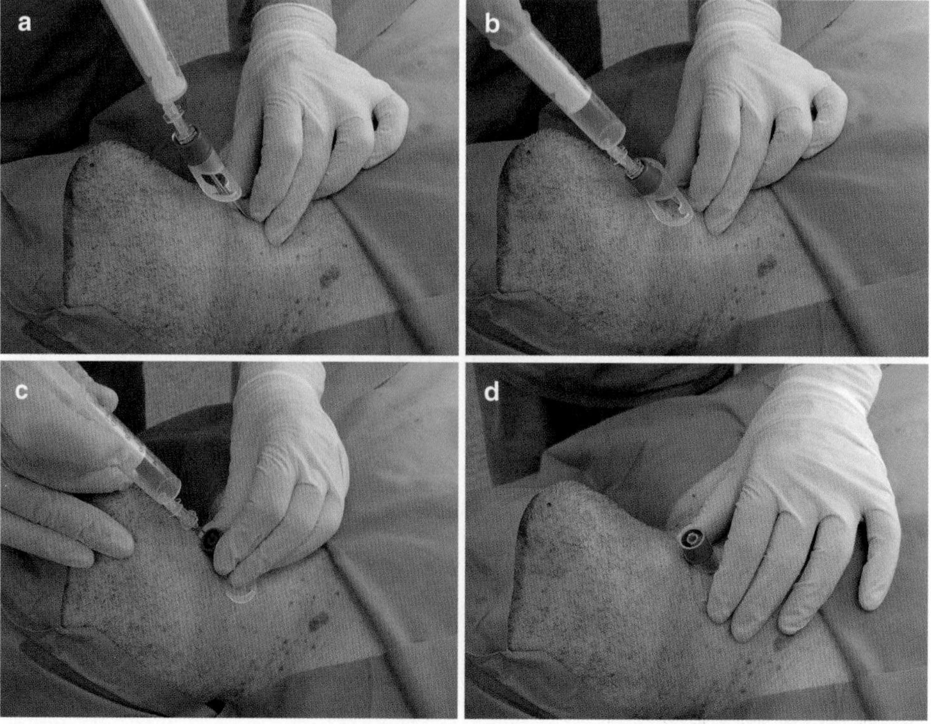

Figure 13.25. (a) Puncture with the Ravussin catheter. The nondominant hand stabilizes the larynx. (b) Upon perceiving the loss of resistance one aspirates into the syringe. The free entry of air confirms the position of the needle tip in the tracheal lumen. (c) One keeps the needle stable and advances the catheter. The trajectory of the catheter is guided by the curvature of the needle. (d) Final placement of the Ravussin catheter in the trachea, ready for jet ventilation.

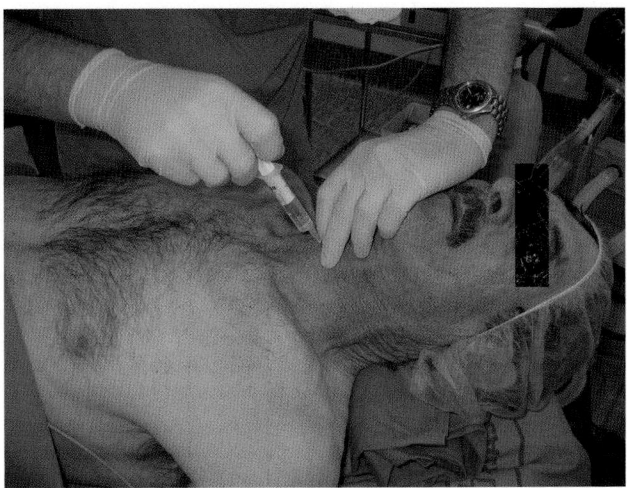

Figure 13.26. Patient awake, not in extremis. While performing injection of local anesthesia in the cricothyroid membrane and tracheal mucosa, the operator should keep the neck extended and the larynx stabilized.

kinking. Extension may need to be limited in patients with cervical trauma or known vertebral lesions.

2. If the patient is not in extremis, the site should be *prepped* with an appropriate skin disinfectant, and *local anesthetic* should be injected (see Figure 13.26).
3. *Locate* and *stabilize* the cricothyroid membrane. In general, right-handed clinicians should perform the procedure from the patient's left side, holding the larynx firmly between the middle finger and thumb of the left hand so as to permit localization of the depression that marks the site of the membrane.
4. *Puncture* the skin in the midline, tilting the catheter hub and syringe toward the patient's chin, with the tip angled dorsally and caudally. The clinician should keep the longitudinal axis of the trachea in mind during the puncture. The straight catheter should enter the skin at a 30° angle to the skin, and the entry point should be superior to the proximal edge of the cricoid cartilage. If using a curved catheter, a wider angle with the skin could be necessary to easily enter the trachea[35].
5. *Aspirate* air during insertion, or after feeling the loss of resistance when the tip of the needle enters the trachea (see Figure 13.27a, b). One author recommends using a 20 cc syringe so that the loss of resistance is more easily appreciated as the catheter is advanced[36]. One can aspirate air into an empty syringe or into a syringe half-filled with IV fluid (see Figure 13.28). The latter option allows the clinician to appreciate bubbling into the syringe as the needle enters the tracheal lumen. If the catheter is not advanced a few millimeters after bubbles first appear, the catheter itself may not have fully penetrated the membrane and it may shear off as it is threaded off the needle. To avoid injuring or even perforating the membranous trachea as the needle is advanced, the syringe should be tipped cephalad so that the needle enters along a shallower angle to the skin.
6. *Slide* the catheter off the needle. The needle must not be withdrawn as the catheter is advanced. It serves as a Seldinger guide for the catheter during placement. The needle and catheter *should never be* advanced together, as this risks tracheal injury or perforation. As the needle is held carefully in place, the catheter should be advanced to the hub.
7. *Aspirate* air after having withdrawn the needle keeping the catheter hub flush to the skin. In a spontaneously breathing patient, reconfirm placement with end-tidal CO_2 (see Figure 13.29)[31].
8. *Secure* the catheter. In emergencies, the catheter is likely to be most secure when firmly held by an assistant (see Figure 13.30)[36]. Frantic efforts to secure the catheter in other ways may be unsuccessful and may delay the initiation of ventilation. If the catheter is not firmly held or otherwise secured, the pressure jets may cause it to be dislodged. In

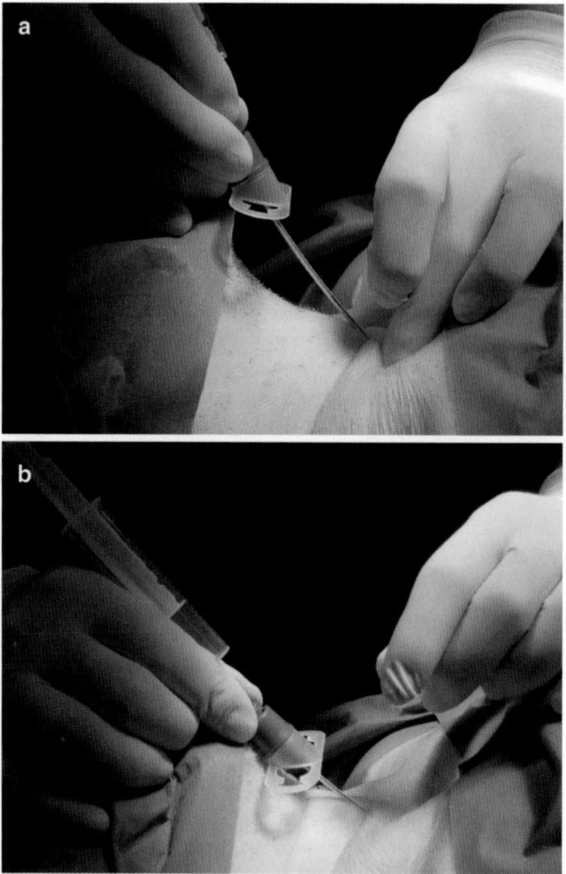

Figure 13.27. (**a**) Aspiration can be done after feeling the loss of resistance when the tip of the needle enters the trachea. (**b**) Always strive to keep the larynx stable, concentrate on the spatial orientation of the trachea, be attentive to the perception of resistance to the needle's advance, and above all be extremely cautious if the needle doesn't advance easily and one experiences difficulty aspirating air.

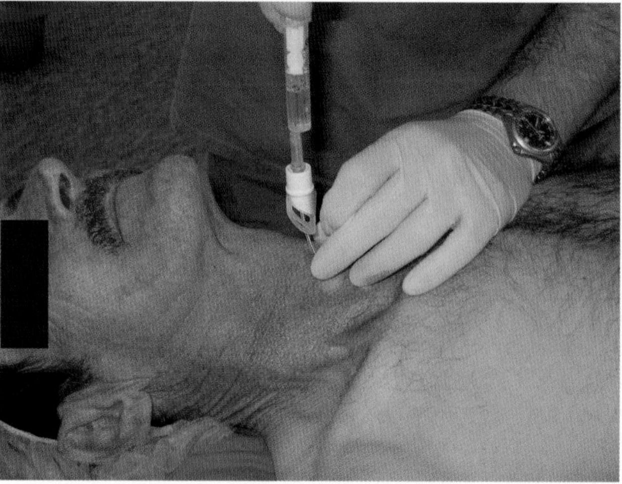

Figure 13.28. Transcricoid puncture in an awake patient before elective transtracheal ventilation. Tracheal entry can be appreciated by air bubbles that enter the fluid-filled syringe. At other times in which a fluid-filled syringe may not be available (e.g., emergencies) tracheal entry can be appreciated by a loss of resistance to aspiration as the needle is advanced. The sensation is comparable to that experienced when blood suddenly fills a syringe that enters a major vessel, such as the internal jugular or femoral vein.

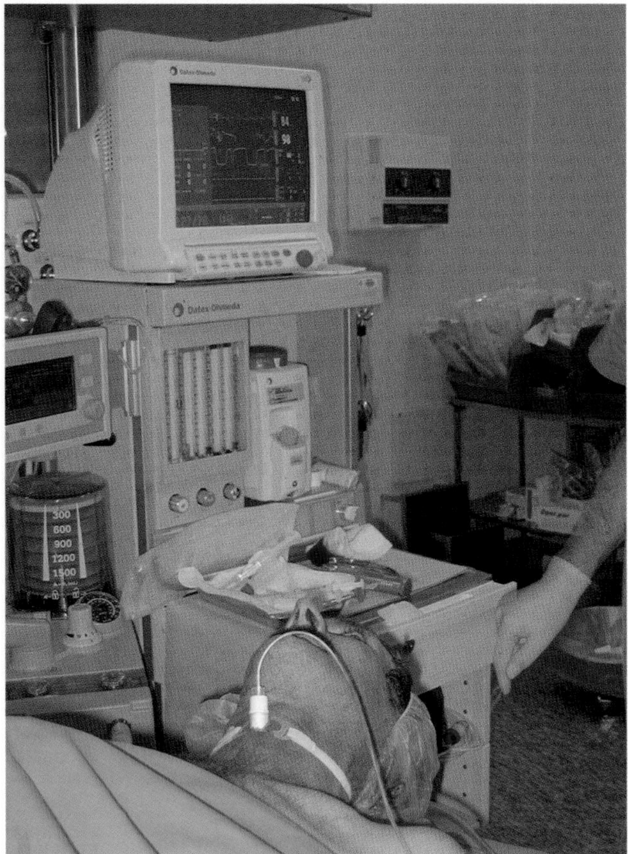

Figure 13.29. Confirming intratracheal catheter placement with capnography: the capnograph is connected to the transtracheal catheter and capnographic tracings are seen on the monitor during the patient's spontaneous respiration.

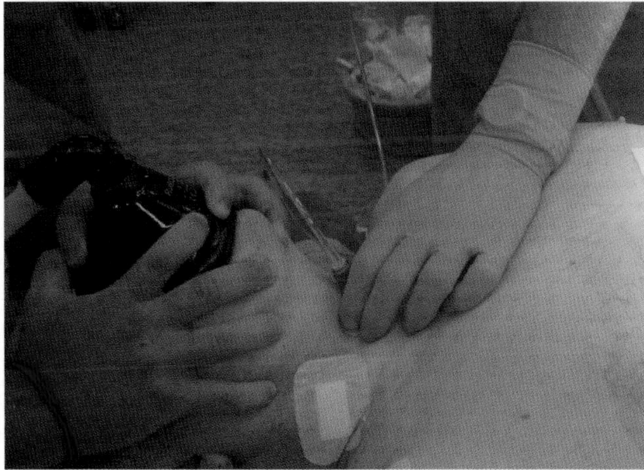

Figure 13.30. TTJV during management of an emergent airway. Also apparent is the difficult mask ventilation, performed in this case with a two-handed mask grip.

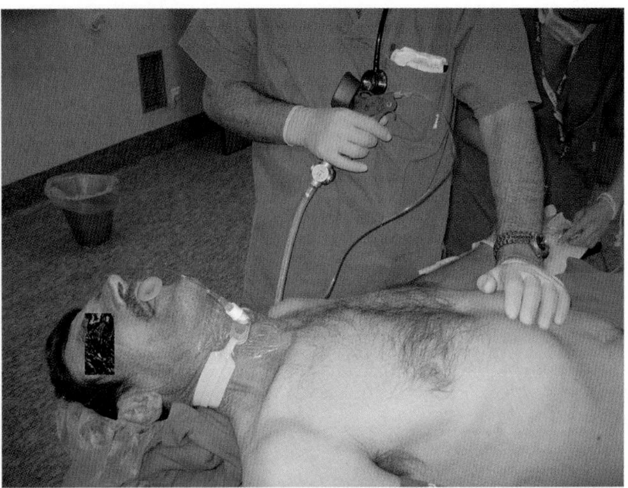

Figure 13.31. During TTJV in an anesthetized patient the upper airway is kept open with an oral airway. At the same time one listens for exhalation, and observes chest rise and fall with each jet insufflation. Palpation is another way to detect entry and exit of gas.

elective situations, the airway should be secured using the simplest technique that is appropriate. Some catheters come with side phalanges that permit a ribbon to be used to anchor the catheter using the circumference of the neck (see Figure 13.31). Others, such as the Cook, should be secured by tying 0-silk around the hub and suturing this to the pre-tracheal skin.

Ventilation Technique

As noted above, low-frequency manual jet injectors are most commonly used when the indication for TTJV is anticipatory management of a difficult airway or rescue of a hypoxic patient. In general, the rule with LFJV is to use low respiratory rates (6–14 breaths/min) with short inspiratory and long expiratory times (high I:E ratios—1:3, 1:4). Driving pressures as low as 7.5–15 psi (0.5–1 bar, 527–1.054 cm H_2O) are sufficient to emergently oxygenate the great majority of patients. Any hypercapnia that develops can be tolerated without significant adverse effects for 10–14 min. Factors such as airway resistance, thoracic compliance, and patient size influence the driving pressure that is required; for this reason it is recommended that one begin with low pressure and increase it according to the clinical response[10]. A manual jet injector must include a pressure regulator (see Figure 13.10a, b), which should be initially set between 15 and 30 psi (1.054–2.109 cm H_2O) in order to reduce the risk of barotrauma[14].

One must closely observe the degree and symmetry of thoracic expansion and retraction, as well as listen for exit of gas through the mouth, or using a stethoscope, through the larynx (see Figure 13.31). Any of the following are very worrisome signs: decreased or asymmetric thoracic expansion, changes in gas outflow, changes in pulmonary or cardiac auscultation, the sensation of crepitus or appearance of subcutaneous emphysema on the neck or over the chest, jugular venous distension, and tracheal shift. One must also maintain a high level of suspicion for barotrauma should there be any unexpected hemodynamic changes, such as hypotension, tachycardia, or bradycardia.

For children between 2 and 10 years of age pressure should be kept at less than 30 psi (<2 atm or 200 kPa, 2,100 cm H_2O). For children less than 2 years of age, a manual bag should be used[34]. Given that pulmonary expansion cannot be reliably predicted from airway pressures in children, there are those who recommend that ventilation be continuously monitored by having the clinician place his or her hand on the patient's chest, in addition to continuously confirming exhalation of gas[37].

Complications

Few serious TTJV complications have been described but certainly such complications are underreported[11]. As with many procedures, TTJV is safest under elective conditions and most dangerous when used during emergencies[17,29]. No data about delayed sequelae have been reported, possibly because injuries related to TTJV often appear immediately. Complications include:

1. *Barotrauma*, which may result from one or more of the following:
   (a) Expiratory phase: exhalation is too brief, leading to progressive gas entrapment. This can occur because of an obstructing mass lesion or inflammatory process, glottic closure, or lack of sufficient time for exhalation (e.g., in emphysematous patients). This is particularly likely to occur when compliance and resistance are high such that more gas enters than leaves leading to elevated peak pressures or pulmonary hyperinflation, which in turn can lead to alveolar rupture[30,38].
   (b) Inspiratory phase: TTJV is administered using excessive driving pressures or inspiratory times, which give rise to very high tidal volumes and peak pressures.
   (c) Insufflated gas dissects through the tissues via the cricothyroid membrane puncture site, sometimes resulting in pulmonary interstitial emphysema. Occasionally this can occur in the post-anesthesia care unit after a paroxysm of coughing[39].
2. *Direct trauma from the needle or catheter tip*. Examples include puncture of the posterior tracheal wall with creation of a tracheo-esophageal fistula, hematoma from a local vascular injury, or hemoptysis.
3. *Extraluminal injection*. The tip of the catheter is placed outside the tracheal lumen or migrates outside the lumen (e.g., if the catheter is not adequately secured) and insufflates the tissues of the neck. Undetected communication with the GI tract can cause massive inflation with risk of gastric rupture[40].
4. *Technical error or equipment malfunction*:
   — Ventilation impossible because of catheter kinking.
   — The catheter is oriented *cephalad* rather than caudally. This occurs in up to 20% of all attempts at tracheal catheterization[41].
   — Failure to place the catheter[30,31].
5. *Local injury*:
   — Tracheal erosion secondary to prolonged ventilation without humidification.
   — Infection at the puncture site[42].
6. *Insufficient ventilation* with a correctly placed catheter:
   — Hypoventilation secondary to an inadequate respiratory rate or driving pressure (minute volume too low).
   — Arterial oxygen desaturation. This may be seen when using low FiO_2 (e.g., during laser surgery because of flammability concerns) or in patients prone to developing atelectasis (e.g., obese patients).

Analysis and Prevention of Complications

In order to be able to obtain the maximum benefit from TTJV we recommend that clinicians take certain precautions to avoid complications that, although infrequent, occur more often than with conventional ventilation[43]. Because the first published work in the 1970s pointed to a high rate of injuries associated with TTJV, the technique was viewed with mistrust. The publications that followed in the 1980s permitted TTJV to be viewed as relatively safe, particularly if used in elective situations[38]. Most of the information about jet ventilation relates to its elective use in the field of perilaryngeal surgery, where it has worked well in conjunction with laser techniques.

Gerig et al. placed 154 transtracheal catheters in elective cases, using a flexible fiberoptic bronchoscope to observe and guide placement. Of the 154, 100 were placed through the cricothyroid membrane, and 54 entered the tracheal lumen between either the cricoid ring and first tracheal ring or the first and second tracheal rings. When the catheter entered through the cricothyroid membrane, it made contact with the membranous trachea in 9% of cases and caused damage to it in 1%. In the 54 cases in which the catheter entered the trachea below the cricothyroid membrane, the respective rates of contact and damage were 18% and 2% (p = n.s.)[44].

Bourgain et al. conducted a multicenter prospective study of 643 patients who underwent elective laryngeal procedures with high-frequency transtracheal jet ventilation. This group was unable to place the catheter in 0.3% of the cases. Of the remaining patients, 8.4% developed subcutaneous emphysema, 2.5% developed pneumomediastinum, and 1% developed pneumothorax. The use of a microprocessor that prevented the initiation of a breath until airway pressure fell below a preset value did not avoid this low incidence of complications[30].

Jaquet et al. published a retrospective study including 534 microlaryngoscopies in which jet ventilation was employed using transtracheal jet ventilation ($n = 265$) or jet ventilation from above through the glottis ($n = 469$). Most complications occurred during jet ventilation. Patients ventilated with transtracheal catheters experienced complications in 7.5% of cases vs. 1.7% of those ventilated with glottic ones. Of four cases with serious barotrauma, three were with transcricoid catheters. It is important to be mindful that these authors were extremely experienced with such modes of ventilation, using the Ravussin cannula which they had designed, an Acutronic jet ventilator rather than a manually cycled one, and a larynx stented in the open position by a rigid laryngoscope or bronchoscope, barotrauma still occurred. (Once the ventilation catheter and laryngoscope were properly positioned, the ventilation frequency was increased to 150–300/min with a driving pressure 1–3 bar [15–45 psi].) The authors note that laryngospasm was an important dynamic cause of expiratory obstruction that resulted in barotrauma. They advise that the airway manager remain vigilant about laryngospasm[39], however any cause of airway outflow obstruction, such as recovery of spontaneous vocal cord movement from insufficient relaxation can produce the same consequences.

It is notable that all these studies refer to the elective OR situation, and that even in these circumstances serious complications occur with some frequency. It is easy to understand that during a respiratory emergency the combination of psychological stress and lack of time makes problems more likely to occur, as is true for any other procedure. In all circumstances, understanding the fundamentals of jet ventilation, together with frequent practice, combine to allow the clinician to safely employ the technique[43].

In addition to being mindful of the contraindications and precautions already discussed, airway managers must take many patient-related factors and practices into account when performing TTJV. First, respiratory and hemodynamic monitoring is critical, and is as much clinical as instrumental. In elective cases, and when possible in emergencies, pulse oximetry, end tidal or transcutaneous capnometry, airway pressure monitoring, rhythm and frequent blood pressure monitoring should be performed. Neuromuscular monitoring should also be considered to ensure adequate relaxation.

In patients with effacement of anatomic landmarks of the neck because of masses, scars, extreme cervical flexion, or previous radiotherapy, transcricoid puncture can be difficult, and dangerous. Clinicians must be especially cautious in these cases and in those that present with glottic or supraglottic airway obstruction. Complete expiratory obstruction is an absolute contraindication to jet ventilation[30].

Inspiratory obstruction is more frequent than expiratory obstruction. When a patient is breathing spontaneously, through a normal airway, and there is incomplete airway obstruction, the upper airway tends to collapse during inspiration. During expiration positive intraluminal pressure tends to expand and open the upper airway. For the reasons described above, TTJV should be administered with fast inspiration at the lowest possible pressure consistent with adequate ventilation followed by slow expiration[39,45].

Trauma patients, especially if they have thoracic injury, should also be considered to be at higher risk for barotrauma. Patients who are obese or who have decreased thoracic compliance will also have greater propensity to hypoventilation and can require higher driving pressures that exceed those recommended for avoiding barotrauma. Patients with COPD, asthma, or other obstructive pulmonary disease, especially when the obstructive pathology is accompanied by increased thoracic distensibility, are prone to developing air trapping and high positive end-expiratory pressures, so, in theory, have a higher risk of barotrauma with TTJV[39]. However, studies have not lent support to the idea that patients with COPD experience more barotrauma complications[46]. Perhaps this is because of the heterogeneity of patients as well as the techniques used and operator experience. Some authors who use HFJV advocate the use of manually controlled breaths with LFJV before initiating high-frequency ventilation in order to avoid peaks in pressure secondary to obstruction of the outflow of gas.

Multiple attempts at cricoid puncture increases the risk that insufflated gases will dissect along the tissue planes of the neck. This highlights the need for careful placement and limited attempts[39]. Although most difficulties with cricothyroid puncture occur in relation to abnormal anatomy, it is important to follow general guidelines about catheter selection and technique in all cases. The catheter itself should be kink-resistant and designed so that it orients itself caudally in the trachea[15,35]. Some authors recommend using a guide in order to assure that the catheter points toward the distal trachea[41]. As noted above, some anesthesiologists perform cricoid puncture under endoscopic guidance with the patient anesthetized[10,30,44], or while protecting the trachea with a rigid bronchoscope[39]. Finally, the catheter must be firmly secured to prevent migration or deformation (see Figure 13.31). The operator or an assistant may even need to hold the catheter firmly against the neck while using the other hand to trigger the ventilator (see Figure 13.30).

As mentioned above, "baro-volutrauma" is the risk most associated with jet ventilation, and airway managers must be vigilant to minimize this risk. Despite numerous case reports, the true incidence of this complication is unknown. It is inevitable that it will occasionally occur[47]. As discussed above, Jaquet et al. reported four cases of serious barotrauma in 1,093 cases. Three of the four occurred with transtracheal catheters[39], a trend that is consistent with other reports that the complication is more frequent with this route than when the trachea is accessed through the glottis[43].

To protect against barotrauma, it is critical to perform careful airway assessment when possible. Airway edema, caused by trauma, infection, or allergic reactions may impede the exit of gas, as may hematoma, abscess, and mass lesions. The size, shape, and location of a mass all affect jet ventilation, as does the existence of associated fibrosis or edema that can reduce the caliber of the airway. In order to mitigate upper airway obstruction, one relies on the maneuvers familiar to any airway manager—placement of oral or nasal airways, mandibular subluxation, chin-lift, and head tilt. If exhalation of gas is not appreciated after opening the airway, jet ventilation must be suspended immediately and other means of accessing the airway must be initiated, such as surgical or dilatational cricothyrotomy[14,39].

Barotrauma during jet ventilation can manifest with alarming rapidity in the form of subcutaneous emphysema, pneumomediastinum, pneumothorax, or even pneumoperitoneum[48]. Subcutaneous emphysema will quickly obscure the surface landmarks and make corrective measures even more challenging. The expectation that one will appreciate classical finding of absent breath sounds on the affected side may be dangerously misleading in the event of a tension pneumothorax. Clinicians may attribute whistling or wheezing-like respiratory sounds to bronchospasm. In fact, these sounds may be made by air dissecting around tissue planes and insufflating the soft tissues of the face, neck, mediastinum, and thorax. Failure to correctly identify these sounds, prevent further tissue insufflation, and decompress involved structures may lead to tension pneumothorax, pneumomediastinum, or other immediately life-threatening events.

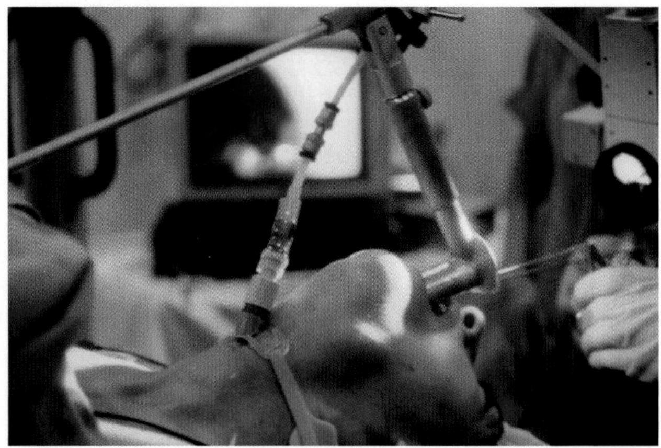

Figure 13.32. Use of high-frequency jet ventilation during laryngeal microsurgery. There must be optimal coordination between the anesthesiologist and the surgeon. Incautious maneuvers may damage the catheter or result in a serious expiratory obstruction. The anesthesiologist must avoid insufflation during periods of critical glottic obstruction (e.g., laryngospasm, hemostatic procedures, etc.).

The anesthesiologist must be vigilant about identifying a catheter that has been displaced, for example, after a paroxysm of coughing. To avoid this some authors administer a dose of local anesthesia through the catheter[14] or advise that the patient be kept at a sufficiently deep anesthetic plane and maintained on a neuromuscular blocker during the surgery. The earliest sign of inadequate muscle relaxation during the application of transtracheal jet ventilation is that the glottic muscles react to the impact of the jet of gas at the carina. This can be observed on the video monitor connected to the surgical microscope before airway pressure increases and even before one can appreciate any evoked motor activity at the forearm. This is a critical piece of information to be aware of during HFJV, because there is very little time to react to any obstruction[43].

Airway pressure monitoring, when coupled with an automatic end-expiratory pressure-triggered ventilation stop, offers additional safety. This feature is available on some ventilators. It protects patients should pulmonary over distension or glottic closure occur. The feature is especially useful in the face of airway obstruction, be it in the proximal airway because of masses and other space-occupying lesions, or because of obstructive bronchial disease in the lungs. Obstruction at either level predisposes to air entrapment[49] and in COPD patients the end-expiratory pressure may not follow pulmonary volumes, and there may be great differences between alveolar and tracheal pressures[50].

Observation of chest wall movement is useful for detecting hypoventilation, and this information should be taken very seriously, especially in an emergency. To exactly quantify the degree of hypoventilation, arterial blood gas, gas exhaled across a catheter, or a transcutaneous CO_2 sensor can be used. Hypoventilation can be corrected by increasing the frequency of ventilation with a manual jet ventilator or by increasing the driving pressure with a high-frequency ventilator.

Desaturation should improve after one corrects any treatable cause of the problem, such as pulmonary edema. If the FiO_2 is less than 100%, increasing it to 100% can improve the saturation, although the normal course of action is to increase the degree of insufflation by adjusting driving pressure and respiratory rate, which can lead to greater alveolar recruitment.

A final note with regard to avoiding complications is that there must be optimal coordination between the anesthesiologist and the surgeon and planning for the immediate postoperative period. Incautious maneuvers may damage the catheter or result in a serious expiratory obstruction (see Figure 13.32). The anesthesiologist must avoid insufflation during periods of critical glottic obstruction (e.g., laryngospasm, hemostatic procedures, etc.). It is advisable that patients be allowed to awaken while being ventilated with a face or laryngeal mask, and that the transcricoid catheter be left in place during the immediate postoperative period[39].

Drawbacks of TTJV with Respect to Surgical or Dilatational Cricothyroidotomy

Although placement of a transcricoid catheter is simpler and faster than either cricothyroidotomy method, TTJV requires a nonstandard ventilation technique using specialized equipment and carries a greater risk of barotrauma on the one hand, or hypoventilation on the other. In addition a thin-walled catheter is more likely to kink and has a greater predisposition to be displaced from the tracheal lumen than does a tube that is equal to or larger than 4 mm ID, and the catheter, unlike contemporary surgical and dilatational cricothyroidotomy tubes (e.g., cuffed Cook Melker tube, Cook Medical, Bloomington IN) does not seal the airway from the pharynx. Without this, there is no barrier against aspiration, nor is tracheobronchial suctioning possible. Only with HFJV, because there is nearly constant efflux of gas, may there be some protection against aspiration[51].

In the final analysis, TTJV is a very useful ventilatory technique that carries a high risk of barotrauma-related morbidity. The risk is low, and generally acceptable, if one:

1. Understands the fundamentals of the technique.
2. Masters the procedure in elective circumstances or in appropriate practice scenarios before using it in an emergency.
3. Monitors ventilation with the necessary vigilance.

Appendix: Approximate Measures of Pressure

1 atm (1bar) = 1 kg/cm2 (1.033 kg/cm2) = 100 kPa (101.3 kPa) = 15 psi (14.69 psi) = 1000 cmH2O = 760 mmHg

Physiology and Mechanism of Action

Tidal volume (V_t), is the sum of the volume of the jet of gas (V_j) that is insufflated from the catheter and the volume of gas entrained by the venturi effect (V_e), minus the gas which escapes from the airway or "spilt volume" (V_s). So, $V_t = (V_j + V_e) - V_s$ (see Figure 13.33).

Generally speaking, V_j increases as driving pressure increases. Manual ventilation at high pressure (>3 bar or 45 psi) using a 14 or 16G catheter can result in flows that exceed 500 cc/s.

V_e is generated by the gas flow that escapes from the catheter at high velocity. This results in negative tracheal pressure relative to the surrounding atmosphere (Venturi effect), which in turn "entrains" or drags adjacent gasses into the airway. V_e theoretically could add significantly to the volume of inspiration contributed by V_j, but in practice, aspiration and entrainment of gas are thought to be minimal with TTJV[52].

V_s results from the increase in intrathoracic pressure that occurs as gas enters the chest during inspiration. This volume of gas is subtracted from the volume that reaches the respiratory tree ($V_j + V_e$) because ventilation occurs in a system that is open proximally. The more compliant the chest wall and/or the lungs, as well as the less resistance offered by the airway, the smaller V_s will be.

The inspiratory phase of TTJV occurs via insufflation of oxygen or air under pressure. Expiration is passive, a function of the elastic recoil of the lungs, pleura, and tracheal wall. Tidal volumes and peak inspiratory pressures observed during manual TTJV or LFJV are similar to those observed with intermittent positive pressure ventilation through an endotracheal tube. In contrast, HFJV administers low tidal volumes with lower corresponding peak inspiratory pressures than LFJV (see Figure 13.34).

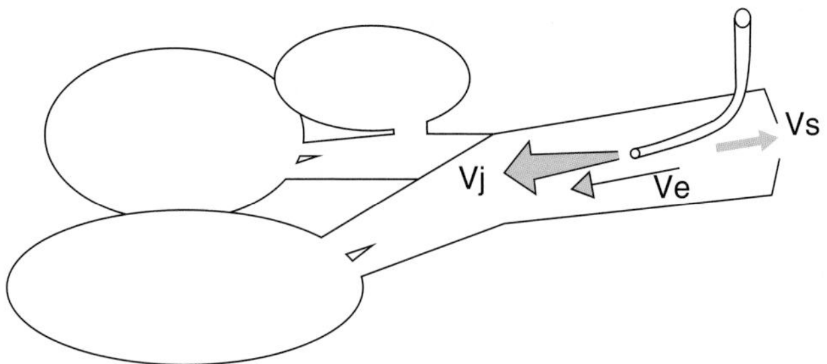

Figure 13.33. Schematic view of the trachea, lung, and transtracheal catheter during inspiration. V_j jet volume; V_e entrainment volume; V_s spilt volume or backflow gas.

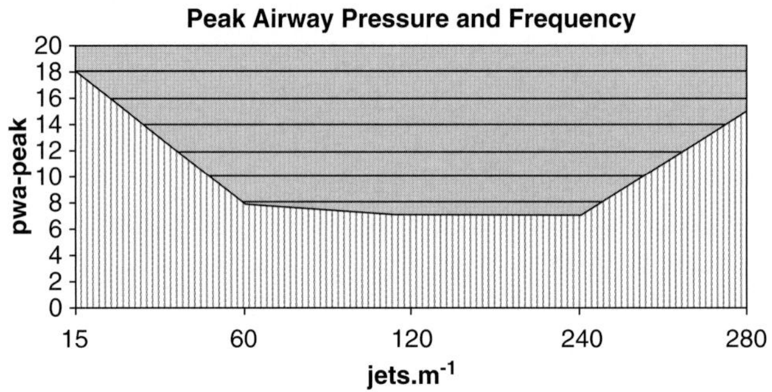

Figure 13.34. This chart shows the U-shaped relationship between frequency of jet insufflation and peak airway pressure (Paw), holding other variables constant. With low frequencies, Paw values are similar to those observed during conventional positive pressure ventilation. With higher frequencies Paw falls, but it increases again when frequency is extremely high.

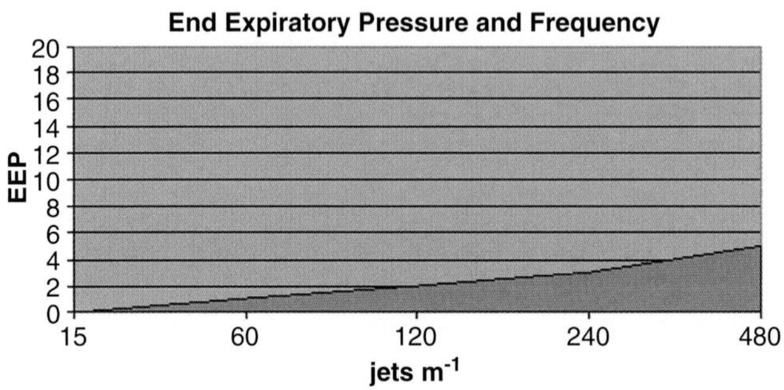

Figure 13.35. This chart shows the relationship between frequency of jet insufflation and end-expiratory pressure (EEP), holding other variables constant. End-expiratory pressure (EEP) rises progressively with as frequency rises.

Peak inspiratory pressure depends on various factors that are amenable to manipulation by the clinician's adjustments to the jet ventilator. These include driving (or working) pressure and inspiratory time, which determine the volume insufflated with each triggering of the ventilator. This pressure is also determined by "fixed" patient and equipment related factors. These include the diameter of the trachea, the diameter and length of the catheter that one has inserted, any obstruction to efflux of gas from the airway, and, as with V_s, pulmonary and chest wall compliance. For example, the pediatric tracheal diameter is smaller than the adult and this predisposes children to having higher tracheal pressures.

The generation of auto-PEEP is often associated with insufficient expiratory time, a function of respiratory rate (see Figure 13.35) and I:E ratio, particularly if it coexists with tracheal, or proximal laryngeal stenosis that limits expiratory flow and gives rise to intrapulmonary gas entrapment. This situation predisposes patients to barotrauma and decreases systemic venous blood return to the heart[17,53–55].

Maintaining One's Skills

When a technique is not incorporated into one's normal practice, it is very improbable that one will be able to employ it correctly in a situation with maximum risk, maximum urgency, and a great deal of psychological stress. In addition, TTJV is unsafe in inexpert hands. The need to resort to the cricothyroid approach is unusual, but it may save a life. Because we are authorized to induce apnea, we are also obliged to prepare ourselves to use TTJV to rescue patients if that becomes necessary.

The first set of recommendations concerns equipment. We must familiarize ourselves with the equipment described above, and have certified, not improvised ventilators, catheters, and tubing. Any ventilator must be equipped with a pressure regulator.

The second set of recommendations relates to training. Airway managers should arrange regular practice, timing the procedure and noting any failures or obstacles to mastering the procedure that arise. We must also bear in mind that procedural skills decay with the passage of time[56,57] so that any skills gained in practice must be periodically refreshed. To this end, training may be carried out in a variety of airway models, including manikins[58], improvised laryngotracheal simulators, pig or goat tracheas, or in the best existing model: human cadavers[59].

The third set of recommendations concerns different ways to maintain one's skills by performing related procedures when indicated. Patients who are to be intubated awake benefit from transcricoid administration of local anesthetic. Anesthesiologists and other airway managers often have the opportunity to assist surgeons during OR tracheotomies, particularly when it is not emergent. Finally, in the ICU or PACU, there are frequent opportunities to practice the tracheal approach by performing dilatational tracheostomy.

The fourth set of recommendations is the most accessible of all: routinely practice identifying the anatomic structures of the anterior neck. During the preoperative airway assessment, or even before performing intubation in the ICU or ED, we typically acquaint ourselves with the anatomy that we will soon manage, becoming familiar with any difficulties that may present themselves. Identifying the landmarks relevant to TTJV and to cricothyroidotomy will make us that much more ready to act in the event that we need to perform these life-saving procedures.

References

1. Reed JP, Kemph JP, Hamelberg W, Hitchcock FA, Jacoby J. Studies with transtracheal artificial resuscitation. Anesthesiology. 1954;15(1):28–41.
2. Flory FA, Hamelberg W, Jacoby JJ, Jones JR, Ziegler CH. Transtracheal resuscitation. J Am Med Assoc. 1956;162(7):625–8.
3. Spoerel WE, Narayanan PS, Singh NP. Transtracheal ventilation. Br J Anaesth. 1971; 43(10):932–9.
4. Klain M, Smith RB. High frequency percutaneous transtracheal jet ventilation. Crit Care Med. 1977;5(6):280–7.
5. Heidegger T, Gerig HJ, Henderson JJ. Strategies and algorithms for management of the difficult airway. Best Pract Res Clin Anaesthesiol. 2005;19(4):661–74.
6. American Society of Anesthesiologists Task Force on Management of the Difficult Airway. Practice guidelines for management of the difficult airway: an updated report by the American Society of Anesthesiologists Task Force on Management of the Difficult Airway. Anesthesiology. 2003;98(5):1269–77.

7. Benumof JL. Management of the difficult adult airway. With special emphasis on awake tracheal intubation. Anesthesiology. 1991;75(6):1087–110.
8. Melker RJ, Kost KM. Percutaneous dilational cricothyrotomy and tracheostomy. In: Hagber C, editor. Benumof's airway management: principles and practice. 2nd ed. Philadelphia: Mosby Elsevier; 2007. p. 640–77.
9. Manoach S, Corinaldi C, Paladino L, Schulze R, Charchaflieh J, Lewin J, et al. Percutaneous transcricoid jet ventilation compared with surgical cricothyroidotomy in a sheep airway salvage model. Resuscitation. 2004;62(1):79–87.
10. Gerig HJ, Schnider T, Heidegger T. Prophylactic percutaneous transtracheal catheterisation in the management of patients with anticipated difficult airways: a case series. Anaesthesia. 2005;60(8):801–5.
11. Boyce JR, Peters GE, Carroll WR, Magnuson JS, McCrory A, Boudreaux AM. Preemptive vessel dilator cricothyrotomy aids in the management of upper airway obstruction. Can J Anaesth. 2005;52(7):765–9.
12. Chandradeva K, Palin C, Ghosh SM, Pinches SC. Percutaneous transtracheal jet ventilation as a guide to tracheal intubation in severe upper airway obstruction from supraglottic oedema. Br J Anaesth. 2005;94(5):683–6.
13. Evans KL, Keene MH, Bristow AS. High-frequency jet ventilation—a review of its role in laryngology. J Laryngol Otol. 1994;108(1):23–5.
14. Gulleth Y, Spiro J. Percutaneous transtracheal jet ventilation in head and neck surgery. Arch Otolaryngol Head Neck Surg. 2005;131(10):886–90.
15. Vadodaria BS, Gandhi SD, McIndoe AK. Comparison of four different emergency airway access equipment sets on a human patient simulator. Anaesthesia. 2004;59(1):73–9.
16. Yealy DM, Stewart RD, Kaplan RM. Myths and pitfalls in emergency translaryngeal ventilation: correcting misimpressions. Ann Emerg Med. 1988;17(7):690–2.
17. Benumof JL, Scheller MS. The importance of transtracheal jet ventilation in the management of the difficult airway. Anesthesiology. 1989;71(5):769–78.
18. Ryder IG, Paoloni CC, Harle CC. Emergency transtracheal ventilation: assessment of breathing systems chosen by anaesthetists. Anaesthesia. 1996;51(8):764–8.
19. Morley D, Thorpe CM. Apparatus for emergency transtracheal ventilation. Anaesth Intensive Care. 1997;25(6):675–8.
20. Cook TM, Nolan JP, Magee PT, Cranshaw JH. Needle cricothyroidotomy. Anaesthesia. 2007;62(3):289–90.
21. Gaughan SD, Ozaki GT, Benumof JL. A Comparison in a lung model of low- and high-flow regulators for transtracheal jet ventilation. Anesthesiology. 1992;77(1):189–99.
22. Bould MD, Bearfield P. Techniques for emergency ventilation through a needle cricothyroidotomy. Anaesthesia. 2008;63(5):535–9.
23. Gaughan SD, Benumof JL, Ozaki GT. Can an anesthesia machine flush valve provide for effective jet ventilation? Anesth Analg. 1993;76(4):800–8.
24. Yildiz Y, Preussler NP, Schreiber T, Hueter L, Gaser E, Schubert H, et al. Percutaneous transtracheal emergency ventilation during respiratory arrest: comparison of the oxygen flow modulator with a hand-triggered emergency jet injector in an animal model. Am J Emerg Med. 2006;24(4):455–9.
25. Schaefer R, Hueter L, Preussler NP, Schreiber T, Schwarzkopf K. Percutaneous transtracheal emergency ventilation with a self-made device in an animal model. Paediatr Anaesth. 2007;17(10):972–6.
26. Hamaekers A, Borg P, Enk D. The importance of flow and pressure release in emergency jet ventilation devices. Paediatr Anaesth. 2009;19(5):452–7.
27. Ravussin P, Freeman J. A new transtracheal catheter for ventilation as resuscitation. Can Anaesth Soc J. 1985;32(1):60–4.
28. Dhara SS, Liu EH, Tan KH. Monitored transtracheal jet ventilation using a triple lumen central venous catheter. Anaesthesia. 2002;57(6):578–81.
29. Patel RG. Percutaneous transtracheal jet ventilation: a safe, quick, and temporary way to provide oxygenation and ventilation when conventional methods are unsuccessful. Chest. 1999;116(6):1689–94.
30. Bourgain JL, Desruennes E, Fischler M, Ravussin P. Transtracheal high frequency jet ventilation for endoscopic airway surgery: a multicentre study. Br J Anaesth. 2001;87(6):870–5.

31. Russell WC, Maguire AM, Jones GW. Cricothyroidotomy and transtracheal high frequency jet ventilation for elective laryngeal surgery. An audit of 90 cases. Anaesth Intensive Care. 2000;28(1):62–7.
32. Boon JM, Abrahams PH, Meiring JH, Welch T. Cricothyroidotomy: a clinical anatomy review. Clin Anat. 2004;17(6):478–86.
33. Gibbs MA, Walls RM. Surgical airway. In: Hagber C, editor. Benumof's airway management: principles and practice. 2nd ed. Philadelphia: Mosby Elsevier; 2007. p. 678–96.
34. Walls RM, Gibbs MA. Surgical airway. In: Katz RL, Patel RV, editors. Seminars in anesthesia, perioperative medicine and pain—the difficult airway, vol. 20(3). Philadelphia: Saunders; 2001. p. 183–92.
35. Sdrales L, Benumof JL. Prevention of kinking of a percutaneous transtracheal intravenous catheter. Anesthesiology. 1995;82(1):288–91.
36. Rosenblatt W, Benumof J. Transtracheal jet ventilation via percutaneous catheter and high pressure source. In: Hagber C, editor. Benumof's airway management: principles and practice. 2nd ed. Philadelphia: Mosby Elsevier; 2007. p. 616–30.
37. Depierraz B, Ravussin P, Brossard E, Monnier P. Percutaneous transtracheal jet ventilation for paediatric endoscopic laser treatment of laryngeal and subglottic lesions. Can J Anaesth. 1994;41(12):1200–7.
38. Weymuller Jr EA, Pavlin EG, Paugh D, Cummings CW. Management of difficult airway problems with percutaneous transtracheal ventilation. Ann Otol Rhinol Laryngol. 1987;96(1 Pt 1):34–7.
39. Jaquet Y, Monnier P, Van Melle G, Ravussin P, Spahn DR, Chollet-Rivier M. Complications of different ventilation strategies in endoscopic laryngeal surgery: a 10-year review. Anesthesiology. 2006;104(1):52–9.
40. Gilbert TB. Gastric rupture after inadvertent esophageal intubation with a jet ventilation catheter. Anesthesiology. 1998;88(2):537–8.
41. Higgs A, Vijayanand P. Prophylactic percutaneous transtracheal catheterisation. Anaesthesia. 2005;60(12):1245–6.
42. Smith RB, Schaer WB, Pfaeffle H. Percutaneous transtracheal ventilation for anesthesia and resuscitation: a review and report of complications. Can Anaesth Soc J. 1975;22(5):607–12.
43. Cozine K, Stone JG, Shulman S, Flaster ER. Ventilatory complications of carbon dioxide laser laryngeal surgery. J Clin Anesth. 1991;3(1):20–5.
44. Gerig HJ, Heidegger T, Ulrich B, Grossenbacher R, Kreienbuehl G. Fiberoptically-guided insertion of transtracheal catheters. Anesth Analg. 2001;93(3):663–6.
45. Farmery AD. Physics and physiology. In: Calder I, Pearce A, editors. Core topics in airway management. Cambridge: Cambridge University Press; 2005. p. 35–42.
46. Desruennes E, Bourgain JL, Mamelle G, Luboinski B. Airway obstruction and high-frequency jet ventilation during laryngoscopy. Ann Otol Rhinol Laryngol. 1991;100(11):922–7.
47. Baer GA. Prevention of barotrauma during intratracheal jet ventilation. Anaesthesia. 1993;48(6):544–5.
48. Craft TM, Chambers PH, Ward ME, Goat VA. Two cases of barotrauma associated with transtracheal jet ventilation. Br J Anaesth. 1990;64(4):524–7.
49. McLeod AD, Turner MW, Torlot KJ, Chandradeva K, Palin C. Safety of transtracheal jet ventilation in upper airway obstruction. Br J Anaesth. 2005;95(4):560–1.
50. Bourgain JL, Desruennes E, Cosset MF, Mamelle G, Belaiche S, Truffa-Bachi J. Measurement of end-expiratory pressure during transtracheal high frequency jet ventilation for laryngoscopy. Br J Anaesth. 1990;65(6):737–43.
51. Klain M, Keszler H, Stool S. Transtracheal high frequency jet ventilation prevents aspiration. Crit Care Med. 1983;11(3):170–2.
52. Baer GA. No need for claims: facts rule performance of jet ventilation. Anesth Analg. 2000;91(4):1040–1.
53. O'Sullivan TJ, Healy GB. Complications of Venturi jet ventilation during microlaryngeal surgery. Arch Otolaryngol. 1985;111(2):127–31.
54. Standiford TJ, Morganroth ML. High-frequency ventilation. Chest. 1989;96(6):1380–9.
55. Young JD. Gas movement during jet ventilation. Acta Anaesthesiol Scand. 1989;33 Suppl 90:S72–4.
56. Prabhu AJ, Correa R, Wong DT, McGuire G, Chung F. What is the optimal training interval for a cricothyroidotomy? Can J Anaesth. 2001;48:A59.

57. Helm M, Gries A, Mutzbauer T. Surgical approach in difficult airway management. Best Pract Res Clin Anaesthesiol. 2005;19(4):623–40.
58. Wong DT, Prabhu AJ, Coloma M, Imasogie N, Chung FF. What is the minimum training required for successful cricothyroidotomy?: a study in mannequins. Anesthesiology. 2003;98(2):349–53.
59. Breitmeier D, Schulz Y, Wilke N, Albrecht K, Haeseler G, Panning B, et al. Cricothyroidotomy training on cadavers—experiences in the education of medical students, anaesthetists, and emergency physicians. Anasthesiol Intensivmed Notfallmed Schmerzther. 2004;39(2):94–100.

14

The Role of Surgical Airway Access

Kerstin M. Stenson

Introduction

Anesthesiologists and head and neck surgeons traditionally have embodied the phenomenon of collegial interactions, and few professional interactions are more rewarding than those that result in successful management of a patient with a difficult airway. In these situations, the difficult airway becomes a shared challenge that demands mutual trust and cooperation between otolaryngologist and anesthesiologist[1]. Pre-intubation communication is mandatory, with arrangements for intubation details and contingency plans outlined. This chapter will focus on how the head and neck surgeon can aid the anesthesiologist during the perioperative care of a patient with a challenging airway.

K.M. Stenson (✉)
Professor of Surgery, Department of Surgery/Section of Otolaryngology—Head and Neck Surgery,
The University of Chicago, Chicago, IL 60637, USA
e-mail: kstenson@surgery.bsd.uchicago.edu

D.B. Glick et al. (eds.), *The Difficult Airway: An Atlas of Tools and Techniques for Clinical Management*,
DOI 10.1007/978-0-387-92849-4_14, © Springer Science+Business Media New York 2013

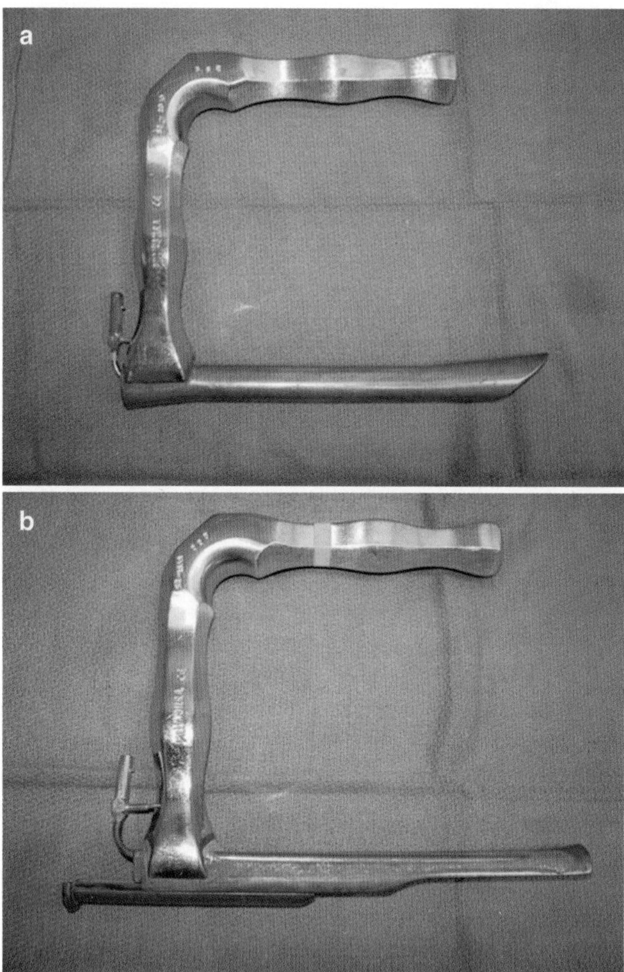

Figure 14.1. (**a**) Anterior commissure laryngoscope, with narrow mid-portion and bell-shaped end to facilitate laryngeal view. (**b**) Jackson-Pilling laryngoscope with removable slide allowing for placement of endotracheal tube or rigid bronchoscope.

Rigid Endoscopy

Laryngoscopy

Occasionally, patients undergoing elective surgery with presumptive normal anatomy can be ventilated by face mask, but are unexpectedly direct laryngoscopy failures, even for experienced anesthesiologists. On other rare occasions, there is a sudden cascade of events such as oral bleeding or emesis that makes mask ventilation and intubation with a Miller or Macintosh blade nearly impossible. In these situations, the use of the anterior commissure or Jackson laryngoscope may be very helpful (Figure 14.1a, b). The design of both of these laryngoscopes was heavily influenced by Chevalier Jackson, known in the Otolaryngology field as the father of modern laryngology and endoscopy. Both instruments consist of a closed tubular structure with distal and recessed lighting that prevents the tongue from obscuring the laryngeal view and allows rigid suctioning. In addition, the ergonomic handles allow for improved leverage and stability for passing an endotracheal tube, bronchoscope, or gum elastic bougie[2–4]. The anterior commissure laryngoscope has an hourglass shape whose narrowest area contacts the constricted area of the dentition when exposing the larynx[5]. It also has an anterior flare and an oval aperture at its tip that proves invaluable for exposing the glottic inlet. The Jackson-Pilling laryngoscope has a

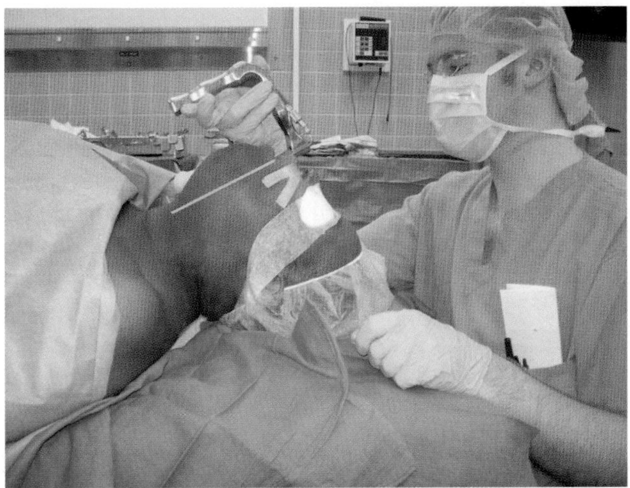

Figure 14.2. Head and neck surgeon using anterior commissure laryngoscope to view larynx. Note the direct line from oropharynx to larynx that is afforded with this rigid tube laryngoscope.

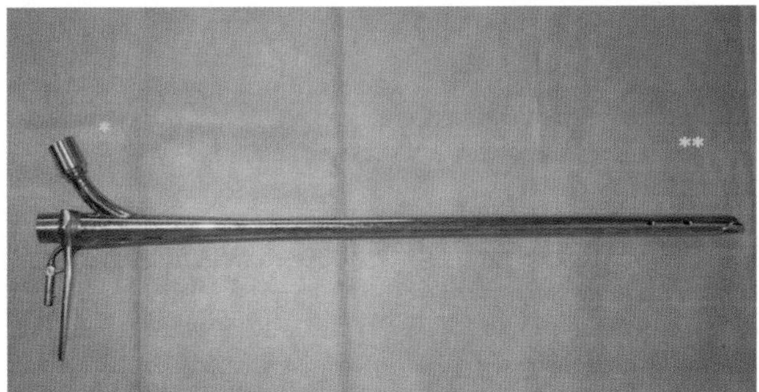

Figure 14.3. Rigid bronchoscope showing ventilator port (*asterisk*) and distal vents (*two asterisks*).

removable lower slide that aids the passage of a rigid bronchoscope if necessary. The laryngoscopy technique involves the paraglossal or retromolar placement of the laryngoscope. A brief intraoral exam is done in order to place the laryngoscope in an area of absent upper dentition. This maneuver facilitates the displacement of the tongue as the laryngoscope is advanced from the corner of the mouth. The larynx is viewed after the neck is extended, bringing the laryngeal and oral axes into alignment[5]. Most otolaryngologists are able to find at least part of the larynx in most patients using this method (Figure 14.2).

Rigid Bronchoscopy

The method of rigid bronchoscopy is attributed to Gustav Killian and Chevalier Jackson who developed this lifesaving technique for retrieval of tracheobronchial foreign bodies[6,7]. Today the indications for rigid bronchoscopy include massive hemoptysis, foreign body retrieval, airway stenosis, laser resections, and pediatric bronchoscopy. The closed-tube design of the rigid bronchoscope includes a proximal ventilator adaptor port and distal vents to facilitate concurrent ventilation with rigid suctioning, foreign body retrieval, or lasering (Figure 14.3). The rigid bronchoscope excels at securing stenotic airways. The broncoscope allows for displacement of soft tissue that may prolapse into the field (sometimes aided by the Jackson laryngoscope, above), and can bridge a malacic or disrupted segment while planning definitive surgical repair. Subglottic or tracheal dilation can also be achieved by sequentially replacing the bronchoscope with the next larger size until an adequate lumen size is achieved. Positive-pressure ventilation is maintained throughout these procedures.

The inherent rigidity of the ventilating bronchoscope makes visualization beyond the segmental bronchial orifices difficult. Likewise, the only contraindication to rigid bronchoscopy is cervical spine disease that prevents proper positioning for bronchoscopy. Newer bronchoscopes may be coupled with coaxial telescopes for improved optical detail. The most common complication after rigid bronchoscopy is subglottic edema which typically can be managed conservatively with racemic epinephrine treatments and systemic steroids.

Cricothyroidotomy

Cricothyroidotomy represents the categorical procedure of choice when there is complete airway obstruction. Some reviews of cricothyroidotomy describe this procedure in a manner that allows for planning, patient positioning, and local or general anesthesia[8]. The reality of most situations that call for a cricothyroidotomy is this: death or irreversible anoxic brain injury will occur if an airway via a cricothyroidotomy is not obtained. *Knowing when* to proceed to cricothyroidotomy following failed laryngoscopy and intubation represents the fundamental tenet in emergent airway management[9]. Patients with falling oxygen saturation who cannot be intubated or ventilated by face mask or a supraglottic airway device should have a cricothyroidotomy performed. Repeat laryngoscopy and intubation attempts are associated with increased complications and may convert a patient from "cannot intubate" to "cannot intubate/cannot ventilate." All surgical and nonsurgical personnel should understand how to perform a cricothyroidotomy.

The clear advantages of cricothyroidotomy consist of speed and the need for minimal equipment: a knife and endotracheal tube are the only prerequisite tools. The procedure is typically performed under less than ideal circumstances and risk of injury to the vocal cords, recurrent laryngeal nerves, esophagus, or vascular structures can be high. Most if not all cricothyroidotomy complications can be repaired. Although, the procedure may be lifesaving, there is recent evidence that a surgical airway is often attempted too late and poorly performed. The National Audit Project of the Royal College of Anaesthetists and the Difficult Airway Society recommended that all anesthesiologists be trained and practiced to retain the skills required to perform an emergency cricothyroidotomy.

The steps involved in performing a cricothyroidotomy are depicted in Figure 14.4a–d in patients with a *palpable* cricoid cartilage[10,11]. A single horizontal incision through the skin and cricothyroid membrane with dilation (if necessary) and insertion of an endotracheal tube provides rapid control. Pressure is applied and hemostasis can be obtained after the patient is resuscitated and stabilized.

It is a familiar observation that patients with emergent airway obstruction also have abnormal laryngeal or neck anatomy. For example, patients who have undergone external beam radiation or surgical ablation for head and neck malignancies often *do not have a palpable cricoid cartilage*. Rapid surgical control of the airway in these patients is handled by making the longest midline vertical incision necessary to palpate the external laryngeal anatomy (Figure 14.5a). When the cricothyroid membrane is palpated, a horizontal incision is made and an endotracheal tube is placed (Figure 14.5b). Occasionally, the thyrohyoid membrane is entered. Here, the thyroid cartilage is retracted forward/anteriorly, the laryngeal inlet is visualized, and an endotracheal tube is inserted.

Conversion of Cricothyroidotomy to Tracheotomy

Some authorities state that because of the complete (and therefore restrictive) cartilaginous ring of the cricoid, a cricothyroidotomy should be converted to tracheotomy to avoid the long-term complication of subglottic stenosis. Conversion is most strongly indicated if there is a high likelihood of long-term ventilation or an associated injury.

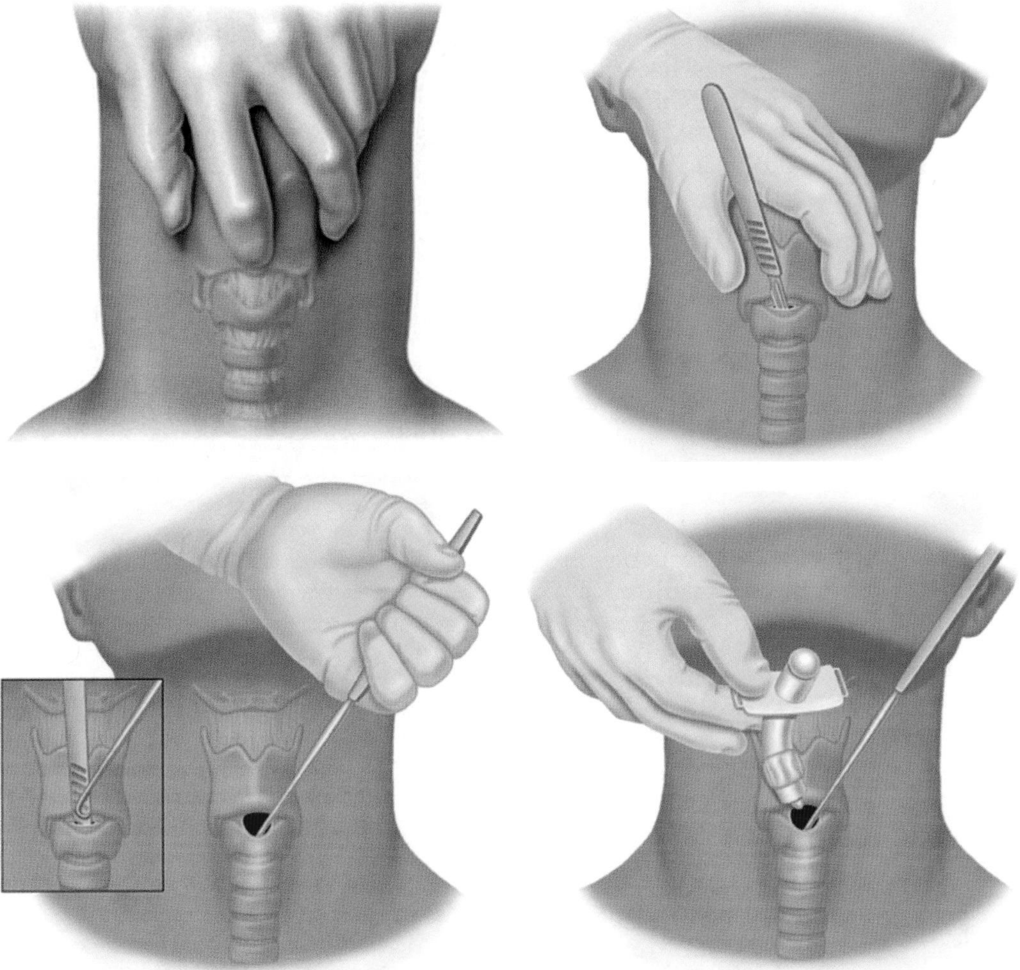

Figure 14.4. Steps of cricothyroidotomy. Step 1: Immobilize the larynx and palpate the cricothyroid membrane with the index finger (Step 1 was published in Color Atlas of Emergency Department Procedures, Custalow, CB. Elsevier Saunders, Philadelphia 2005. Copyright ©2005 Elsevier). Step 2: Make a horizontal stab incision through both skin and cricothyroid membrane. Step 3: Stabilize the larynx by placing a cricoid hook under the cricoid cartilage Step 4: Insert the tracheotomy or endotracheal tube into the trachea (Steps 2–4 reprinted with permission of Custalow, CB. Emergent surgical cricothyroidotomy (cricothyroidotomy). In: UpToDate, Basow, DS (Ed), UpToDate, Waltham, MA 2010).

More recent studies indicate that the incidence of subglottic stenosis after unconverted cricothyroidotomy is low overall, and is less frequent if the patient has no laryngotracheal inflammation[12,13]

Cricothyroidotomy by Nonsurgical Personnel

It is incumbent upon surgical, emergency medicine, and anesthesia training programs to provide instruction in the cricothyroidotomy procedure. Several studies have shown that minimal training allows the non-surgeon to perform cricothyroidotomy effectively and successfully[14–17]. In elective situations for general preparedness, it is advised that the surgeon and anesthesiologist palpate the cricothyroid membrane on *every* patient going to the operating room. This exam takes seconds, provides immediate practical reinforcement of the patient's anatomy, and allows the team to precisely visualize the location of the cricothyroid membrane in the event of a perioperative emergency.

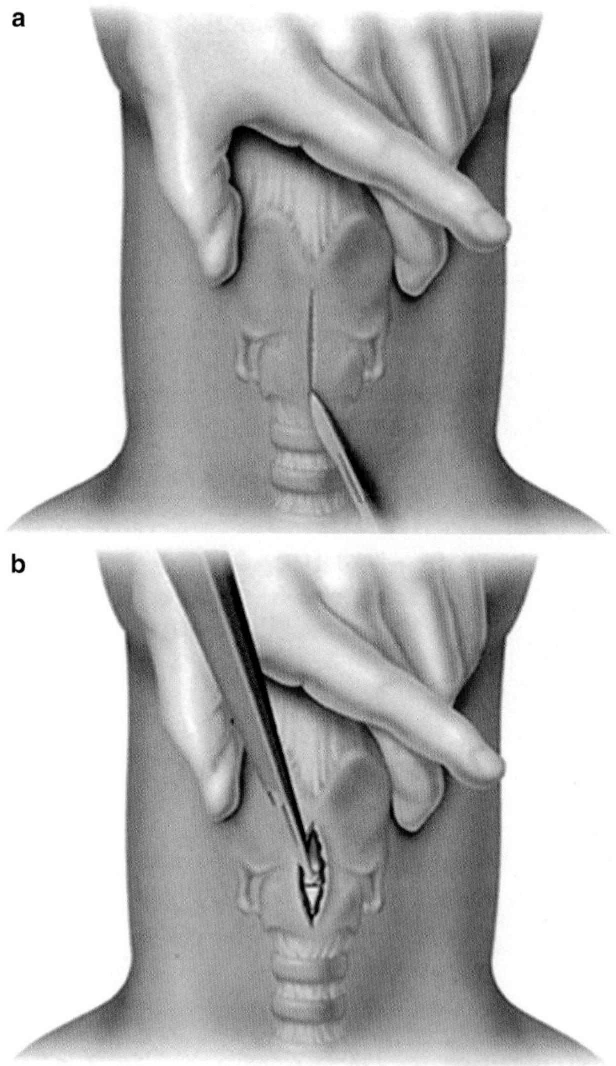

Figure 14.5. Long midline vertical incision (**a**) followed by horizontal incision (**b**) thru cricothyroid membrane in patients with difficult to palpate landmarks (this figure was published in Color Atlas of Emergency Department Procedures, Custalow, CB. Elsevier Saunders, Philadelphia 2005. Copyright ©2005 Elsevier). (**a**) Midline vertical incision. (**b**) Horizontal incision through cricothyroid membrane.

Emergency cricothyroidotomy remains the final airway route for the "cannot intubate cannot ventilate" circumstance. One alternative percutaneous method to access the cricothyroid membrane utilizes the Seldinger/dilational technique. Although most physicians can be taught surgical cricothyroidotomy, the dilational technique is a well-known one that is familiar to most anesthesiologists. The percutaneous cricothyroidotomy devices (see Figure 14.6) require minimal or no dissection and may be a more straightforward choice for anesthesiologists in a life-or-death scenario.

Tracheotomy

The main indications for urgent or emergent tracheotomy include obstructing laryngeal tumors or laryngeal trauma (Figure 14.7). Emergency tracheotomy generally has a higher incidence of complications[10,18] and is often difficult due to the patient's air hunger and

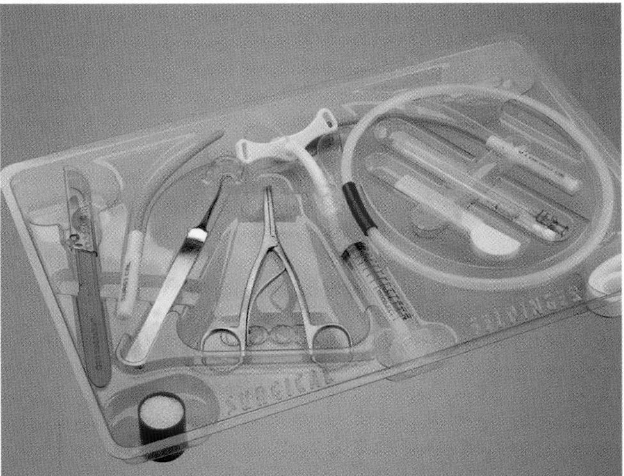

Figure 14.6. The Melker Percutaneous Cricothyroidotomy Kit consists of a scalpel, needle, syringe, guide wire, dilator, and tracheostomy tube. In addition, a tracheal dilator and tracheal hook are available should they be required. A skin incision is made over the cricothyroid membrane, a needle with a catheter on it is passed through the membrane, oriented in a caudal direction. Attached to the needle is a syringe partially filled with saline. Aspiration of a continuous stream of air confirms tracheal placement of the needle. The needle is removed, leaving the catheter in situ. A guide wire is advanced through the catheter. The dilator is inserted into the tracheostomy tube and both dilator and tracheostomy tube are advanced over the guide wire with a corkscrew motion. If significant resistance is encountered, the tracheal dilator can be employed (but this is rarely required). Confirmation of tracheal placement by auscultation and capnography is mandatory (permission for use granted by Cook Medical Incorporated, Bloomington, Indiana).

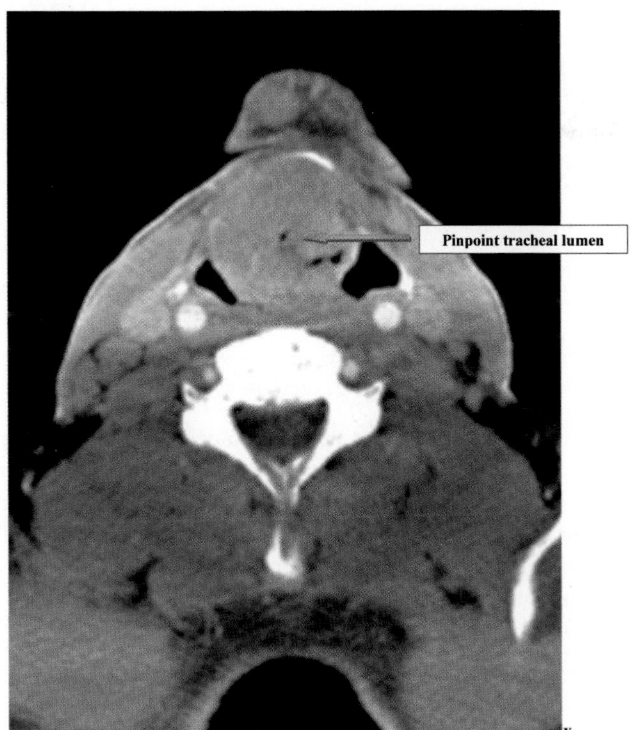

Figure 14.7. CT scan of a patient with large laryngeal tumor. The arrow marks the pinpoint tracheal lumen.

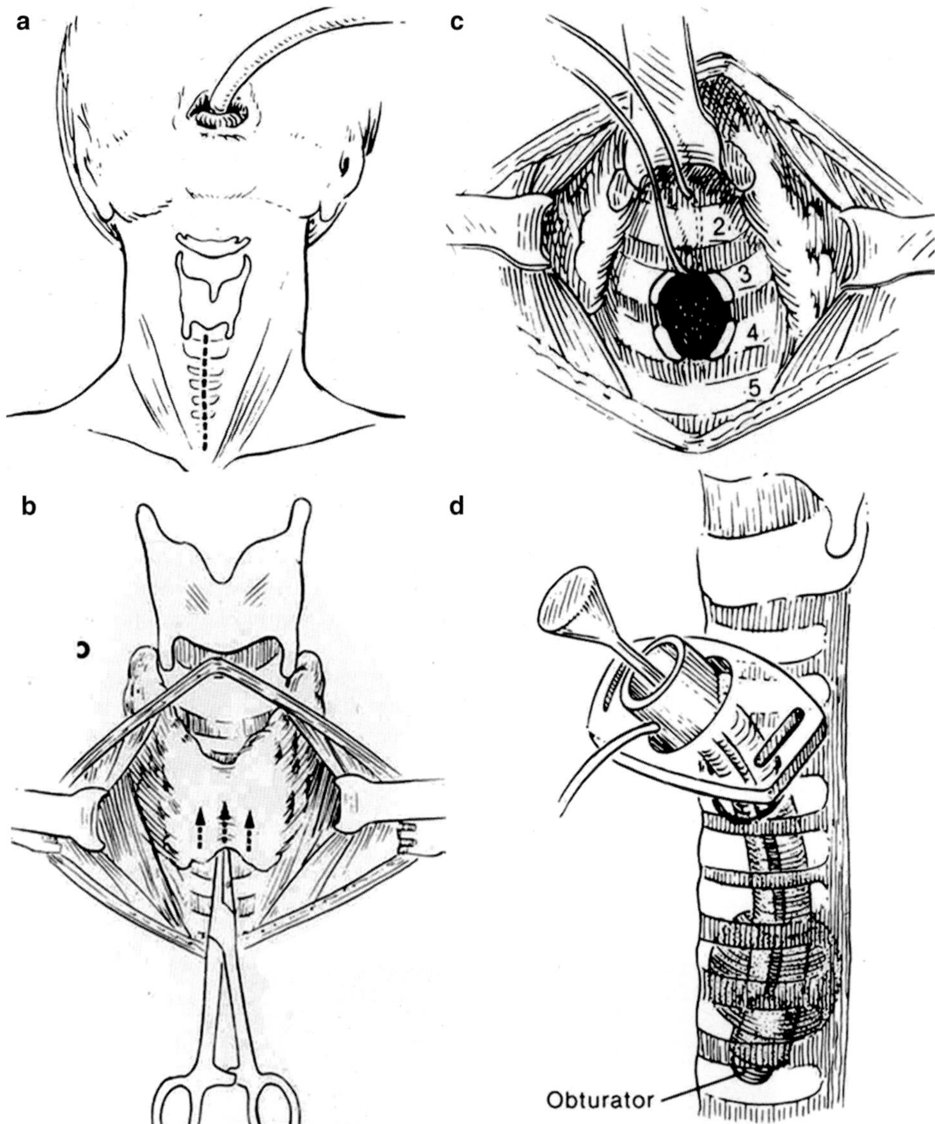

Figure 14.8. Steps of tracheotomy. (**a**) Step 1: Vertical incision (**b**) Step 2: Retract strap muscles and transect thyroid isthmus. (**c**) Step 3: Cricoid retracted and 2nd or 3rd tracheal ring removed. (**d**) Step 4: Trach tube guided into opening with obturator (this figure was published in Atlas of Laryngeal Surgery, Charles W. Cummings, copyright Elsevier Health Sciences, 1984).

agitation coupled with their desire to sit upright. As with any operative procedure, it is critical for the surgeon and anesthesiologist to communicate directly and rapidly prior to the intervention. Administration of general anesthesia may result in total airway obstruction[19]. A vertical incision is utilized by the most skilled surgeon available. Figure 14.8 illustrates the steps involved in performing a tracheotomy.

Based upon their study of 90 patients undergoing awake tracheotomy, Altman et al. recommended the following[20]:

1. Upright position of the patient to aid in secretion management and prevention of tongue prolapse.
2. Minimal or total avoidance of intravenous anesthetic, analgesic, or anxiolytic as these substances suppress the respiratory drive.
3. No transtracheal local anesthetic to avoid coughing and further agitation.

4. The use of a liberal/large incision and the cricoid hook.
5. The availability of a "finder" needle (a 10 cc syringe half-filled with saline coupled to a 18-gauge needle). Air bubbles seen on aspiration with the syringe indicate tracheal placement of the needle.

Complications of tracheotomy include stenosis, hemorrhage, pneumothorax or pneumomediastinum, tracheoesophageal fistula, recurrent laryngeal nerve injury, cardiac arrest, pulmonary edema, tube obstruction, or tube displacement[21–23]. Stenosis may reflect preoperative damage to the trachea in patients who have a history of prolonged intubation. Intraoperative or postoperative hemorrhage often can be prevented by careful surgical technique. Even slow "oozing" postoperatively can lead to death from airway obstruction if not recognized secondary to an occlusive clot in the airways. Tracheo-innominate fistula is a rare but devastating complication more likely to occur in patients with tracheotomy lower than the third tracheal ring. This may be seen in patients who are septic, on steroids, malnourished and possibly those with excessive cuff inflation and often follows a less impressive "herald bleed." The lifesaving maneuver involves retrosternal digital compression of the innominate artery while a cardiovascular surgeon is readied.

The pathophysiology of pneumothorax or pneumomediastinum results from the tremendous negative intrathoracic pressures that are generated when a patient breathes against an obstructed glottis. The patients, soft tissue becomes susceptible to dissection of air along the pleural planes through the tracheostomy skin incision. Pneumomediastinum may lead to pleural rupture and pneumothorax. Pneumothorax can also result from a displaced or improperly placed tracheotomy tube, ruptured bleb, laceration of pleural domes, or high-positive pressures during ventilation. If the tracheotomy is made too low, there is increased chance of displacement and creation of a false passage. If the tracheotomy is made too high, the end of the tracheotomy tube can erode through the common tracheoesophageal wall, creating a fistula. A tracheoesophageal injury can also occur acutely during the procedure, especially if the patient is agitated or the dissection is difficult.

The tracheotomy tube can become obstructed by blood, inspissated secretions, a tissue flap as a result of a false passage, or by an overinflated cuff[24]. It is critical that the inner tracheotomy tube and trachea are visualized with a flexible laryngoscope or bronchoscope to aid in diagnosis of tube obstruction and malpositioning.

Extraordinary Circumstances

Lost airway during anesthesia induction[1]. Patients may arrive to the operating room with various states of airway obstruction, ranging from an obvious acute airway emergency to more nuanced situations, such as patients with oropharyngeal bleeding or facial trauma. Sofferman et al. outlines several considerations that the otolaryngologist/head and neck surgeon and anesthesiologist must understand in order to maximize patient safety and facilitate securing the airway. These include:

1. NPO vs. full-stomach status.
2. Adult, infant, or child.
3. Underlying cardiorespiratory function and extent of relative hypoxia or hypercarbia.
4. Tolerance of supine position.
5. Status of cervical spine.
6. Mandible stability/position.
7. Oropharyngeal bleeding and airway patency.
8. Patient anxiety or agitation which is often a consequence of hypoxemia.
9. Level and severity of obstruction.

Although often implicitly understood by teams that frequently work together, these factors must be explicitly discussed along with contingencies should they be required. Cricothyroidotomy *may* be deferred if the surgeon and anesthesiologist both trust the

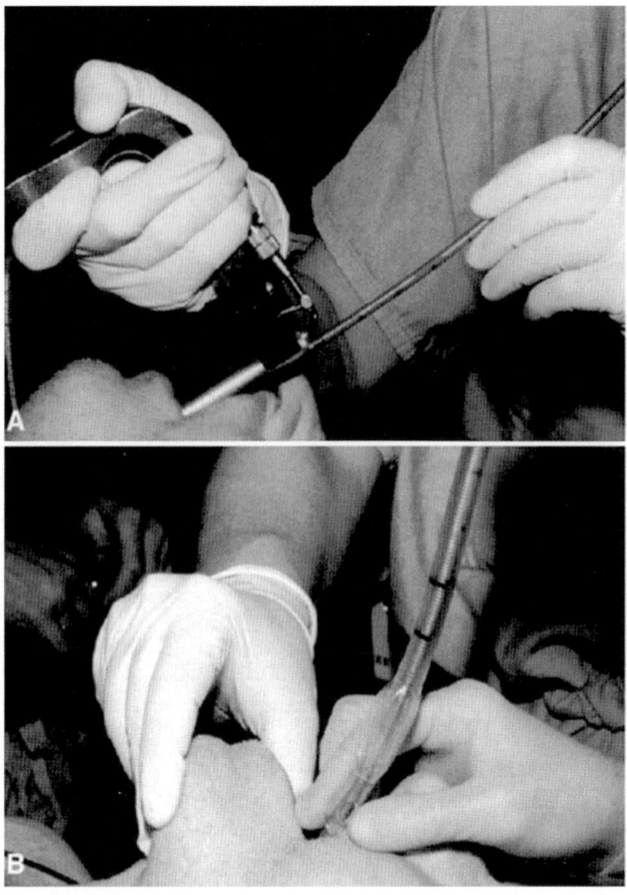

Figure 14.9. Gum Elastic Bougie inserted into trachea via anterior commissure laryngoscope and intubation over same bougie as a guide (from Sofferman R, Johnson D, Spencer R. Lost airway during anesthesia induction: alternatives for management. Laryngoscope. 1997;107:1476–1482).

alternative method or technology and application thereof. One such example is the use of the anterior commissure laryngoscope with semirigid gum elastic bougie[1]. As mentioned above, the design of the anterior commissure laryngoscope can often permit visualization of at least the posterior larynx. Once this is in view, the bougie can be inserted into the trachea and an endotracheal tube passed over it to secure the airway (Figure 14.9). A rare complication that can occur during elective or emergency tracheotomy is loss of the airway during insertion of the tracheotomy device. A false passage, usually anteriorly, can occur due to altered anatomy (see below), obesity, or low tracheotomy site. McGuire et al. recommend preoperative placement of a jet-ventilation airway exchange catheter through the endotracheal tube via a bronchoscope port adaptor if the patient is having an elective tracheotomy[25]. In more urgent situations, the authors recommend jet ventilation via a large-bore intravenous catheter placed through the trachea at the level of the sternal notch. Great care must be exercised to avoid barotrauma. In addition, a sternotomy or emergency cardiopulmonary bypass can be undertaken.

Altered Anatomy. Older patients with kyphoses or those with congenital cervical spine abnormalities present particularly difficult airway challenges to the anesthesiologist and surgeon. Due to the abnormally low position of the larynx, these types of patients often require sternotomy for tracheotomy[26]. In these situations, it is safer to perform a cricothyroidotomy. The cricothyroidotomy site is stomatized to the surrounding skin edges and maintained as long as the patient requires. Any potential damage to the subglottis is prevented by the use of a small tracheotomy tube with the minimal required cuff pressures.

Patients with morbid obesity present an additional challenge for airway management. Those patients with poorly or uncontrolled obstructive sleep apnea are candidates for tracheotomy, either as a separate procedure or in conjunction with other surgeries. Increased cervical girth, due to thick layers of subcutaneous fat, interferes with proper tracheotomy tube positioning. This problem is managed by debriding the fat of the subcutaneous and perifascial adipose tissue, and thinning the fat layers adjacent to the strap muscles[27]. These maneuvers allow the skin edges to be tacked down to the stoma. Because the tracheotomy is stomatized, a standard tracheotomy, rather than a custom length tube, can be inserted and maintained using customary post-tracheotomy care.

Conclusion

We live in a time in which extraordinary techniques for managing patients with airway challenges have become routine. Nonetheless, we must remain steadfast in our commitment to patient well-being through communication, flexibility, and preparedness.

References

1. Sofferman R, Johnson D, Spencer R. Lost airway during anesthesia induction: alternatives for management. Laryngoscope. 1997;107:1476–82.
2. Davies R, Balachandran S. Anterior commissure laryngoscope. Anaesthesia. 2003;58:721–2.
3. Zeitels S. Chevalier Jackson's contributions to direct laryngoscopy. J Voice. 1998;12:1–6.
4. Riazi S, Karkouti K, Heggie J. Case report: management of life-threatening oropharyngeal bleeding with recombinant factor VIIa. Can J Anaesth. 2006;53:881–4.
5. Holinger P. An hour-glass anterior commissure laryngoscope. Laryngoscope. 1960;70:1570–1.
6. Conacher I, Curran E. Local anaesthesia and sedation for rigid bronchoscopy for emergency relief of central airway obstruction. Anaesthesia. 2004;59:290–2.
7. Wain J. Rigid bronchoscopy: the value of a venerable procedure. Chest Surg Clin N Am. 2001;11:691–9.
8. Linscott M, Horton W. Management of upper airway obstruction. Otolaryngol Clin North Am. 1979;12:351–73.
9. Rodricks MB, Deutschman CS. Emergent airway management. Crit Care Clin. 2000;16: 389–409.
10. Weymuller E. Acute airway management. In: Cummings CW, editor. Otolaryngology-head and neck surgery. 2nd ed. St. Louis, MO: CV Mosby Publishing Co; 1986. p. 2382–95.
11. Burkey B, Esclamado R, Morganroth M. The role of cricothyroidotomy in airway management. Clin Chest Med. 1991;12:561–71.
12. DeLaurier G, Hawkins M, Treat R, et al. Acute airway management. Role of cricothyroidotomy. Am Surg. 1990;56:12–5.
13. Gillespie M, Eisele D. Outcomes of emergency surgical airway procedures in a hospital-wide setting. Laryngoscope. 1999;109:1766–9.
14. Isaacs J, Pedersen A. Emergency cricothyroidotomy. Am Surg. 1997;63:346–9.
15. DiGiacomo J, Angus L, Simpkins C, et al. Safety and efficacy of the rapid four-step technique for cricothyroidotomy using a Bair claw [letter]. J Emerg Med. 2001;20:303–4.
16. Davis D, Bramwell K, Hamilton R, et al. Safety and efficacy of the rapid four-step technique for cricothyroidotomy using a Bair Claw. J Emerg Med. 2000;19:125–9.
17. Hatton K, Price S, Craig L, et al. Educating anesthesiology resident to perform percutaneous cricothyroidotomy, retrograde intubation, and fiberoptic bronchoscopy using preserved cadavers. Anesth Analg. 2006;103:1205–8.
18. Wenig B, Applebaum E. Indications for and techniques of tracheotomy. Clin Chest Med. 1991;12:545–53.
19. Moorthy S, Gupta S, Laurent B, et al. Management of airway in patients with laryngeal tumors. J Clin Anesth. 2005;17:604–9.
20. Altman K, Waltonen J, Kern R. Urgent surgical airway intervention: a 3 year county hospital experience. Laryngoscope. 2005;115:2101–4.

21. Burtner D, Goodman M. Anesthetic and operative management of potential upper airway obstruction. Arch Otolaryngol. 1978;104:657–61.
22. Goldenberg D, Gov Ari E, Golz A, et al. Tracheotomy complication: a retrospective study of 10020 cases. Otolaryngol Head Neck Surg. 2000;123:495–500.
23. Myers E, Carrau M. Early complications of tracheotomy. Clin Chest Med. 1991;12:589–95.
24. Saini S, Taxak S, Singh M. Tracheostomy tube obstruction caused by an overinflated cuff. Otolaryngol Head Neck Surg. 2000;122:768–9.
25. McGuire G, El-Beheiry H, Brown D. Loss of the airway during tracheostomy: rescue oxygenation and re-establishment of the airway. Can J Anaesth. 2001;48:697–700.
26. Patel K, Zdanski C. Cricothyroidotomy vs. sternal tracheotomy for challenging airway anatomy. Laryngoscope. 2008;118:1827–9.
27. Gross N, Cohen J, Anderson P, et al. "Defatting" tracheotomy in morbidly obese patients. Laryngoscope. 2002;112:1940–4.

15

Evaluation and Management of the Difficult Pre-Hospital Airway

Janis P. Tupesis and Nathan Van Dyk

J.P. Tupesis (✉)
Department of Emergency Medicine, University of Wisconsin School of Medicine and Public Health, Madison, WI 53792, USA
e-mail: jtupesis@medicine.wisc.edu

N. Van Dyk
Emergency Department, Vista East Medical Center, Waukegan, IL 60085, USA

D.B. Glick et al. (eds.), *The Difficult Airway: An Atlas of Tools and Techniques for Clinical Management*, DOI 10.1007/978-0-387-92849-4_15, © Springer Science+Business Media New York 2013

Introduction

Airway management in the pre-hospital setting poses a unique set of challenges. While elective management of a patient's airway is typically performed in a controlled environment by experienced clinicians, circumstances in the pre-hospital setting are often much different than those in the operating room or even the Emergency Department. As seen in Figures 15.1 and 15.2, patient care happens in a wide variety of surroundings including accident scenes, private residences, and in Emergency Medical Service vehicles. Often, there are challenges to the rapid establishment of an adequate airway in ill or injured patients. This can include entrapped or difficult to access patients, unsafe or hostile settings, and psychomotor challenges such as having to perform procedures in the back of a moving ambulance or helicopter. In addition, pre-hospital airway management often happens in the setting of an acute, decompensated medical condition coupled with an increased risk of regurgitation with impaired protective reflexes. In contrast to the controlled inpatient location, patients are frequently in a state of cardiovascular collapse, respiratory distress, or suffering from polytrauma. It is estimated that difficult intubating conditions are encountered in approximately 7–10% of patients requiring airway management in the pre-hospital setting[1,2]. It is unclear whether these numbers are truly reflective of the dimension of the problem. In recent studies evaluating the incidence of adverse events during pre-hospital airway management by paramedics in patients with severe head injuries, it was noted that complications frequently occur. In one study, 31 (57%) of 54 patients demonstrated desaturation during rapid sequence intubation (RSI). Six (19%) patients experienced marked bradycardia (HR <50 beats/min) during these desaturation events[3]. It is in this context that we wish to discuss the evaluation, approach, and management of the difficult airway.

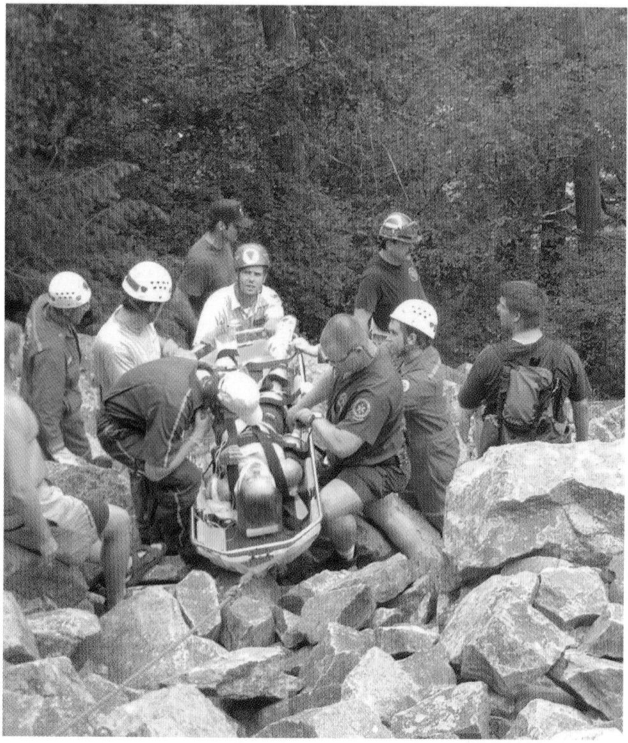

Figure 15.1. EMS pre-hospital patient management (courtesy: Dr. Mike Abernethy).

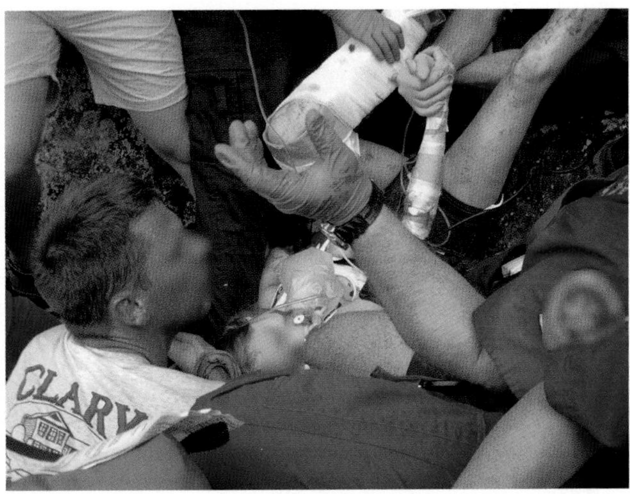

Figure 15.2. EMS pre-hospital patient care (courtesy: Dr. Mike Abernethy).

Emergency Medical Services Systems

In order to appreciate these clinical challenges, one has to have a basic understanding of the different levels of care of Emergency Medical Services (EMS). A broad range of practitioners provide pre-hospital airway management in the United States. The amount of training varies from the Emergency Medical Technician-Basic (EMT-Basic) to the physician (Emergency Medicine) level, as seen in Figure 15.3. The most common level of training for an ambulance crew in a metropolitan EMS system is EMT-Basic or Emergency Medical Technician-Paramedic (EMT-Paramedic). An EMT-Basic will have approximately 120 h of classroom training learning such skills as scene assessment, clinical operations, and the approach to the injured patient. They typically will have the skill set necessary to provide basic airway interventions including manual repositioning of the airway, removal of foreign bodies from the mouth, suctioning of the oropharynx, and the use of oropharyngeal and nasopharyngeal airway adjuncts to improve bag-mask ventilation (BMV)[4]. With additional training and experience, these providers can become paramedic EMTs. With this training they gain skills in management of orthopedic injuries, management of burns, spinal cord injury management along with triage and treatment of patients in mass casualty incidents. An EMT-Paramedic will have at least 1,000 h of classroom training and their skill set will encompass advanced airway maneuvers including orotracheal intubation and the use of supraglottic devices, as seen in Figures 15.4 and 15.5. However, there is a great deal of variability from jurisdiction to jurisdiction in regard to the training protocols used and the standing medical order sets that delineate what types of airway modalities are used. While some EMS systems limit their pre-hospital providers to endotracheal intubation (ETI) and rescue airway techniques, some advanced EMT Paramedics are trained to use RSI, Bipap/CPAP or perform surgical airway interventions[5].

Helicopter EMS programs are frequently staffed by critical care registered nurses with airway skills similar to advanced paramedics. Board certified emergency medicine physicians staff a few helicopter EMS programs in the U.S. and many parts of Europe. Some ground-based EMS programs also have the ability to deploy physicians. The term Basic Life Support (BLS) generally refers to the EMT-Basic level, and the term Advanced Life Support (ALS) generally refers to the EMT-Paramedic level. This, along with different pre-hospital protocols for airway management (different devices, approaches, ability to perform RSI), make it difficult to have a standardized approach to EMS pre-hospital airway management. In this context—the approach, management, and indications for pre-hospital airway management are discussed below.

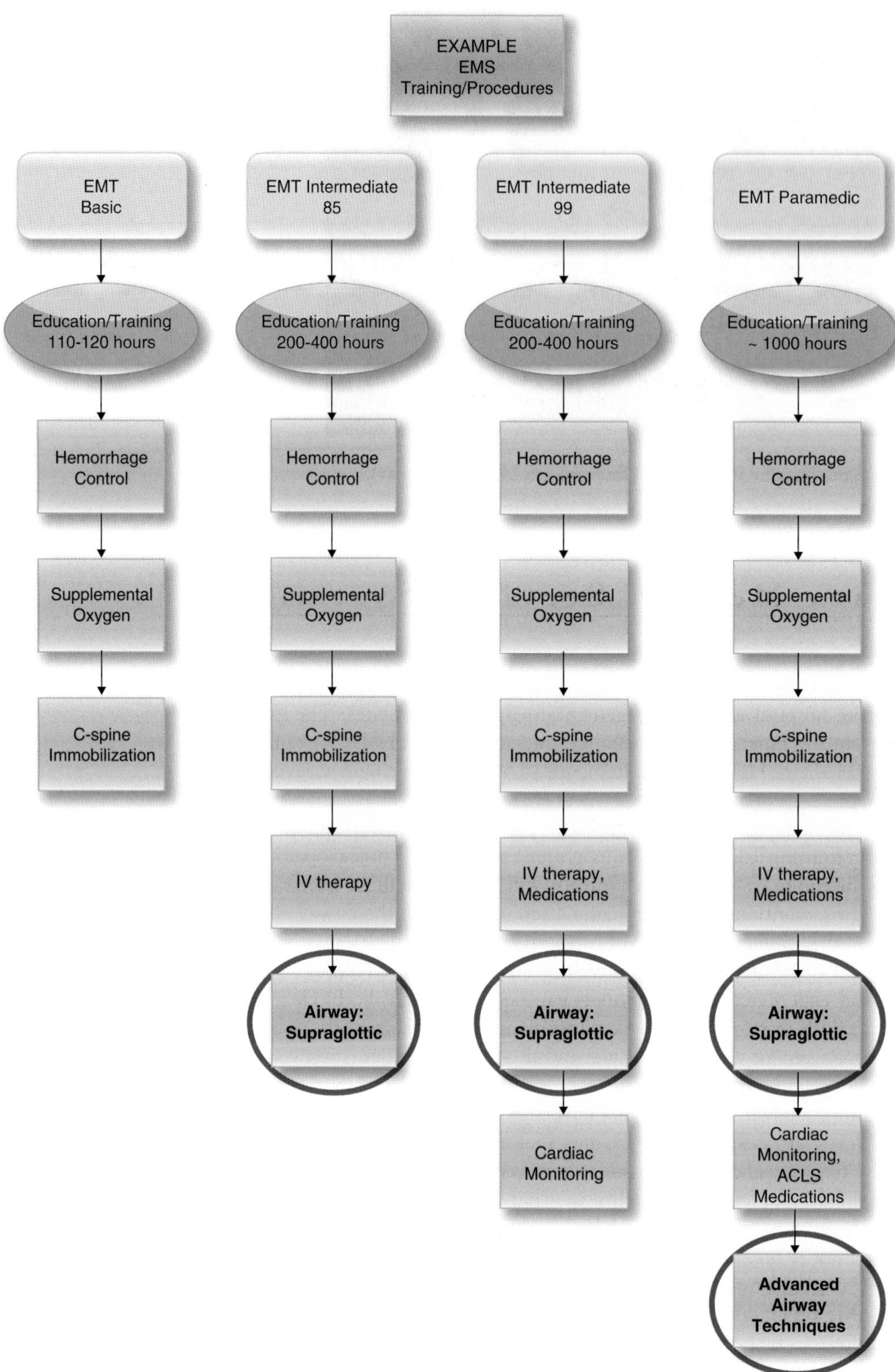

Figure 15.3. Example—EMS training and procedure competency.

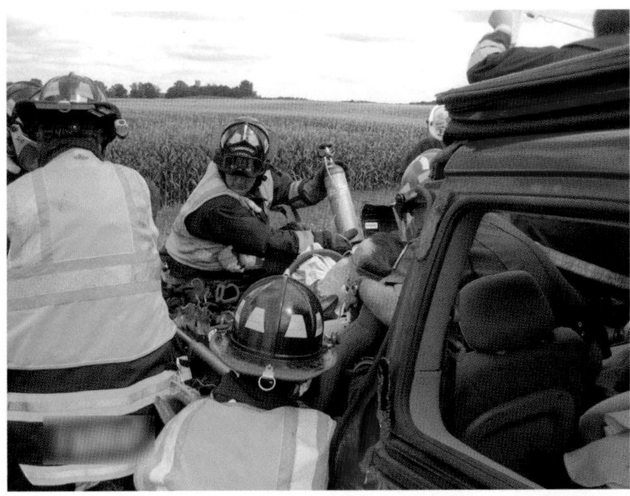

Figure 15.4. Difficult airway management in the field—EMT paramedics (courtesy: Dr. Mike Abernethy).

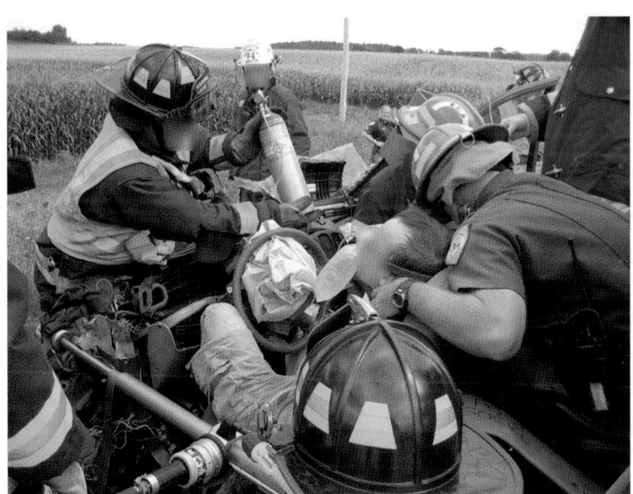

Figure 15.5. Difficult airway in a confined space—EMT paramedics (courtesy: Dr. Mike Abernethy).

Evaluation and Approach

Indications for intubation in the pre-hospital setting are similar to those in other situations. They include physiologic derangements that lead to ventilatory failure or failure to oxygenate with associated hypoxemia. Other indications for airway management in the pre-hospital setting focus on the patient's ability to maintain or protect a patent airway. These often include altered mental status with a loss of gag/cough reflex and acute airway obstruction (ex: traumatic head injury, pooling of secretions in the posterior oropharynx). Another factor that must be considered is the possibility that the patient's condition may change or deteriorate suddenly or during the time required to transport the patient to the receiving facility. The risks of securing the airway prior to transport need to be weighed against the possibility that there will be a change in the patient's clinical status en route, necessitating airway management in a much more difficult setting (ambulance/helicopter). If airway compromise is likely, securing the airway prior to departure may well be the safest course of action.

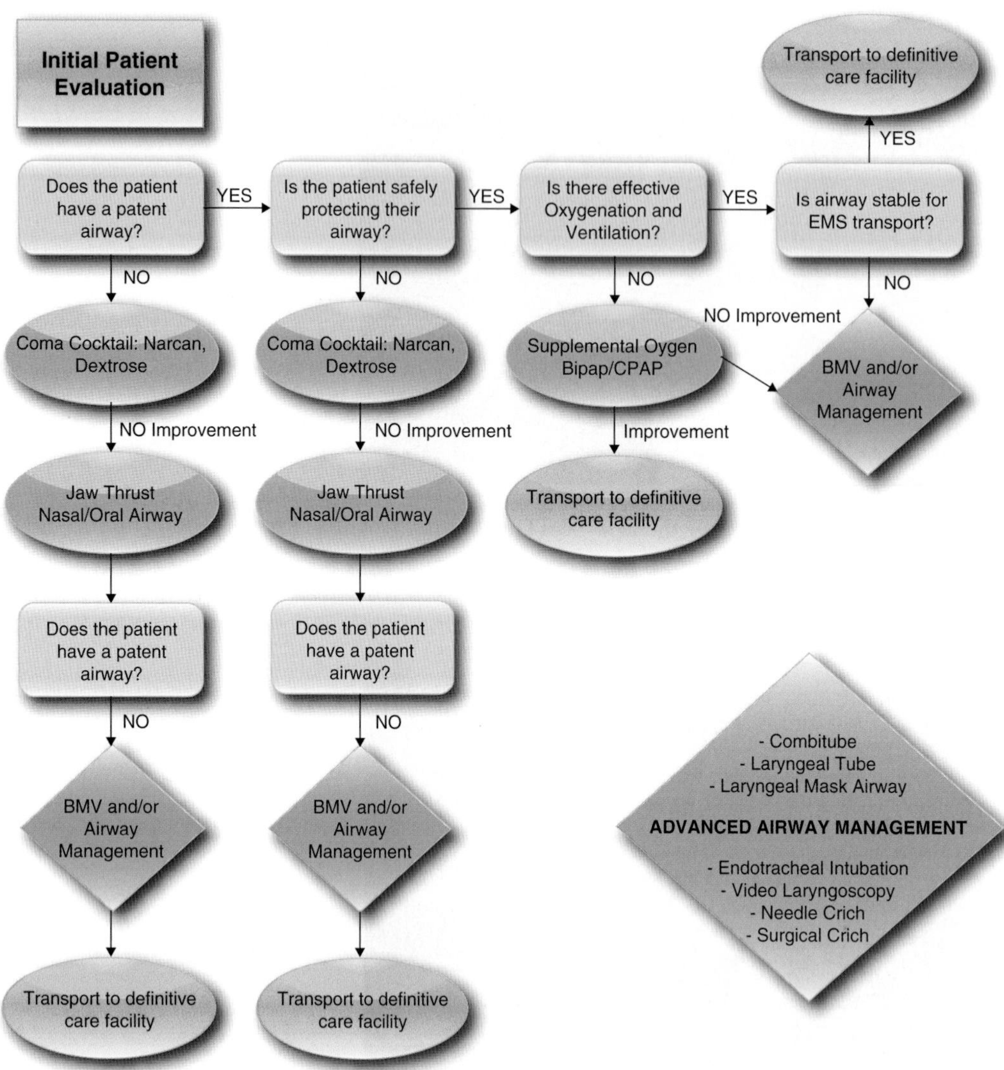

Figure 15.6. Pre-hospital difficult airway algorithm.

Predicting a difficult airway in the pre-hospital setting is more challenging than for an elective intubation in the hospital. In the vast majority of cases time will not permit a formal evaluation of the airway. Typically, the patient will not be able to cooperate with an examination and will be unable to give a detailed medical history. In contrast to an elective, inpatient airway procedure—the pre-hospital airway will not have ideal conditions such as a fasting state by the patient, premedication, ideal patient positioning, adequate lighting and equipment, and assistance from other medical professionals. Most importantly, however, there is frequently little time to prepare, plan, and discuss therapeutic interventions and limited options for backup. As thorough an examination as time permits should be made to determine if predictors of a difficult airway, including either ventilation or intubation are present. Even under optimal conditions all pre-hospital airways should be considered difficult and contingency plans should be made in advance regarding rescue airway devices. The decision to undertake intubation in the field needs to be weighed carefully versus rapid transport to a more controlled setting.

Management

As with conventional airway management, there are many different options in the pre-hospital setting. As discussed in previous chapters, decisions regarding airway management require an organized, algorithmic approach based on the patient assessment and clinical status. An algorithmic approach to the pre-hospital airway is given above, as seen in Figure 15.6. It is very similar to other difficult airway algorithms, but takes into consideration the possibility of acutely reversible causes of ventilatory failure, the possibility of injury to the cervical spine and the importance of transport of the patient for definitive care.

Patient Positioning

As seen in Figures 15.7 and 15.8, many times the easiest way to help a patient maintain a patent airway is simple positioning. Maneuvers such as a jaw-thrust will often help establish a patent upper airway. This is especially true in patients in the pre-hospital setting that are supine and have an altered level of consciousness or have lost their protective airway reflexes (e.g., patients with drug overdoses or hypoglycemia) and patients that have

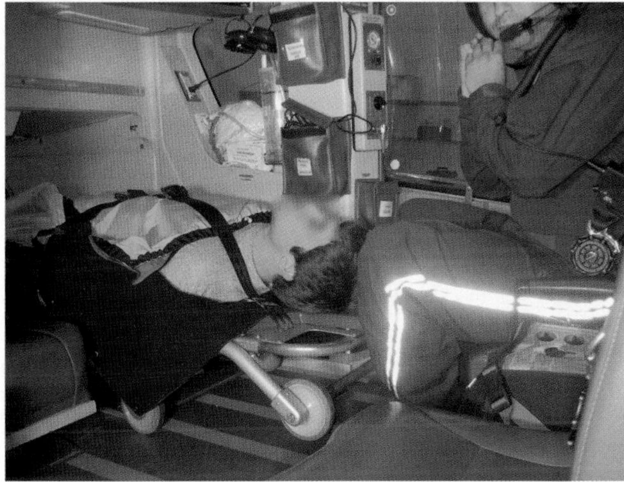

Figure 15.7. Patient positioning without airway intervention (courtesy: Dr. Mike Abernethy/UW Medflight).

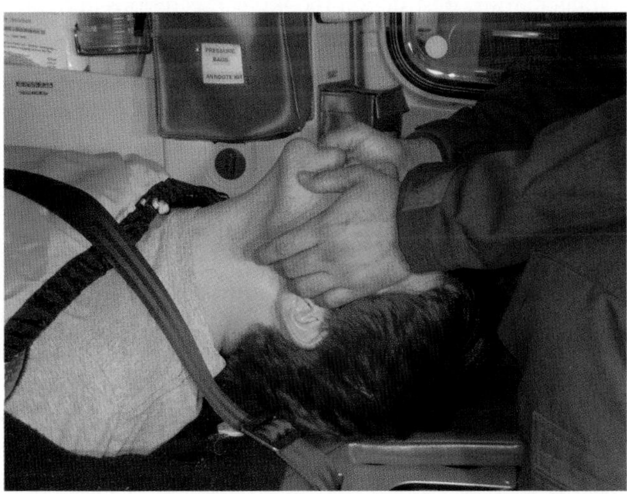

Figure 15.8. Jaw-thrust maneuver (courtesy: Dr. Mike Abernethy/UW Medflight).

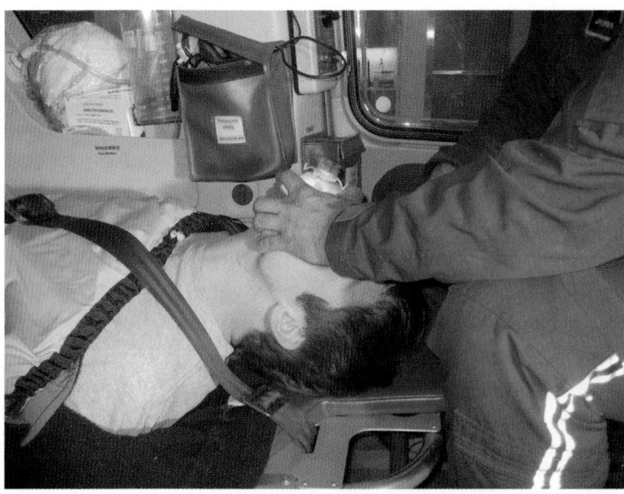

Figure 15.9. A proper sized mask is selected (courtesy: Dr. Mike Abernethy/UW Medflight).

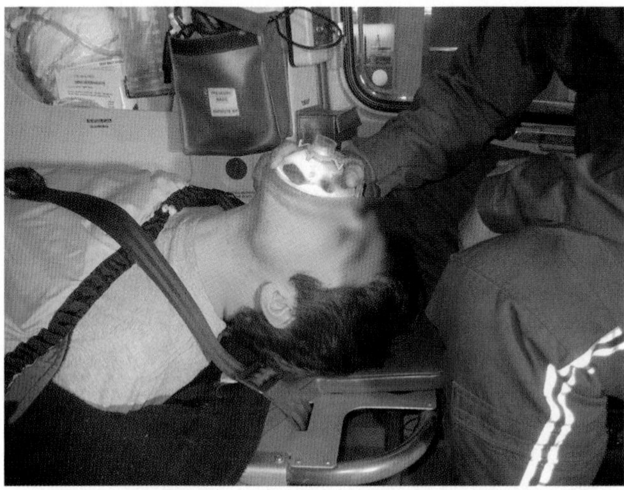

Figure 15.10. A tight seal is achieved as the chin is drawn up into the mask (courtesy: Dr. Mike Abernethy/UW Medflight).

evidence of mild upper airway obstruction (pooling of secretions in the posterior oropharynx). The jaw-thrust maneuver is most easily done by placing the index and middle fingers at the angle of the mandible. The mouth is then opened by exerting an anterior force on the angle of the mandible—lifting the entire mandible and moving the base of the tongue away from the posterior oropharynx, thereby opening a passage to the hypopharynx. This method is simple, safe, noninvasive and requires no specialized equipment. In addition, all levels of EMS personnel are familiar with this airway technique. Disadvantages include the difficulty in maintaining this technique for a long period of time and its inability to protect from aspiration. Though this technique does not significantly move the head or neck, cervical spine precautions still need to be utilized in patients with possible cervical spine injury and facial trauma.

Bag-Mask Ventilation

If a patient does not respond to optimal positioning maneuvers and does not begin breathing spontaneously, bag-mask ventilation (BMV) should be initiated, as seen in Figures 15.9 and 15.10. Although not a definitive airway, it is a crucial emergency skill

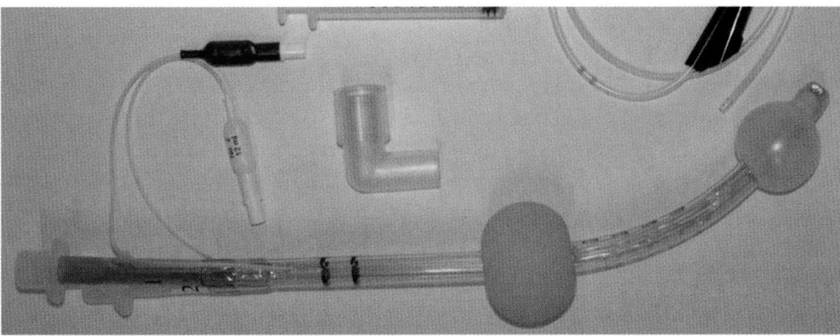

Figure 15.11. Combitube.

that allows for effective oxygenation and ventilation until a more definitive airway can be established. BMV requires an appropriately sized mask and proper positioning of the patient with a jaw-thrust and a chin lift as allowed by c-spine immobilization. Ideally, both nasal and oral airways should be placed to help facilitate optimal air exchange. BMV can be a difficult skill to teach and maintain[6], and suboptimal BMV technique can lead to ineffective oxygenation and ventilation, increased gastric insufflation and aspiration. Recent data even indicate that passive oxygen administration might be preferable to BMV in certain situations[7]. If BMV is unsuccessful, steps should be taken to establish a more definitive airway. Once this decision has been made, the next step is to decide what airway modality will be used. This will often depend on the experience of the pre-hospital provider, the availability of airway adjuncts and other rescue airway devices, the transport time to the closest hospital and the pre-hospital protocols for the given EMS system. Options can include placement of supraglottic devices such as a Combitube or LMA, or definitive airway management by ETI.

Combitube™ (See also Chap. 12)

The Combitube (Figure 15.11; Tyco-Kendall-Sheridan, Mansfield, MA), one of the first supraglottic[1] airway devices, is still used in many EMS systems. Its benefits include a technique that is easily taught and performed, the ability to place it in difficult circumstances (nonideal patient positioning, obese patients, patients that need cervical spine immobilization) and its high success rate for oxygenation/ventilation[8]. It also has the benefit of providing some protection again aspiration because it has an inflated cuff sealing off the esophagus. This is important for a patient population that is almost always non-fasted. The Combitube has been shown to be effective as a primary and rescue airway in the pre-hospital setting. Numerous studies have shown it to be useful when it comes to ease of placement and efficacy of oxygenation and ventilation in pre-hospital cardiac arrest[9–12]. Complication and success rates with the Combitube are generally acceptable for a rescue airway device. However, there are still complications noted in the literature. Cases of subcutaneous emphysema, pneumomediastinum, pneumoperitoneum, and esophageal injuries have been reported[13]. Furthermore, in some reports the success rates for intubation with an ETT were better than for Combitube placement[14,15].

When used in the pre-hospital setting, both balloons of the Combitube are checked for air leaks and a small amount of water-soluble lubricant is applied to each balloon and the distal end of the device if possible. The patient is placed in a sniffing position as the situation allows. The device is inserted following the curvature of the patient's airway and esophagus until the black line on the device is even with the patient's incisors or anterior

[1]The Combitube is more appropriately regarded as an "extraglottic" airway device though we are herein referring to as a "supraglottic" device for the purposes of not introducing a new category.

alveolar ridge, and the larger balloon is in the hypopharynx. The distal end of the device resides in the esophagus greater than 95% of the time with blind placement. The inventor recommends the use of the 37 Fr (SA) size for adults less than 6 ft in height (< 180 cm), in conjunction with a laryngoscope to retract the tongue, minimize the force exerted on the posterior pharynx and facilitate pharyngeal placement of the device. A laryngeal view is not required. The blue balloon port labeled #1 (the larger more proximal balloon) is insufflated with 85–100 mL of air to achieve a pharyngeal seal. The white port to the distal balloon is the then insufflated with 5–15 mL of air to achieve an esophageal seal.

Ventilation is initially attempted through the longer blue tube ("#1 lumen"), and auscultation is performed. If capnography is positive, breath sounds are present, and there is absence of gastric insufflation, the device has been typically positioned in the esophagus and ventilation is continued through the blue tube. (If the open end of the Combitube has been positioned in the esophagus, a gastric tube can be passed through the second lumen to decompress the stomach.) Though relatively rare, if lung inflation does not result from ventilation through the longer blue lumen, it should be attempted through the white lumen ("#2") as the distal end of the device is probably in the trachea. With the proper confirmatory findings ventilation may be continued through the white tube as the patient is transported to a higher level of care or preparations are made for a surgical airway in the field if satisfactory oxygenation cannot be maintained.

LMA™ (See also Chap. 7)

The Laryngeal Mask Airway™ (LMA, LMA North America, San Diego, CA) is a supraglottic device that has slowly gained acceptance in the pre-hospital setting. While initially used as a rescue device, it has become a primary airway device in some BLS and ALS systems in lieu of both noninvasive ventilation/BMV and ETI, as seen in Figures 15.12 and 15.13. While the LMA is not a definitive airway, its ease of use and effectiveness has proven attractive for use in certain pre-hospital scenarios. In the latest Advanced Cardiac Life Support guidelines on CPR and Emergency Cardiac Care, the American Heart Association and the International Liaison Committee on Resuscitation regard the LMA, the Combitube and the endotracheal tube as advanced airway devices. The LMA has been shown to be a reasonable alternative to ETI by paramedics, both by decreasing time to ventilation and increasing success rates in securing an airway in a real-time model[16]. When compared to BMV and Combitube in models of cardiopulmonary resuscitation, the insertion time of the LMA was significantly less[17]. Similarly, the use of LMAs vs. ETTs by paramedics in a pediatric arrest model led to more rapid establishment of effective ventilation with fewer complications[18]. More recently, the role of the intubating LMA (ILMA) has been evaluated in the pre-hospital setting. As with the standard LMA, the ILMA is emerging as an alternative to standard methods of ETI. Both in manikin models and real-time clinical scenarios, pre-hospital providers and emergency physicians were able to successfully use the ILMA to rapidly establish a definitive airway after receiving appropriate training[19–21]. The ILMA also provides an airway modality that has been shown to be easier and quicker to place in patients whose necks were stabilized with manual in-line traction[22].

As in the controlled hospital setting, the properly sized LMA is *completely* deflated and the cuff is slightly lubricated. If possible, the patient is ideally placed in the sniffing position. The index and long finger of the operator's dominant hand are positioned in the sulcus where the cuffed portion of the LMA meets the tube. Following the curvature of the airway anatomy the LMA is gently, but firmly inserted to the proper depth. First slight pressure is exerted against the hard palate, then the soft palate and finally the posterior pharynx as the LMA is guided into place. The cuff is then inflated to form a proper seal over the glottic opening. Placement is confirmed by observation for chest rise, auscultation of the axillae and epigastrium, and capnography.

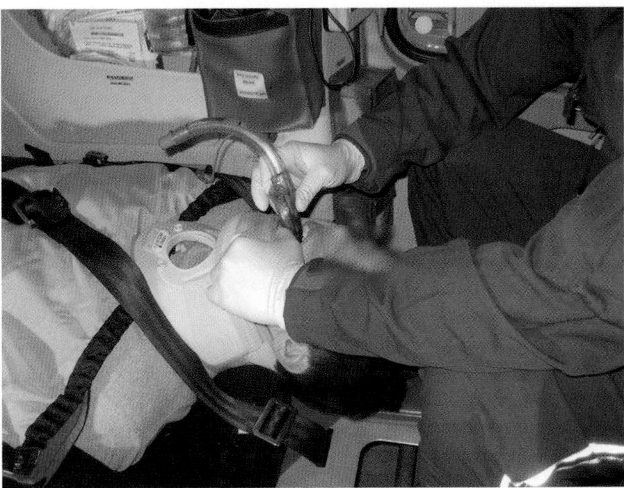

Figure 15.12. LMA insertion with c-collar in place (courtesy: Dr. Mike Abernethy/UW Medflight).

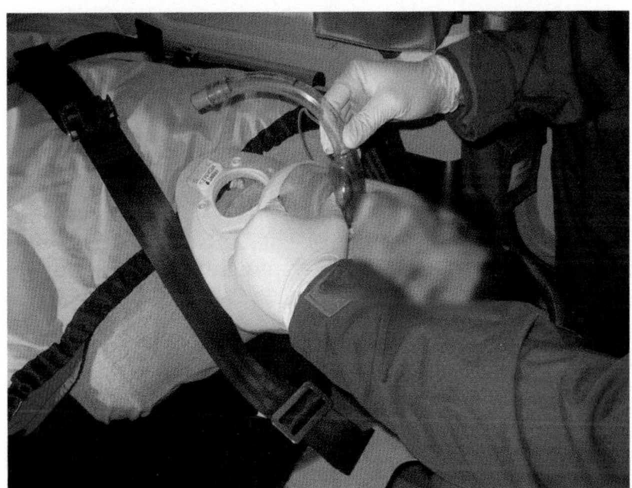

Figure 15.13. Closer view of LMA insertion (courtesy: Dr. Mike Abernethy/UW Medflight).

Laryngeal Tube™ (See also Chap. 12)

The Laryngeal Tube Airway (LT, VBM Medizintechnik, Germany, also referred to as the King LT Airway®) is a newer supraglottic device that is similar in concept to the Combitube, but somewhat less complicated to use. As seen in Figure 15.14, the device is inserted in a similar fashion to a Combitube, but the manufacturer advises a lateral "rotated" approach until the distal end of the device begins to negotiate the curve from the oral to pharyngeal and esophageal axis at which point the device is rotated back to a midline position. The device is advanced until the base of the connector is aligned with the upper incisors or the alveolar ridge. Inflation causes the tube to "sit" in optimal position. Unlike the Combitube, this device can only be placed in the esophagus and is shaped to make tracheal entry unlikely. After insertion there is only one tube for ventilation and one port to inflate. For pre-hospital use the balloons are initially inflated with the maximum volume permitted (60–90 mL of air depending on the size of the device), and then deflated to the lowest pressure that assures an adequate seal. The distal cuff is somewhat larger than that of the Combitube and is supposed to prevent tracheal placement of the device. After proper placement has been confirmed a lubricated gastric tube (up to 18fr) may be placed through the smaller esophageal port to decompress the stomach.

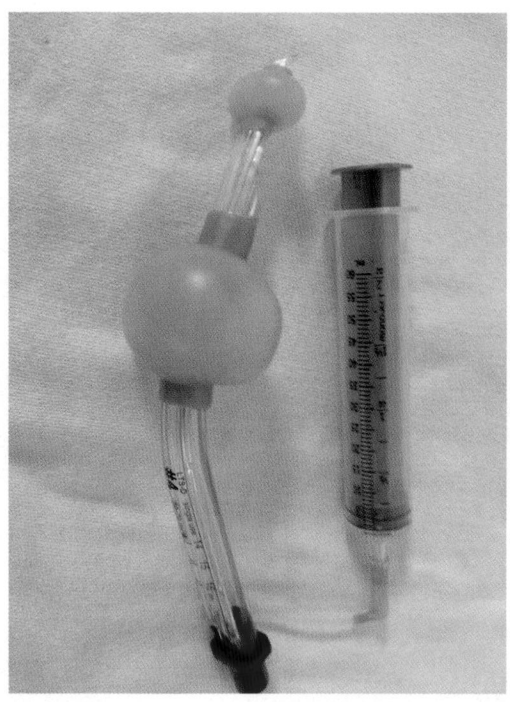

Figure 15.14. King LT (courtesy: Dr. Janis Tupesis).

Though a relatively new device, there is a growing body of literature supporting the use of the LT in the pre-hospital setting. In both a simulated setting and a small pilot study with EMS personnel, the LT showed promise as a quick, easy, and effective airway adjunct[23–25]. Both studies noted that the simplicity of use and the ability to place the device rapidly made it an attractive choice for expeditious airway management. In more recent studies, the efficacy and ease of placement of the LT were studied in difficult airway models and compared to successful placement of both endotracheal tubes and Combitubes. In these studies, success rates for placement of the LT were significantly higher than for either the ETT or the Combitube, while placement times were significantly less[26].

Glottic Devices

Endotracheal Intubation

Endotracheal intubation (ETI) via direct laryngoscopy has been the cornerstone of pre-hospital airway management for years. Tracheal intubation with a cuffed endotracheal tube remains the gold standard for securing the patient's airway in the pre-hospital setting. Most EMS systems have ETI as part of their airway management algorithm as the most frequent "definitive" airway in this setting. The evaluation of the patient and decisions regarding airway management are similar to those in the OR and ED setting. If the patient is unresponsive and the jaw relaxed, ETI without pharmacologic supplementation is the airway modality of choice. If the patient is conscious, combative or otherwise labile, drug assisted intubation is generally preferred. Despite being the pre-hospital "gold standard" of airway management for years, challenges remain.

External laryngeal manipulation (ELM) is one of the most effective and immediately available interventions presently employed in the out-of-hospital setting to facilitate a difficult intubation[27]. When a limited view is obtained at laryngoscopy (CL grade 2 or higher), it may be of great benefit for the laryngoscopist to employ ELM to improve the laryngeal view. Using the right hand, and with the cricoid pressure released to improve laryngeal mobility, the larynx is externally manipulated by the operator of the laryngoscope while simultaneously viewing the glottic opening. Classically a backwards, upwards, and rightward pressure or "BURP"[28] force is employed. Essentially, laryngoscopy becomes a bimanual procedure wherein the right hand corrects what has been distorted by the left[29].

In our experience we have found that manipulation in any direction has the possibility of improving the view, and we recommend that if the initial BURP maneuver does not successfully improve the view of the laryngeal inlet, alternative manipulation of the larynx should then be employed. An assistant can be directed to maintain the position of the larynx once the view has been optimized, and the primary operator can proceed with orotracheal intubation in the usual fashion.

Another option is to first have the assistant place their thumb and index finger externally over the larynx and the laryngoscopist can then manipulate the assistant's hand and the larynx as a single unit. Once the view has been optimized, the intubator can then pass the tube while the assistant maintains the larynx in a stable position. This "tri-manual" technique eliminates the need for the laryngoscopist to provide verbal instructions to the assistant to direct the manipulation of the larynx.

RSI, the use of neuromuscular blocking agents combined with a sedative to facilitate orotracheal intubation is not a common practice in most EMS systems in the United States. The complete and flaccid paralysis provided by these agents clearly improves intubating conditions and increases the chance for first pass success while lessening the chance for complications[30,31]. Yet, controversy exists regarding the use of these potentially dangerous agents in the out-of-hospital setting by personnel with less training and less opportunity for skill maintenance than that afforded to hospital-based clinicians who employ these drugs on a routine basis.

There is a valid concern that the administration of a paralytic drug may convert a patient able to breathe spontaneously to one who can neither be intubated nor ventilated. If a rescue device or surgical technique is not rapidly successful, there is the risk of iatrogenic hypoxia leading to a potentially lethal outcome for the patient[32].

Despite these challenges, there are examples of RSI being successfully employed by paramedics in the pre-hospital setting on a large scale and on a long-term basis in Kings County WA[33]. There are three likely contributors to this achievement. First, the medics in this system receive extended training in advanced airway management, including the use of neuromuscular blocking agents and surgical techniques (approximately 2.5 times the overall training hours mandated by the NHTSA). Second, RSI is the standard procedure employed for orotracheal intubation in the out-of-hospital setting, and it is routinely employed throughout the system. Finally a rigorous continuous quality improvement program helps to ensure system-wide skill maintenance. From evaluating the King County experience described above, it appears that RSI can be used safely in the pre-hospital environment, but it is clear that the decision to employ this technique must be made on an individual system-by-system basis. It is also clear that significant resources must be allocated to this endeavor to ensure the adequate training of the EMS providers and to develop a continuous quality improvement program that fosters skill maintenance.

Eschmann Endotracheal Tube Introducer/Gum Elastic Bougie

While there is a significant amount of information regarding the use of the Gum Elastic Bougie (GEB) by both anesthesiologists and emergency physicians, there is limited data as to their role in the pre-hospital setting. In a study by Heegaard et al., the authors evaluated the effectiveness of the endotracheal tube introducer vs. standard ETI in the pre-hospital setting[34]. Despite a small study size, the authors found that after a short training period, success rates for first intubation attempts and total intubation time were similar. Of note, the study also found that the GEB group had a higher percentage of difficult laryngeal views (grade 3 and 4). In a much larger pre-hospital study, the GEB was recommended as the first alternative airway technique in the case of difficult intubation. The authors found success rates of 78% with GEB in this patient population (limited c-spine mobility, morbid obesity, facial trauma) and proposed it as a useful adjunct in the management of the difficult pre-hospital airway[35].

Similar to hospital-based airway assessment, when a grade 2 or 3 CL view is obtained with direct laryngoscopy, a GEB may be helpful in establishing an airway in the pre-hospital setting. Under direct visualization the curved tip of the GEB is guided under the epiglottis, and the glottic opening is "felt" for and the introducer is advanced to 25 cm. With practice the operator can come to appreciate the subtle sensation of the tip of the GEB "clicking" over the anterior tracheal rings. If this sensation is not felt, the device may still be in the trachea, and placement can be confirmed by gently advancing the device until resistance at the level of the narrower distal airways is felt. If such resistance is not felt by 45 cm the endotracheal tube introducer is most likely in the esophagus. After placement of the device in the trachea, and while under direct visualization with the laryngoscope still in place, an assistant loads an endotracheal tube over the GEB and then takes control of its proximal end as it re-emerges from proximal end of the ETT. The primary operator then advances the endotracheal tube over the GEB into the trachea under direct visualization. Occasionally the tip of the tube will impinge upon the structures of the glottic opening and tracheal intubation is impeded. This can be overcome by withdrawing the endotracheal tube a few centimeters, rotating it 90° clockwise or counter clockwise and re-advancing the ETT.

Blind Nasotracheal Intubation

Blind Nasotracheal Intubation (BNI) is infrequently practiced in the pre-hospital setting. With the advent of direct laryngoscopy and alternative/advanced airway techniques, fewer emergency physicians and pre-hospital EMS systems are using BNI. In a recent study of over 600 intubations at a large Level 1 trauma center, only 8 were performed using the BNI technique of which only two were successful[36]. However, it remains a viable option in certain difficult airway situations. BNI has several drawbacks that make it unappealing as a primary intubating technique. First, it typically takes longer and has a higher failure rate that direct laryngoscopy and intubation. Second, it is contraindicated in a large segment of patients in the pre-hospital setting (e.g., combative patients, patients with distorted upper airway anatomy, or patients with facial trauma). Third, it has a higher complication rate than standard intubation techniques. Finally, like other techniques, practice is essential for optimal success.

There have been several small studies that have evaluated the safety and efficacy of BNI in the pre-hospital setting. O'Brien et al. found that BNI is a safe initial field airway approach in spontaneously breathing patients in whom there are no contraindications. They found similar success rates in placing the endotracheal tube in medical and trauma patients, with an overall success rate of 71%[37]. More recent studies showed that the use of endotracheal tubes with distal directional controls is associated with a higher success rate for BNI than are conventional endotracheal tubes[38].

Needle Cricothyroidotomy

Needle cricothyroidotomy and open/surgical cricothyroidotomy in the pre-hospital setting are exceedingly rare events. As some EMS systems allow it to be used as a rescue technique for failed intubation, it will be briefly discussed below. Needle cricothyroidotomy is available as an alternative to an open surgical airway, and it is the surgical airway of choice in children under 8 years. Indications are a failed airway or predicted inability to perform a tracheal intubation when it is indicated. Contraindications include upper airway obstruction, which can lead to barotrauma if the patient cannot adequately exhale, and the ability to secure a less invasive airway.

The cricothyroid membrane is palpated and then punctured with the largest intravenous cannula available. The tip of the needle is angled approximately 45° caudad, and air is continually aspirated from a syringe containing saline. This will result in bubbling that makes tracheal placement more apparent. After advancing the needle 2–3 mm further after tracheal entry to be sure that the entire cannula is within the trachea, it is advanced off of the needle into the trachea with its hub advanced to the skin. Ideally adults should be jet ventilated with the lowest pressure required to achieve chest expansion, allowing sufficient time for the lungs to recoil. This approach provides the ability to deliver up to 50 psi (3,515 cm H_2O, 350 kappa) of 100% oxygen to adults and 1–2 psi per kilogram for children, but barotrauma including rapidly progressive subcutaneous emphysema, can occur very quickly making further surgical access virtually impossible. An insecure catheter or connection can also rapidly produce a disastrous outcome. Thus a luer-lok adapter is highly desirable however in its absence, a 3 cc syringe and an ETT connector that will allow connection to an Ambu bag can be used. It is difficult to generate sufficient pressure without specialized equipment (e.g., a jet ventilator system). Complications include vocal cord injury, esophageal puncture, tears of the posterior membranous trachea, pneumothorax, bleeding, and infection at the site.

Cricothyroidotomy (See Chap. 14)

The simplest method of performing a cricothyroidotomy involves locating the cricothyroid membrane between the thyroid and cricoid cartilages, preparing the anterior neck in an aseptic fashion as time allows. If the landmarks are easily identified, a transverse stab incision is made into the cricothyroid membrane with a #11 scalpel to the full width of the blade. The scalpel is then reversed and the handle is placed into the wound and rotated 90° to dilate the opening. Next the operator's little finger is placed into the wound to further dilate the opening and the tracheal rings are palpated to confirm entry into the trachea. A 6.0–7.0 cuffed ETT is then placed into the trachea and the cuff is inflated. Placement is confirmed by observation of the chest rising, auscultation at the axillae and the epigastrium, and preferably continuous waveform capnography.

Prior to the use of rescue airway devices and RSI protocols, the rates of pre-hospital cricothyroidotomy were surprisingly high. While the rates of surgical airway management in the Emergency Department are typically less than 1%, studies in the 1980s and early 1990s found that rates of pre-hospital cricothyroidotomy were between 2 and 14%[39–41]. Although the rates of the procedure varied, the authors noted that it was frequently being done in massively injured patients, with the majority of patients not surviving to hospital discharge. Indications for cricothyroidotomy were massive facial trauma, patient entrapment, suspected cervical spine injury, and failed oral intubation. More recently, Gerich et al. evaluated the efficacy of a protocol involving the use of midazolam (10–30 mg) and fentanyl (250–500 μg) by a trauma resident and experienced paramedic avoiding the use of paralytic agents. The rationale is difficult to understand since these drugs are likely to produce apnea and even greater hemodynamic instability that more conventional RSI. Nonetheless, they found that successful tracheal intubation was performed in 97% of the patients, with only 2% of the patients requiring surgical airway management[1].

Video Laryngoscopy (See also Chap. 6)

Over the course of the last several years, video laryngoscopy (VL) has become a useful tool in the management of the difficult airway in the emergency setting (see Figures 15.15 and 15.16). Not requiring a direct line of sight to the posterior oropharynx, VL can be useful in patients who are obese, have cervical spine pathology, or who have facial trauma. More recently, the case for use of VL as an adjunct for emergency airway management outside of the hospital has been made. Multiple studies have shown that pre-hospital providers can become proficient in this useful airway technique both in simulated and real patient encounters[2,3,42]. In two recent studies by Aziz[43] and Narang[42], the authors compare timing

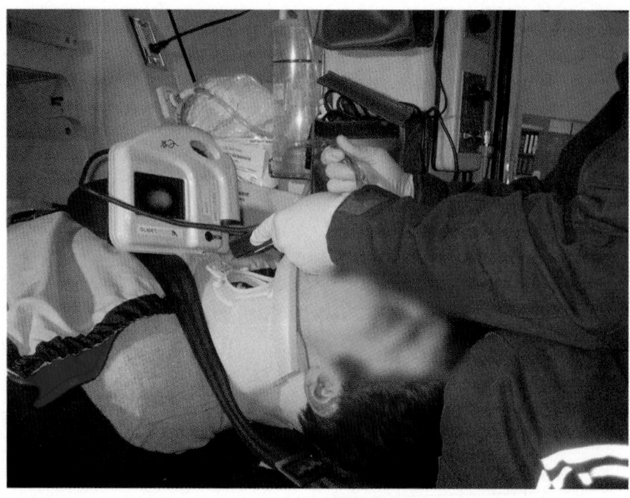

Figure 15.15. Side view of videolaryngoscopy in simulated trauma patient (courtesy: Dr. Mike Abernethy/UW Medflight).

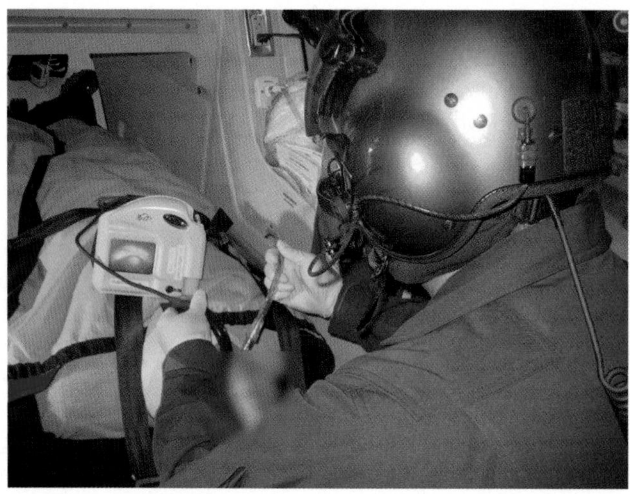

Figure 15.16. Operators view during videolaryngoscopy in simulated trauma patient (courtesy: Dr. Mike Abernethy/UW Medflight).

and success of VL to standard ETI by paramedic students and emergency medicine residents in high fidelity difficult airway simulations. Both groups found that VL provided a better view of the cords and a higher success rate of ETI in the simulated difficult airway scenarios. Similarly, in a large study evaluating tracheal intubation in the Emergency Department, VL had a higher overall success rate and a lower number of esophageal intubations[44]. These authors also found that VL had a higher first attempt success rate when compared to direct laryngoscopy, making it an interesting option to consider for further research in the pre-hospital setting.

The technique of VL in the pre-hospital setting is the same as in any other setting, but is somewhat dependent upon the exact device being used. Angulated laryngoscopes such as the McGrath and GlideScope as well as the channeled devices like the AWS and the Airtraq® are placed in the midline; by contrast, those with traditional Macintosh style blades such as the Storz C-MAC, McGrath Mac, and GlideScope Direct are placed along the right side of the tongue which is deflected to the left. The sequential landmarks of uvula, epiglottis, and glottic opening are visualized. With angulated devices, the use of a stylet is recommended by the manufacturers. A stylet is regarded as optional with the Storz

C-MAC, the McGrath Mac, and the GlideScope Direct and not required for the channeled devices. A definite benefit of these devices for trauma patients is that special positioning is generally not required and the airway manager can approach the patient from positions other than the head of the bed. Unfortunately, bright sunlight can cause visual interference depending on the device and the display unit. This can be overcome, at least in part, by shading the unit with a sheet or large towel. Some devices are more susceptible to fogging; secretions and blood in the oropharynx may also interfere with the view obtained to a greater extent than with direct laryngoscopy. The required mouth opening depends upon the device, but must be adequate to accommodate the blade and permit manipulation of the ETT.

Conclusion

Difficult airway management in the pre-hospital setting can pose a significant challenge. Many times decisions need to be made without the benefit of an adequate patient history or physical exam. In the United States, pre-hospital EMS systems vary in their approach to training, education, recertification, and "airway protocols" used. This has led to wide discrepancies in the standardization of emergency airway management. With the continued development of airway devices that are easier and quicker to place and refined protocols for advanced airway management by pre-hospital providers, the management of the difficult airway in this setting continues to evolve.

References

1. Gerich TG, et al. Pre-hospital airway management in the acutely injured patient: the role of surgical crichothyrotomy revisited. J Trauma. 1998;45(2):312–4.
2. Adnet F, et al. Survey of out-of-hospital emergency intubations in the French pre-hospital medical system: a multicenter study. Ann Emerg Med. 1998;32(4):454–60.
3. Sakles J, et al. Training with video imaging improves the initial intubation success rates of paramedic trainees in an operating room setting. Ann Emerg Med. 2001;37(1):46–50.
4. United States Department of Transportation. National Highway Traffic Safety Administration. EMT-Basic: National Standard Curriculum.
5. United States Department of Transportation. National Highway Traffic Safety Administration. EMT-Paramedic: National Standard Curriculum.
6. Cummins R, et al. Ventilation skills of emergency medical technicians: a teaching challenged for emergency medicine. Ann Emerg Med. 1986;15:1187–92.
7. Bobrow et al. Passive oxygen insufflation is superior to bag-valve-mask ventilation for witnessed ventricular fibrillation out-of-hospital cardiac arrest. Ann Emerg Med. Online: 7 Aug 2009.
8. Staudinger T, et al. Emergency intubation with the combitube: comparison with the endotracheal airway. Ann Emerg Med. 1993;22(10):1573–5.
9. Lefrancois D, et al. Use of the esophageal tracheal combitube by basic emergency medical technicians. Resuscitation. 2002;52:77–83.
10. Davis D, et al. The combitube as a salvage airway device for paramedic rapid sequence intubation. Ann Emerg Med. 2003;42(5):697–704.
11. Tanigawa K, et al. Chose of airway devices for 12,020 cases of nontraumatic cardiac arrest in Japan. Prehosp Emerg Care. 1998;2(2):96–100.
12. Rumball CJ, et al. The PTL, Combitube, laryngeal mask and oral airway: a randomized pre-hospital comparative study of ventilatory effectiveness and cost-effectiveness in 470 cases of cardiorespiratory arrest. Prehosp Emerg Care. 1997;1(1):1–10.
13. Vezina MC, et al. Complications associated with the esophageal-tracheal Combitube® in the pre-hospital setting. Can J Anesth. 2007;54(2):124–8.
14. Ochs M, et al. Successful pre-hospital airway management by EMT-Ds using the combitube. Prehosp Emerg Care. 2000;4:333–7.
15. Calkins T, et al. Success and complication rates with pre-hospital placement of an esophageal-tracheal combitube as a rescue airway. Prehosp Disaster Med. 2006;23:97–100.

16. Deakin C, et al. Securing the pre-hospital airway: a comparison of laryngeal mask insertion and endotracheal intubation by UK paramedics. Emerg Med J. 2005;22:64–7.
17. Doerges V, et al. Airway management during cardiopulmonary resuscitation—a comparative study of bag-valve-mask, laryngeal mask airway and combitube in a bench model. Resuscitation. 1999;41:63–9.
18. Chen L, Hsiao A. Randomized trial of endotracheal tube versus laryngeal mask airway in simulated pre-hospital pediatric arrest. Pediatrics. 2008;122:e294–7.
19. Levitan R, et al. Use of the intubating laryngeal mask airway by medical and nonmedical personnel. Am J Emerg Med. 2000;18(1):12–6.
20. Timmerman A, et al. Intubating laryngeal mask airway for difficult out-of-hospital airway management: a prospective evaluation. Br J Anesth. 2007;99(2):286–91.
21. Frascone RJ, et al. Successful training of HEMS personnel in laryngeal mask airway and intubating mask airway placement. Air Med J. 2008;27(4):185–7.
22. Komatsu R, et al. Comparison of the intubating laryngeal mask airway and laryngeal tube placement during manual in-line stabilization of the neck. Anaesthesia. 2005;60:113–7.
23. Russi C, et al. The laryngeal tube device: a simple and timely adjunct to airway management. Am J Emerg Med. 2005;25:263–7.
24. Russi C, et al. A pilot study of the King LT supralaryngeal airway use in a rural Iowa EMS system. Int J Emerg Med. 2008;1:135–8.
25. Jokela J, et al. Laryngeal tube and intubating laryngeal mask insertion in a manikin by first-responder trainees after a short video-clip demonstration. Prehosp Disaster Med. 2009; 24(1):63–6.
26. Russi C, et al. A comparison of the King-LT to endotracheal intubation and combitube in a simulated difficult airway. Prehosp Emerg Care. 2008;12(1):35–41.
27. Benumof JL, Cooper SD. Quantitative improvement in laryngoscopic view by optimal external laryngeal manipulation. J Clin Anesth. 1996;8:136.
28. Knill RL. Difficult laryngoscopy made easy with a "BURP". Can J Anaesth. 1993;40:279.
29. Alexander R. More on BURP. Can J Anaesth. 1994;41(1):74.
30. Perry JJ, Lee J, Wells G. Are intubation conditions using rocuronium equivalent to those using succinylcholine? Acad Emerg Med. 2002;9:813.
31. Li J, Murphy-Lavoie H, Bugas C, et al. Complications of emergency intubation with and without paralysis. Am J Emerg Med. 1999;17:141.
32. Pace SA, Fuller FP. Out-of-hospital succinylcholine-assisted endotracheal intubation by paramedics. Ann Emerg Med. 2000;35:568.
33. Warner K, Sharar S, Copass M, Bulger E. Prehospital management of the difficult airway: a prospective cohort study. J Emerg Med. 2009;36(3):257–65.
34. Heegard W, et al. Use of the endotracheal tube introducer as an adjunct for oral tracheal intubation in the pre-hospital setting. Air Med J. 2003;22(1):28–31.
35. Jabre P, et al. Use of gum elastic bougie for pre-hospital difficult intubation. Am J Emerg Med. 2005;23(4):552–5.
36. Sakles J, et al. Airway management in the emergency department: a one-year study of 610 tracheal intubations. Ann Emerg Med. 1998;31(3):325–32.
37. O'Brien D, et al. Pre-hospital blind nasotracheal intubation by paramedics. Ann Emerg Med. 1989;18(6):612–7.
38. O'Connor R, et al. Paramedic success rates for blind nasotracheal intubation is improved with the use of an endotracheal tube with directional tip control. Ann Emerg Med. 2000;36(4):328–32.
39. Cook S, et al. Pre-hospital cricothyrotomy in air medical transport: outcome. J Air Med Transp. 1991;10(12):7–9.
40. Xeropotamos NS, et al. Pre-hospital surgical airway management: 1 year's experience form the Helicopter Emergency Medical Service. Injury. 1993;24(4):222–4.
41. Fortune J, et al. Efficacy of pre-hospital surgical crichothyrotomy in trauma patients. J Trauma. 1997;42(5):832–8.
42. Narang A, et al. Comparison of intubation success of video laryngoscopy versus direct laryngoscopy in the difficult airway using high-fidelity simulation. Simul Healthc. 2009;4(3):160–5.
43. Aziz M, et al. Video laryngoscopy with the macintosh video laryngoscope in simulated pre-hospital scenarios by paramedic students. Prehosp Emerg Care. 2009;13(2):251–5.
44. Sakles J, Mosier J, Chiu S, Keim S. Tracheal intubation in the emergency department: a comparison of Glidescope video laryngoscopy to direct laryngoscopy in 822 intubations. J Emerg Med. 2012;42(4):400–5.

16

Extubation of the Difficult Airway

Louise Ellard and Richard M. Cooper

Introduction

Even though tracheal extubation is more likely to be associated with airway complications[1], most literature surrounding management of the difficult airway is focused on intubation. The American Society of Anesthesiologists practice guidelines for management of the difficult airway recommend that the anesthesiologist should have a pre-formulated strategy for extubating such patients[2]. The ASA Closed Claims Analysis supports the need for such a strategy[3].

L. Ellard
Department of Anesthesia and Pain Management, Toronto General Hospital, Toronto, ON, Canada, M5G 2C4

R.M. Cooper (✉)
Departments of Anesthesia and Anesthesia and Pain Management, University of Toronto, Toronto General Hospital, Toronto, ON, Canada, M5G 2C4
e-mail: richard.cooper@uhn.on.ca

D.B. Glick et al. (eds.), *The Difficult Airway: An Atlas of Tools and Techniques for Clinical Management*, DOI 10.1007/978-0-387-92849-4_16,

This chapter aims to:

- Summarize the complications associated with tracheal extubation and reintubation
- Discuss the stratification of risk associated with extubation
- Provide strategies to manage extubation of the difficult airway

Extubation fails when an attempt to remove a tracheal tube is unsuccessful, requiring the patient to be reintubated. This may be accompanied by an unsuccessful attempt to reintubate the trachea. Any reintubation should be considered to be more difficult than the original intubation as it is more likely to be associated with haste, hemodynamic instability, hypoxia, and/or acidosis as well as airway edema and bleeding from the initial intubation (especially if the initial intubation was difficult).

It is reasonable to consider the failed extubation in two separate clinical settings: the intensive care unit (ICU), where such failures are relatively common, and the operating room or post-anesthesia care unit (PACU), where they are far less frequent. In the ICU, a "trial of extubation" is sometimes attempted in order to minimize the risks, discomfort, and expense of prolonged intubation, and the incidence of reintubation is on the order of 6–20%[4–6]. Although complications associated with the extubation of postoperative patients may be more frequent, they rarely require reintubation. Combining the results of four large studies involving over 150,000 postsurgical patients, the incidence of reintubation ranged from 0.09 to 0.19%[7–10].

Complications, including hypertension, tachycardia, coughing, aspiration, and airway obstruction can be associated with *any* extubation. Airway obstruction may be further complicated by negative pressure pulmonary edema. However, most of the discussion of this chapter will relate to issues of oxygenation and ventilation with the extubation of more challenging airways and strategies designed to increase the probability of safe and successful extubation.

Summary of Extubation Problems

The causes of a failed extubation can generally be classified as a failure of oxygenation, ventilation, inadequate clearance of pulmonary secretions, or loss of airway patency. Airway obstruction can be the result of laryngeal edema, tracheobronchial injury, vocal cord injury, laryngospasm, macroglossia, or swelling external to the airway. These in turn can have many etiologies, including those related to the patient, the surgical procedure, or the original airway management. Airway edema is reported to occur in 2–37% of ICU patients following "prolonged intubation"[11]. Airway injuries may occur from the lips to the distal trachea or main stem bronchi. Glottic or tracheal injury may occur despite a good laryngeal view[12,13] or during awake flexible bronchoscopic intubation[14]. The trachea can be injured by the ETT or its introducer or by ischemic compression by the cuff on the tracheal mucosa. Airway injuries are presumed to be less likely if intubation is easy; however the ASA Closed Claims Analysis revealed that 58% of airway trauma[15] and 80% of laryngeal injuries were associated with "non-difficult" intubations[16]. Even when direct laryngoscopy provides a satisfactory glottic view[12] or intubation is facilitated by fiberoptic visualization[14], airway injury can occur and go unsuspected until after the endotracheal tube is removed. Glottic immobility may result from injury to the recurrent laryngeal nerve (RLN) or the arytenoid cartilages[17–26]. Arytenoid injury may be more common than the literature would have us believe[17,27] and has resulted from seemingly uneventful intubations[21,24,28]. Vocal cord paralysis results from injury to the vagus or one of its branches (see Table 16.1), which can occur as a surgical complication, usually associated with neck, thyroid, or thoracic surgery. The left RLN can also be compressed by thoracic tumors, aortic aneurysmal dilatation, or left atrial enlargement. In addition, the anterior division of the RLN can be compressed by an overinflated endotracheal tube cuff[29].

Table 16.1. Clinical features associated with injury to various branches of the vagus nerve.

Injured nerve	Anatomical change	Clinical features
External branch superior laryngeal nerve (unilateral)	Shortened, adducted vocal fold with a shift of epiglottis and anterior larynx toward the affected side	Breathy voice, no obstruction
External branch superior laryngeal nerve (bilateral)	Epiglottis overhangs making the vocal folds difficult to visualize. If seen, they are bowed	Hoarseness with reduction in volume and range of voice but no obstruction
RLN (unilateral)	Vocal fold assumes a fixed paramedian position	Hoarse voice. Weak cough. Possibly marginal airway
RLN (bilateral)	Vocal folds in fixed paramedian position	Inspiratory stridor. Surgical airway usually necessary[105]

Macroglossia may complicate surgery performed in the sitting, prone, or "park-bench" positions[30–33] or with steep or prolonged Trendelenburg positioning. Other causes include angioedema[34], extreme volume overloading, or tongue trauma, particularly when the patient has a coagulopathy. Lam and Vavilala postulate that in most cases, macroglossia results from venous compression leading to arterial insufficiency and a subsequent reperfusion injury[32]. If macroglossia occurs or progresses after extubation, it can lead to partial or complete airway obstruction making reintubation necessary but control of the airway may be difficult or impossible to achieve[31].

Risk Stratification of Extubation

Two questions should be considered prior to extubating any patient:

1. Is this patient at greater risk of failing extubation?
2. If reintubation is required, is it likely to be difficult? (see Table 16.2)

If the answer to both of these questions is "yes" then the patient represents a high-risk extubation. Figure 16.1 proposes a decision matrix to stratify the risk of the extubation of a given patient.

A patient may be at greater risk of failing extubation if they have marginal physiological reserve. In addition, paradoxical vocal cord motion (PVCM), COPD, obesity, sleep apnea, tracheomalacia, Parkinson's disease, rheumatoid arthritis, and acute burns or smoke inhalation all predispose to an increased risk of reintubation being required. Table 16.2 lists features that should highlight the possibility of increased difficulty of reintubation.

Surgical Procedures Associated with High-Risk Extubations

ENT Surgery

The reintubation rate appears to be significantly higher (1–3%) following a variety of head and neck procedures[35–39] including panendoscopy[7].

Laryngeal Surgery

Patients undergoing panendoscopy (laryngoscopy, bronchoscopy, and esophagoscopy) are at an increased risk of postoperative airway obstruction and are approximately 20 times as likely to require reintubation compared with other surgical procedures particularly if a biopsy is taken[7]. Most of the reintubations occurred within 1 h of extubation and were generally attributed to coexisting COPD.

Table 16.2. Features increasing the difficulty of reintubation.

Difficult initial intubation or advanced airway equipment necessary, e.g. bronchoscopic intubation
Subsequent events that may have changed the anatomy/ease of intubation
Airway edema
Airway trauma (e.g. from surgery such as panendoscopy or from initial intubation)
Recurrent laryngeal nerve injury
Tracheomalacia
Extrinsic compression, e.g. neck hematoma
Limited access to the airway
Intermaxillary fixation (jaws wired shut)
Cervical spine instability or immobilization
Chin-to-chest "guardian suture" to prevent traction on a new tracheal anastomosis
Confining space limiting access, e.g. PACU bay, ICU, or patient room

INCREASED LIKLIHOOD OF REINTUBATION REQUIRED?		INCREASED RISK OF DIFFICULT REINTUBATION? NO	YES
	NO	Low risk	Intermediate - high risk
	YES	Intermediate risk	High risk

Figure 16.1. This is an extubation risk stratification table based upon the likelihood of reintubation being required and the anticipated difficulty achieving this. Patients at low risk for both are regarded as "low risk extubations"; patients more likely to require reintubation are an intermediate-risk; patients in whom this is likely to be difficult are an intermediate-high risk; and those who have an increased risk failing extubation and in whom reintubation would be difficult are the highest risk patients.

Thyroid Surgery

A variety of airway injuries can be associated with thyroidectomies, including superior and RLN injuries, wound hematoma, and tracheomalacia. RLN injury is far more likely to occur with thyroid surgery for cancer than benign disease[38]. Local hemorrhage or hematoma occurs postoperatively in 0.1–1.6% of patients undergoing thyroid surgery[38,40–43]. Tracheomalacia is rare following thyroidectomy, even in patients with significant retrosternal tracheal compression[43–48] and when present, usually it does not become apparent until after the ETT is removed and spontaneous ventilation has resumed[49].

Deep Neck Infections

Infections involving the submandibular, sublingual, submental, prevertebral, and retropharyngeal spaces present significant airway management challenges, and continued postoperative intubation is usually necessary. Potter et al. retrospectively compared the outcomes of 34 patients in whom a tracheostomy was performed with 51 patients who remained intubated following surgical drainage[50]. All patients had undergone surgical

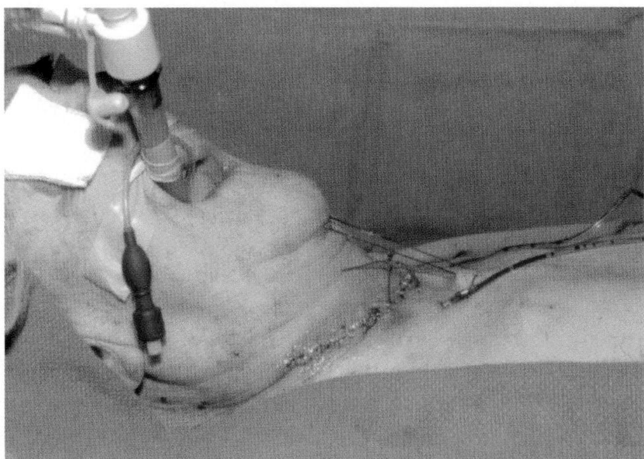

Figure 16.2. The patient has recently undergone a cricotracheal resection and to minimize tension on the anastomoses, the chin-to-chest distance is reduced with a "guardian suture" preventing cervical extension. This patient had undergone a Bailey Maneuver, exchanging the ETT for an LMA prior to emergence. This was intended to permit assessment of spontaneous breathing prior to emergence and reduce coughing on awakening. The photograph was provided courtesy of Dr. Patrick Gullane, University Health Network, Toronto and is reprinted with permission from Elsevier from "Extubation and reintubation of the difficult airway." In: Hagberg CA, editor. Airway management. 3rd ed.; 2012.

drainage for impending airway compromise and required airway support postoperatively. Two deaths occurred, one resulting from an unintended extubation and the other from post-extubation laryngeal edema and the inability to reestablish the airway. The latter patient was noted to have a cuff-leak prior to extubation, and signs of obstruction developed 30 min after the endotracheal tube was removed. Surgical drainage rarely results in immediate airway improvement and reintubation or an emergent surgical airway if required may be complicated by edema, tissue distortion, and urgency.

Tracheal Resection

Patients presenting for surgical tracheal resection present three distinct challenges for the anesthesiologist during the extubation phase:

1. An early extubation[51–55] is desirable to avoid positive pressure on the anastomosis and the presence of a foreign body in the airway.
2. A cough-free extubation is ideal to avoid disruption of the new anastomosis.
3. If reintubation is required, access is limited due to the guardian suture between the chin and chest[52,53] (Figure 16.2) and the anesthesiologist must ensure that the endotracheal tube cuff is not inflated in the region of the new anastomosis.

UPPP

A variety of surgical procedures have been employed to treat obstructive sleep apnea (OSA) including uvulopalatopharyngoplasty (UPPP)[56]. A retrospective review of 101 UPPP procedures identified an early postoperative respiratory complication rate of 10%[57]. Ten of 11 patients required reintubation with one death resulting from airway obstruction. These patients often fall in the high risk "box" in the decision matrix—the combination of obesity, sleep apnea, and airway surgery increases the risk of reintubation being required, and also the likelihood that reintubation may be difficult.

Cervical Spine Surgery

Cervical spine procedures may be complicated by vocal cord paralysis or airway obstruction. The anterior surgical approach requires tracheal and esophageal retraction toward the opposite side to permit exposure which can cause edema. Vocal cord dysfunction was seen in 5% of 411 patients undergoing anterior cervical discectomy and fusion[58]. Emery et al. studied the records of 133 patients who underwent anterior cervical corpectomies with arthrodesis between 1974 and 1989[37]. They identified 7 patients (5.3%) who required postoperative reintubation and attempted to identify the common features causing postoperative airway compromise. The authors believe that preexisting pulmonary disease, moderate or severe preoperative myelopathy, extensive multilevel decompression with prolonged surgery, and tissue retraction were risk factors for postoperative airway obstruction but there were no controls[37]. They recommended 1–3 days of elective intubation postoperatively, a "cuff leak" test and direct laryngoscopy at extubation. Extubation criteria following anterior cervical spine surgery were discussed at length on The Society for Airway Management Online Forum in January-February 2011. Groups that perform this surgery frequently, generally extubate their patients at the conclusion of the surgery, except when the blood loss is high (>500 mL), the surgery is prolonged (>5 h) or involves greater than three levels, the airway was difficult or would be expected to be difficult or comorbidities exist, such as severe cervical myelopathy, obesity, or OSA. Patients with multiple risk factors are cared for in an ICU setting and are extubated over an airway exchange catheter (AEC).

Patients undergoing posterior cervical surgery have a lower risk of requiring reintubation (1.1–1.7%)[59,60] but reintubation may be very difficult due to macroglossia, significant retropharyngeal or hypopharyngeal swelling[59], and fixation of the cervical spine. Similarly, patients in cervical immobilization devices for spinal cord protection require careful extubation planning since reintubation may be difficult and rapid surgical access may be virtually impossible. Several of the strategies described below should be given serious consideration.

Posterior Fossa Surgery

Posterior fossa surgery can cause cranial nerve injury, vocal cord paralysis, brainstem or respiratory control center injury[61–65], and macroglossia[31,32]. Gorski suggested that tolerance of the endotracheal tube and the absence of a gag reflex on oral suctioning should arouse suspicion of such an injury[62]. Damage to the cardiovascular and respiratory control centers from edema, ischemia, or compression may result in a loss of respiratory drive or airway obstruction.

Carotid Endarterectomy

Carotid endarterectomy can result in neck swelling, hematoma, or nerve injury. The rate of postoperative wound hematoma is approximately 5–7.1%[66,67] across several large studies. It may be difficult to clinically differentiate between bleeding and edema and wound evacuation does not always solve the problem. In the New York Carotid Artery Surgery study, cranial nerve palsies occurred in 514/9,308 patients (5.5%), involving most commonly the hypoglossal nerve (170) producing tongue deviation to the operative side, a branch of the facial nerve (126) resulting in a lip/facial droop, glossopharyngeal nerve (41), or a branch of the vagus producing vocal cord paresis (31)[66].

Maxillofacial Surgery

Maxillary and mandibular surgery can produce significant facial swelling; however the airway is usually spared. Meisami et al. performed MRI scans 24 h after maxillary and/or mandibular surgery in 40 patients. Despite significant facial swelling seen in almost all patients, none exhibited soft-tissue swelling from the base of the tongue to the glottis[68].

However, complete airway obstruction following elective orthognathic surgery has been reported. Dark and Armstrong described a case involving a young woman who underwent seemingly uneventful mandibular and maxillary osteotomies with submental liposuction. Immediately following extubation, she developed airway obstruction requiring reintubation. Extensive edema from the tongue to the trachea, maximal at the level of the hyoid, was demonstrated on CT[69]. If reintubation is required in these patients, this can be complicated if intermaxillary fixation has been employed.

Medical Conditions Associated with High-Risk Extubations

Paradoxical Vocal Cord Motion

With PVCM, adduction of the true vocal cords occurs on inspiration, expiration, or both. The false vocal cords and the posterior laryngeal wall may further contribute to the airway obstruction[70–73]. Patients with PVCM have a functional rather than anatomical problem and intubation is no more difficult. Extubation, on the other hand, carries a significant risk of requiring reintubation. PVCM may be associated with psychosocial disorders, stress, exercise, gastroesophageal reflux, irritant exposure, or airway manipulation. Regional anesthesia avoids airway intervention, but does not ensure that PVCM will not occur due to the stress-related nature of this condition. Consideration of deep extubation in these patients seems prudent.

Tracheomalacia

Tracheomalacia describes dynamic airway obstruction due to the posterior tracheal wall bulging anteriorly when the intratracheal pressure is reduced or the intrathoracic pressure is increased[27]. This may be congenital[74] or result from extrinsic compression by an intrathoracic goiter[75] or other mass[76]. Severe COPD, prolonged intubation or relapsing polychondritis can also lead to tracheomalacia. In susceptible patients, it is advisable to confirm or exclude the diagnosis during spontaneous breathing prior to emergence.

Parkinson's Disease

Patients with Parkinson's disease (PD) may exhibit laryngeal tremor, vocal fold bowing, and abnormal glottic opening and closing[77]. Extubation is more likely to fail due to involvement of the upper airway and susceptibility to aspiration. It is important to be aware that the unintended perioperative withholding of anti-Parkinsonian medications can produce dramatic unintended effects. This is reinforced by a case report describing a patient who developed airway obstruction and acute respiratory acidosis requiring intubation *preoperatively* due to the withholding of five doses of his anti-Parkinson's medications during fasting[78].

Rheumatoid Arthritis

The three main areas of concern to the anesthesiologist in a patient with rheumatoid arthritis (RA) are the cervical spine, the temporomandibular joint (TMJ), and the cricoarytenoid joints[79,80]. Patients with RA have an increased risk of failing extubation and increased difficulty associated with reintubation. Extubation may fail due to airway obstruction from cricoarytenoid arthritis or secondary to trauma following a difficult intubation in an airway that is already narrowed. Reintubation may be difficult due to a fixed or unstable cervical spine or because mouth opening is limited due to TMJ involvement. Autopsy studies suggest that 30–50% of patients with RA have significant cervical spine involvement and that the cricoarytenoids are involved in 26–86% of patients with RA[81,82].

Obstructive Sleep Apnea and Obesity

Obese patients and those with OSA can also represent "high-risk" extubations. In the ASA Closed Claims Analysis of Adverse Respiratory Events, for claims specifically relating to extubation, 12 of the 18 were obese and 5 of these patients had been diagnosed with OSA[3]. OSA is associated with a risk of airway obstruction following surgery[83] and reintubation may be difficult due to a higher incidence of difficult direct laryngoscopy[84] as well as the potential for gastroesophageal reflux and accelerated arterial oxygen desaturation[85,86] due to a decreased functional residual capacity.

Burns

Reintubation risk is high in burn patients who are known to exhibit bronchorrhea, impaired clearance of secretions, laryngeal and supraglottic edema, increased carbon dioxide production, and progressive acute respiratory distress syndrome. In addition, it may be difficult to secure the ETT due to involvement of the adjacent skin increasing the risk of unintentional extubation[87].

Strategies to Manage Extubation of the Difficult Airway

When a patient is identified as being a "high-risk extubation" a pre-formulated strategy should be in place with the following aims:

(a) To minimize the chances that reintubation will be required
(b) To allow oxygenation and/or ventilation throughout attempts to resecure the airway
(c) To ensure that reintubation, if required, is successful

Throughout this discussion, several prerequisite factors are assumed prior to considering extubation including full recovery of strength and consciousness, reversal of neuromuscular blockade, ability to maintain satisfactory gas exchange, and intact protective airway reflexes.

Step one is a focused examination ensuring that extubation is optimally timed. Once the aforementioned prerequisites are met, consider a bronchoscopic examination and a cuff leak test. Bronchoscopic assessment with an endotracheal tube in situ is of limited value but it helps exclude tube entrapment and occult clots ("coroner's clot") behind the soft palate or adjacent to the glottis, or supraglottic edema. An alternative is exchange of the ETT to a supraglottic airway (SGA) to allow laryngeal and subglottic bronchoscopic examination. This permits assessment of vocal cord movement, tracheal integrity, and increases the chance of a cough-free emergence. This is discussed below. The cuff leak test was proposed to identify patients with sufficient airway swelling to compromise safe extubation. The concept is that if air does not escape around the deflated cuff when the ETT is occluded and the patient exhales, significant airway swelling is likely present. Despite its intuitive appeal, the results of studies are conflicting and in some studies, the cuff leak test failed to predict those patients who subsequently developed stridor following extubation[11,88,89] or required reintubation. Deem argued that absence of a cuff leak may unnecessarily delay extubation while a large cuff leak may produce false reassurance that there will be no difficulties[89].

Step two involves gathering equipment and expertise that may be required if reintubation becomes necessary. Contrary to the initial management of a patient with a difficult airway, under urgent circumstances, methods that have previously been successful may not be available or appropriate. For example, flexible bronchoscopic intubation in an agitated, hypoxic patient with secretions or blood in the airway may be difficult or impossible.

Intermaxillary fixation requires that wire cutters be immediately available and that personnel know which wires to cut, should this be necessary. Consideration of extubation over an AEC or flexible bronchoscope is part of this step (see below). While reintubation is unlikely to be required, it must have a high probability of success.

Step three involves post-extubation monitoring in an appropriate location, for as long as reintubation risk remains high. This could extend for several days in some instances. In certain clinical situations, such as obesity and/or sleep apnea, step-down to nasal-CPAP[83,86,90,91] may be considered.

Exchange for a Supraglottic Airway

During emergence from general anesthesia, most patients tolerate a SGA better than an ETT, with less coughing and pressor responses[92–97]. Prior to exchange, the patient must be at a sufficient depth of anesthesia to avoid coughing, breath holding, and laryngospasm. This technique is useful but can jeopardize a secure airway if not properly executed and should be practiced on routine airways[98] prior to its use in higher-risk extubations. Bailey and others recommend that the SGA be inserted prior to removal of the ETT, with the purported advantage of reducing the risk of losing the airway following tracheal extubation[96,99] (see Chap. 7). Replacement with a SGA provides an excellent means of performing a bronchoscopic assessment of glottic and subglottic anatomy and function. After the substitution is performed, bronchoscopic confirmation of appropriate placement should be made. Then, muscle relaxation can be reversed and spontaneous ventilation allowed to resume, while maintaining the appropriate depth of anesthesia. A bronchoscope passed through the SGA can be used to assess vocal cord movement, and appearance to exclude, for example, PVCM or tracheomalacia. During this examination, the view is protected from oral secretions, the oxygen concentration can be adjusted as required, and inadequate ventilation can be supplemented. This technique is particularly useful in patients with recurrent post-extubation stridor or for those undergoing thyroidectomy when either tracheomalacia or vocal cord paralysis is suspected[43,100].

Extubation over a Flexible Bronchoscope

Examination using a flexible bronchoscope (FB) can also take place via the ETT without substitution for a SGA. After suctioning the oropharynx, the FB is passed through the ETT to a position above the carina and the ETT cuff is deflated slowly to minimize coughing. The ETT is withdrawn into the oropharynx with subsequent, very gradual withdrawal of the FB to a supraglottic region. Once the patient is comfortable, the FB is further withdrawn to a position just above the vocal cords. Even with such a deliberate technique, excessive secretions, coughing, swallowing, or poor tolerance frequently frustrates the exercise with insufficient opportunity to visualize the structures of interest. If significant abnormalities are noted, and the view has not been lost, it is possible to immediately reinsert the bronchoscope and advance the ETT.

Airway Exchange Devices and Jet Ventilation via These Devices

There are a number of products designed as AECs that can be used to facilitate a "reversible extubation." These long hollow catheters usually have end and/or distal side holes, connectors for jet and/or manual ventilation, distance and radiopaque markers, and can be connected to a capnograph to confirm placement and provide respiratory monitoring (Figure 16.3). When used to facilitate extubation, the AEC is introduced through the endotracheal tube, such that the distance markings on the two devices are aligned. Then the endotracheal tube is carefully withdrawn. Spontaneous breathing may take place around the device and most patients will be able to talk or cough with an AEC in situ. They must be properly secured to ensure that they do not come out prematurely

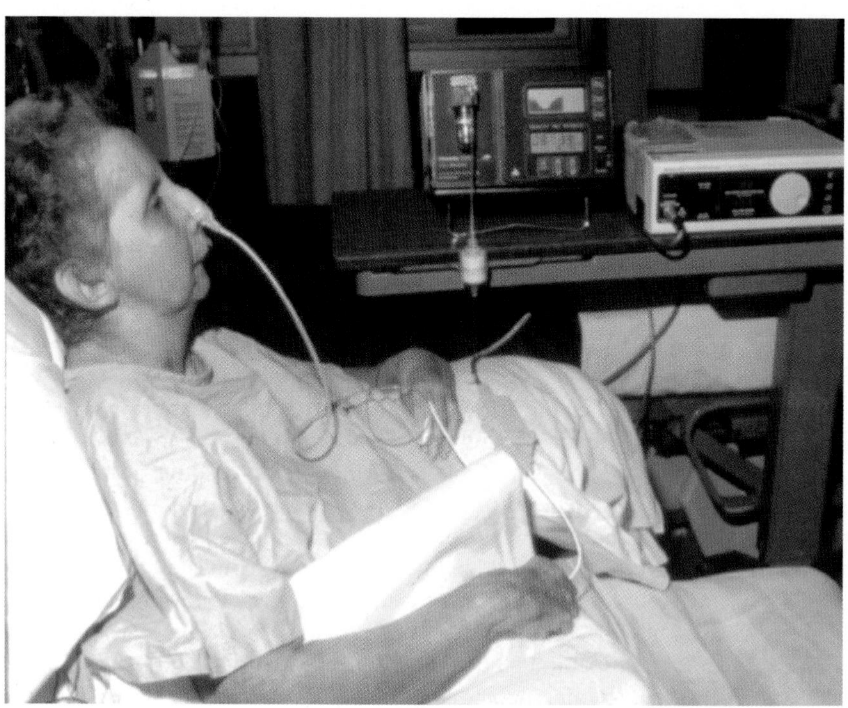

Figure 16.3. An airway exchange catheter (AEC) is connected to a capnograph. Because the AEC is in the mid- or distal trachea, very little dead space is aspirated and the continuous values closely correlate with arterial pCO_2.

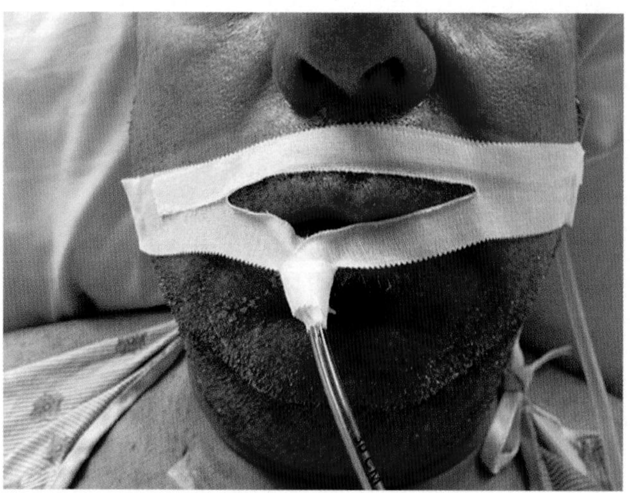

Figure 16.4. It is challenging to secure an AEC, particularly when it replaces an oral ETT. This photograph demonstrates secure fixation in the center of the mouth. If secured via the nares, care must be taken to avoid contact and pressure on the nasal ala. Reprinted with permission from Elsevier from "Extubation and reintubation of the difficult airway." In: Hagberg CA, editor. Airway management. 3rd ed.; 2012.

(Figure 16.4). If reintubation is required, an ETT is advanced over the AEC. This can be assisted by gentle laryngoscopy or indirect laryngoscopy[101]. Even if the larynx cannot be seen, tongue retraction may still prove very helpful. It is wise to delegate someone to secure the AEC during the reintubation. It is best to minimize the size discrepancy between the internal diameter of the ETT and the external diameter of the AEC by choosing a larger diameter tube exchanger and/or a smaller diameter ETT. This decreases the risk of the leading edge of the ETT getting caught on glottic structures. If resistance is encountered, ETT rotation may successfully release the tube from the pyriform fossa or arytenoid cartilage. These devices increase the probability that a reintubation will succeed; in addition, if difficulty is encountered the device can provide a conduit for oxygen insufflation. From an institutional database, Mort identified 354 patients over a 9-year period who were extubated over an AEC in the OR, PACU, or ICU. The AEC was left in place until the need for reintubation was considered unlikely. Two groups emerged: those who required reintubation while the AEC was still in place and another group who required reintubation within 7 days but after the AEC had been removed. The mean AEC dwell time was 3.9 h (range 5 min to 72 h). In the AEC group, 47/51 patients were successfully reintubated, 87% on the first attempt. Three of the four failures in this group were due to inadvertent removal of the AEC. By contrast, of the 37 patients requiring reintubation without the aid of an AEC, the first pass success rate was only 14% with mild and severe hypoxia seen in 50% and 19%[102]. Reintubation in all cases was attempted by an attending anesthesiologist or anesthesia resident under direct supervision. Although reintubation over an AEC does not guarantee first-pass success, this strategy was strikingly more effective (87% vs. 14% first pass success) with far fewer life-threatening complications. In most reports, the AEC is tolerated well enough to remain in place until reintubation appears unlikely. Carinal irritation, the principal cause of patient intolerance, should prompt a reassessment of the insertion depth. If irritation persists despite appropriate depth, tolerance can be improved by instilling lidocaine through the device. Specialized AECs are available for conversion of a double lumen tube to a single lumen tube and vice versa.

Features of the different devices are summarized in Table 16.3.

Oxygenation

Options for oxygenation with an AEC in place, assuming the chosen device has the necessary connections (see Table 16.3), are insufflation, bag-to-catheter ventilation, or jet ventilation. Bag-to-catheter ventilation is achieved using the provided 15 mm connector. Insufflation is achieved using low flow oxygen (i.e., 1–3 L/min) to a 15 mm connector on the AEC (Figure 16.5). For jet ventilation, a luer-lock adaptor on the AEC is connected to a manual jet ventilator (Figure 16.6). Barotrauma, in some cases fatal, has been reported with insufflation or jet ventilation through AECs[103]. The need for jet ventilation should always be weighed against its possible risks. Insertion depth should be confirmed, the catheter secured to prevent migration and, where possible, a capnograph trace should be obtained to confirm intra-tracheal placement of the AEC before applying oxygen insufflation or jet ventilation. Furthermore, the lowest possible flows and driving pressures should be used, the duration of inspiration should be minimized, and complete exhalation ensured prior to the next jet. The catheter should be in the mid-trachea, avoiding direct mucosal contact and far enough from the carina that distal migration does not occur but not so proximal that jet ventilation results in the catheter's ejection from the glottis. The objective of oxygenation/ventilation through such a device is the correction of life-threatening hypoxemia.

Conclusion

The ASA Task Force, the Canadian Airway Focus Group, and The Difficult Airway Society[104] have recommended that each anesthesiologist have a pre-formulated strategy for extubation of the difficult airway. The need for reintubation cannot always be predicted and reintubation will almost certainly be more difficult than the original intubation. This chapter proposes a decision "matrix" aimed at identifying patients in whom special extubation precautions are warranted. A variety of strategies can be used including exchange for a SGA, use of a flexible bronchoscope, or an AEC for patients that fall into high-risk extubation groups.

Table 16.3. Airway exchange catheters.

Name and company	Dimensions and durometry	Unique features
Sheridan TTX tracheal tube exchanger (Hudson Respiratory care Inc., Temulca, CA)	2.0 mm OD 3.3 mm OD 4.8 mm OD 5.8 mm OD Available in two lengths (56 and 81 cm) 85 shore[a]	Thermolabile—softens with heat Radiopaque stripe and distance markings Single distal end hole, no side holes No connectors for oxygenation
Sheridan JETTX exchanger	Single OD, suitable for ETTs greater than 6.5 mm ID 100 cm long	Single distal end hole Proximal slip-fit connector that can attach to a jet ventilator via a luer-lock
JEM Endotracheal Tube Changer (Instrumentation Industries, Bethel Park, PA)	Available in nine sizes 85 shore	Thermolabile—softens with heat Radiopaque stripe and distance markings Single distal end hole, no side holes No connectors for oxygenation
Cook airway exchange catheter (Cook Critical Care, Bloomington, IN)	8.0 Fr (2.7 mm OD) 11 Fr (3.7 mm OD) 14 Fr (4.7 mm OD) 19 Fr (6.3 mm OD) 83 cm long (except 8 F which is 45 cm long) 85 shore	Radiopaque stripe and distance markings between 15 and 30 cm from the distal end Two distal side-holes and an end-hole Two types of proximal connectors (15 mm connector and luer-lock jet ventilation attachment) secured and released by a patented Rapi-Fit® adapter
Arndt Airway Exchange Catheter (Cook Critical Care, Bloomington, IN)	14 Fr (4.7 mm OD) with distal taper 70 cm long	Kit includes an extra stiff Amplatz guidewire with positioning marks + AEC + rapi-fit adaptor and bronchoscopic port Bronchoscopy occurs via the existing airway device; the flexible end of the Amplatz guidewire is then introduced through the working channel and advanced to the carina before removing the bronchoscope. Next, the AEC is advanced over the guidewire to the appropriate depth, determined by aligning the distance markings on the existing airway with that of the AEC; the original airway is carefully removed and its replacement is advanced over the AEC[106]
Endotracheal ventilation catheter (ETVC) (Cardiomed International Inc., Lindsay, ON, Canada)	12 Fr (4 mm OD) 85 cm long 85 shore	Radiopaque stripe along its entire length with distance markings at 4 cm intervals Proximal male hose barb with threaded adapter welded into the catheter that does not restrict the catheter's inner diameter. The threaded adapter connects to a removable luer-lock adapter One distal end hole and eight helically arranged side holes to minimize catheter whip and jet ventilation pressures Oxygen insufflation is achieved by connecting the male component of the ETVC to an oxygen flow meter at low flows (1–2 L/min), titrated to the arterial saturation

[a]Shore is the measure of durometry or hardness of a plastic or rubber

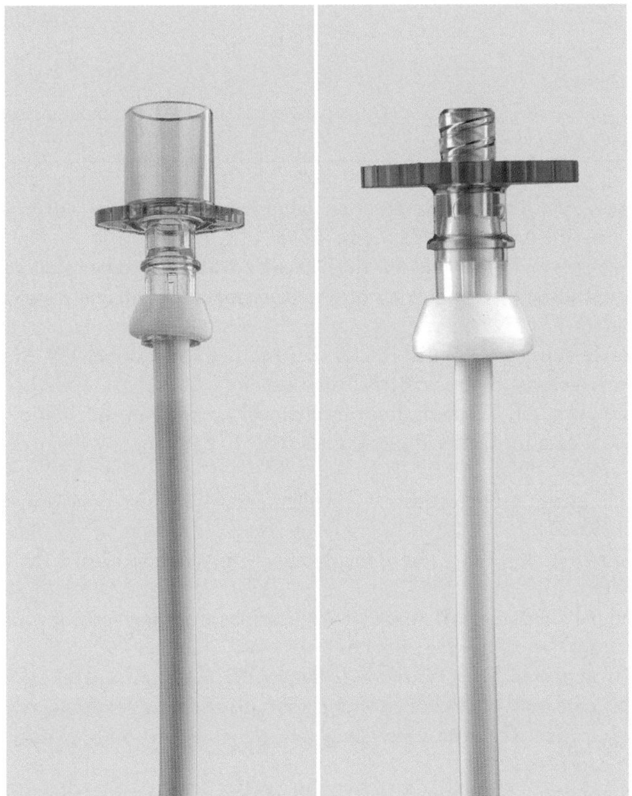

Figure 16.5. A Cook AEC is shown with a 15 mm Rapi-Fit™ adapter (*right*) and a jet adapter (*left*). High resistance will be encountered with bag-device ventilation because of the catheter length and inner diameter; however it can provide some oxygen and ventilation. This device is not ideal for jet ventilation because of the limited number of distal holes resulting is greater catheter whip and injection velocity. The photograph was provided by Cook and is reprinted from "Extubation and reintubation of the difficult airway." In: Hagberg, editor. Airway management. 3rd ed.; 2012 with permission of the publisher.

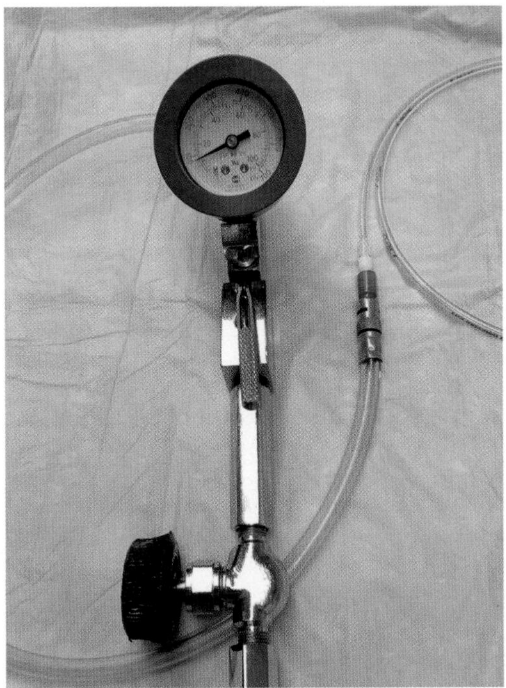

Figure 16.6. An ETVC (Cardiomed International) exchange catheter is connected with its luer-lock adapter to a hand-held jet injector with a pressure-reducing valve.

References

1. Asai T, Koga K, Vaughan RS. Respiratory complications associated with tracheal intubation and extubation. Br J Anaesth. 1998;80(6):767–75.
2. Practice Guidelines for Management of the Difficult Airway. An updated report by the American Society of Anesthesiologists Task Force on Management of the Difficult Airway. Anesthesiology. 2003;98(5):1269–77.
3. Peterson GN, Domino KB, Caplan RA, Posner KL, Lee LA, Cheney FW. Management of the difficult airway: a closed claims analysis. Anesthesiology. 2005;103(1):33–9.
4. Marini JJ, Wheeler AP. Weaning from mechanical ventilation. In: Marini JJ, Wheeler AP, editors. Critical care medicine: the essentials, vol. 1. Baltimore: Williams & Wilkins; 1997. p. 173–95.
5. Epstein SK. Putting it all together to predict extubation outcome. Intensive Care Med. 2004;30(7):1255–7.
6. Lavery GG, McCloskey BV. The difficult airway in adult critical care. Crit Care Med. 2008;36(7):2163–73.
7. Hill RS, Koltai PJ, Parnes SM. Airway complications from laryngoscopy and panendoscopy. Ann Otol Rhinol Laryngol. 1987;96(6):691–4.
8. Mathew JP, Rosenbaum SH, O'Connor T, Barash PG. Emergency tracheal intubation in the postanesthesia care unit: physician error or patient disease? Anesth Analg. 1990;71(6):691–7.
9. Rose DK, Cohen MM. The airway: problems and predictions in 18,500 patients. Can J Anaesth. 1994;41(5 Pt 1):372–83.
10. Lee PJ, MacLennan A, Naughton NN, O'Reilly M. An analysis of reintubations from a quality assurance database of 152,000 cases. J Clin Anesth. 2003;15(8):575–81.
11. Kriner EJ, Shafazand S, Colice GL. The endotracheal tube cuff-leak test as a predictor for postextubation stridor. Respir Care. 2005;50(12):1632–8.
12. Mencke T, Echternach M, Kleinschmidt S, et al. Laryngeal morbidity and quality of tracheal intubation: a randomized controlled trial. Anesthesiology. 2003;98(5):1049–56.
13. Maktabi MA, Smith RB, Todd MM. Is routine endotracheal intubation as safe as we think or wish? Anesthesiology. 2003;99(2):247–8.
14. Maktabi MA, Hoffman H, Funk G, From RP. Laryngeal trauma during awake fiberoptic intubation. Anesth Analg. 2002;95(4):1112–4.
15. Cheney FW, Posner KL, Caplan RA. Adverse respiratory events infrequently leading to malpractice suits. A closed claims analysis. Anesthesiology. 1991;75(6):932–9.
16. Domino KB, Posner KL, Caplan RA, Cheney FW. Airway injury during anesthesia: a closed claims analysis. Anesthesiology. 1999;91(6):1703–11.
17. Tolley NS, Cheesman TD, Morgan D, Brookes GB. Dislocated arytenoid: an intubation-induced injury. Ann R Coll Surg Engl. 1990;72(6):353–6.
18. Weber S. Traumatic complications of airway management. Anesthesiol Clin North America. 2002;20(3):265–74.
19. Hoffman HT, Brunberg JA, Winter P, Sullivan MJ, Kileny PR. Arytenoid subluxation: diagnosis and treatment. Ann Otol Rhinol Laryngol. 1991;100(1):1–9.
20. Appukutty J. Post-intubation cricoarytenoid joint dysfunction. Br J Anaesth. 2008;100(1):141; author reply 141.
21. Debo RF, Colonna D, Dewerd G, Gonzalez C. Cricoarytenoid subluxation: complication of blind intubation with a lighted stylet. Ear Nose Throat J. 1989;68(7):517–20.
22. Close LG, Merkel M, Watson B, Schaefer SD. Cricoarytenoid subluxation, computed tomography, and electromyography findings. Head Neck Surg. 1987;9(6):341–8.
23. Dudley JP, Mancuso AA, Fonkalsrud EW. Arytenoid dislocation and computed tomography. Arch Otolaryngol. 1984;110(7):483–4.
24. Frink EJ, Pattison BD. Posterior arytenoid dislocation following uneventful endotracheal intubation and anesthesia. Anesthesiology. 1989;70(2):358–60.
25. Tan V, Seevanayagam S. Arytenoid subluxation after a difficult intubation treated successfully with voice therapy. Anaesth Intensive Care. 2009;37(5):843–6.
26. Paulsen FP, Rudert HH, Tillmann BN. New insights into the pathomechanism of postintubation arytenoid subluxation. Anesthesiology. 1999;91(3):659–66.
27. Gaissert HA, Burns J. The compromised airway: tumors, strictures, and tracheomalacia. Surg Clin North Am. 2010;90(5):1065–89.
28. Usui T, Saito S, Goto F. Arytenoid dislocation while using a McCoy laryngoscope. Anesth Analg. 2001;92(5):1347–8.

29. Cavo Jr JW. True vocal cord paralysis following intubation. Laryngoscope. 1985;95(11): 1352–9.
30. Drummond JC. Macroglossia, Deja Vu. Anesth Analg. 1999;89(2):534.
31. Kuhnert S, Faust RJ, Berge KHMD, Piepgras DG. Postoperative macroglossia: report of a case with rapid resolution after extubation of the trachea. Anesth Analg. 1999;88(1):220–3.
32. Lam AM, Vavilala MS. Macroglossia: compartment syndrome of the tongue? Anesthesiology. 2000;92(6):1832–5.
33. Spiekermann BF, Stone DJ, Bogdonoff DL, Yemen TA. Airway management in neuroanaesthesia. Can J Anaesth. 1996;43(8):820–34.
34. Kyrmizakis DE, Papadakis CE, Liolios AD, et al. Angiotensin-converting enzyme inhibitors and angiotensin II receptor antagonists. Arch Otolaryngol Head Neck Surg. 2004;130(12):1416–9.
35. Levelle JP, Martinez OA. Airway obstruction after bilateral carotid endarterectomy. Anesthesiology. 1985;63(2):220–2.
36. Tyers MR, Cronin K. Airway obstruction following second operation for carotid endarterectomy. Anaesth Intensive Care. 1986;14(3):314–6.
37. Emery SE, Smith MD, Bohlman HH. Upper-airway obstruction after multilevel cervical corpectomy for myelopathy. J Bone Joint Surg Am. 1991;73(4):544–51.
38. Lacoste L, Gineste D, Karayan J, et al. Airway complications in thyroid surgery. Ann Otol Rhinol Laryngol. 1993;102(6):441–6.
39. Venna RP, Rowbottom JR. A nine year retrospective review of post operative airway related problems in patients following multilevel anterior cervical corpectomy. Anesthesiology. 2002;95:A1171.
40. Rosato L, Avenia N, Bernante P, et al. Complications of thyroid surgery: analysis of a multicentric study on 14,934 patients operated on in Italy over 5 years. World J Surg. 2004; 28(3):271–6.
41. Harding J, Sebag F, Sierra M, Palazzo FF, Henry J-F. Thyroid surgery: postoperative hematoma—prevention and treatment. Langenbecks Arch Surg. 2006;391(3):169–73.
42. Bononi M, Bonapasta SA, Scarpini M, et al. Incidence and circumstances of cervical hematoma complicating thyroidectomy and its relationship to postoperative vomiting. Head Neck. 2010;32(9):1173–7.
43. Palazzo F, Allen J, Greatorex R. Laryngeal mask airway and fibre-optic tracheal inspection in thyroid surgery: a method for timely identification of tracheomalacia requiring tracheostomy. Ann R Coll Surg Engl. 2000;82(2):141–2.
44. Ayabe H, Kawahara K, Tagawa Y, Tomita M. Upper airway obstruction from a benign goiter. Surg Today. 1992;22(1):88–90.
45. Shen W, Kebebew E, Duh Q, Clark O. Predictors of airway complications after thyroidectomy for substernal goiter. Arch Surg. 2004;139(6):656–9; discussion 659–60.
46. Abraham D, Singh N, Lang B, Chan W, Lo C. Benign nodular goitre presenting as acute airway obstruction. ANZ J Surg. 2007;77(5):364–7.
47. Abrams JTMD, Horrow JCMD, Bennett JADDSMD, Van Riper DFMD, Storella RJP. Upper airway closure: a primary source of difficult ventilation with sufentanil induction of anesthesia. Anesth Analg. 1996;83(3):629–32.
48. Cook TM, Morgan PJ, Hersch PE. Equal and opposite expert opinion. Airway obstruction caused by a retrosternal thyroid mass: management and prospective international expert opinion. Anaesthesia. 2011;66(9):828–36.
49. Palazzo FF, Allen JG, Greatorex RA. Respiratory complication after thyroidectomy and the need for tracheostomy in patients with a large goitre. Br J Surg. 1999;86(7):967–8.
50. Potter JK, Herford AS, Ellis III E. Tracheotomy versus endotracheal intubation for airway management in deep neck space infections. J Oral Maxillofac Surg. 2002;60(4):349–54.
51. Gaissert HA, Honings J, Grillo HC, et al. Segmental laryngotracheal and tracheal resection for invasive thyroid carcinoma. Ann Thorac Surg. 2007;83(6):1952–9.
52. Pearson FG, Gullane P. Subglottic resection with primary tracheal anastomosis: including synchronous laryngotracheal reconstructions. Semin Thorac Cardiovasc Surg. 1996;8(4):381–91.
53. Pinsonneault C, Fortier J, Donati F. Tracheal resection and reconstruction. Can J Anaesth. 1999;46(5 Pt 1):439–55.
54. Sandberg W. Anesthesia and airway management for tracheal resection and reconstruction. Int Anesthesiol Clin. 2000;38(1):55–75.

55. Saravanan P, Marnane C, Morris EAJ. Extubation of the surgically resected airway—a role for remifentanil and propofol infusions: [Extubation de voies aeriennes resequees chirurgicalement—un role pour les perfusions de remifentanil et de propofol]. Can J Anesth. 2006;53(5):507–11.
56. Szokol JW, Wenig BL, Murphy GS, Drezek E. Life-threatening upper airway obstruction after tongue base surgery. Anesthesiology. 2001;94:532–4.
57. Haavisto L, Suonpaa J. Complications of uvulopalatopharyngoplasty. Clin Otolaryngol. 1994;19(3):243–7.
58. Morpeth J, Williams M. Vocal fold paralysis after anterior cervical diskectomy and fusion. Laryngoscope. 2000;110(1):43–6.
59. Lee YH, Hsieh PF, Huang HH, Chan KC. Upper airway obstruction after cervical spine fusion: role of cervical fixation angle. Acta Anaesthesiol Taiwan. 2008;46(3):134–7.
60. Epstein NE, Hollingsworth R, Nardi D, Singer J. Can airway complications following multilevel anterior cervical surgery be avoided? J Neurosurg. 2001;94(2 Suppl):185–8.
61. Artru AA, Cucchiara RF, Messick JM. Cardiorespiratory and cranial-nerve sequelae of surgical procedures involving the posterior fossa. Anesthesiology. 1980;52(1):83–6.
62. Gorski DW, Rao TL, Scarff TB. Airway obstruction following surgical manipulation of the posterior cranial fossa, an unusual complication. Anesthesiology. 1981;54(1):80–1.
63. Howard R, Mahoney A, Thurlow AC. Respiratory obstruction after posterior fossa surgery. Anaesthesia. 1990;45(3):222–4.
64. Thompson JW, Newman L, Boop FA, Sanford RA. Management of postoperative swallowing dysfunction after ependymoma surgery. Childs Nerv Syst. 2009;25(10):1249–52.
65. Dohi S, Okubo N, Kondo Y. Pulmonary oedema after airway obstruction due to bilateral vocal cord paralysis. Can J Anaesth. 1991;38(4):492–5.
66. Greenstein AJ, Chassin MR, Wang J, et al. Association between minor and major surgical complications after carotid endarterectomy: results of the New York Carotid Artery Surgery study. J Vasc Surg. 2007;46(6):1138–44.
67. Ferguson GG, Eliasziw M, Barr HWK, et al. The North American Symptomatic Carotid Endarterectomy Trial: surgical results in 1415 patients. Stroke. 1999;30(9):1751–8.
68. Meisami T, Musa M, Keller MA, Cooper R, Clokie CM, Sandor GK. Magnetic resonance imaging assessment of airway status after orthognathic surgery. Oral Surg Oral Med Oral Pathol Oral Radiol Endod. 2007;103(4):458–63.
69. Dark A, Armstrong T. Severe postoperative laryngeal oedema causing total airway obstruction immediately on extubation. Br J Anaesth. 1999;82(4):644–6.
70. Christopher KL, Wood RP, Eckert RC, Blager FB, Raney RA, Souhrada JF. Vocal-cord dysfunction presenting as asthma. N Engl J Med. 1983;308(26):1566–70.
71. Tousignant G, Kleiman SJ. Functional stridor diagnosed by the anaesthetist. Can J Anaesth. 1992;39(3):286–9.
72. Sukhani R, Barclay J, Chow J. Paradoxical vocal cord motion: an unusual cause of stridor in the recovery room. Anesthesiology. 1993;79(1):177–80.
73. Arndt GA, Voth BR. Paradoxical vocal cord motion in the recovery room: a masquerader of pulmonary dysfunction. Can J Anaesth. 1996;43(12):1249–51.
74. Masters IB, Chang AB, Patterson L, et al. Series of laryngomalacia, tracheomalacia, and bronchomalacia disorders and their associations with other conditions in children. Pediatr Pulmonol. 2002;34(3):189–95.
75. Bailey B. Laryngoscopy and laryngoscopes—who's first?: the forefathers/four fathers of laryngology. Laryngoscope. 1996;106(8):939–43.
76. Triglia JM, Nicollas R, Roman S, Kreitman B. Tracheomalacia associated with compressive cardiovascular anomalies in children. Pediatr Pulmonol Suppl. 2001;23:8–9.
77. Gan EC, Lau DP, Cheah KL. Stridor in Parkinson's disease: a case of 'dry drowning'? J Laryngol Otol. 2010;124(6):668–73.
78. Fitzpatrick AJ. Upper airway obstruction in Parkinson's disease. Anaesth Intensive Care. 1995;23(3):367–9.
79. Matti MV, Sharrock NE. Anesthesia on the rheumatoid patient. Rheum Dis Clin North Am. 1998;24(1):19–34.
80. Wattenmaker I, Concepcion M, Hibberd P, Lipson S. Upper-airway obstruction and perioperative management of the airway in patients managed with posterior operations on the cervical spine for rheumatoid arthritis. J Bone Joint Surg Am. 1994;76(3):360–5.

81. Kohjitani A, Miyawaki T, Kasuya K, Mishima K, Sugahara T, Shimada M. Anesthetic management for advanced rheumatoid arthritis patients with acquired micrognathia undergoing temporomandibular joint replacement. J Oral Maxillofac Surg. 2002;60(5):559–66.
82. Kolman J, Morris I. Cricoarytenoid arthritis: a cause of acute upper airway obstruction in rheumatoid arthritis. Can J Anaesth. 2002;49(7):729–32.
83. Rennotte MT, Baele P, Aubert G, Rodenstein DO. Nasal continuous positive airway pressure in the perioperative management of patients with obstructive sleep apnea submitted to surgery. Chest. 1995;107(2):367–74.
84. Juvin P, Lavaut E, Dupont H, et al. Difficult tracheal intubation is more common in obese than in lean patients. Anesth Analg. 2003;97(2):595–600.
85. Benumof JL, Dagg R, Benumof R. Critical hemoglobin desaturation will occur before return to an unparalyzed state following 1 mg/kg intravenous succinylcholine. Anesthesiology. 1997;87(4):979–82.
86. Isono S. Obstructive sleep apnea of obese adults: pathophysiology and perioperative airway management. Anesthesiology. 2009;110(4):908–21.
87. Mlcak RP, Suman OE, Herndon DN. Respiratory management of inhalation injury. Burns. 2007;33(1):2–13.
88. Engoren M. Evaluation of the cuff-leak test in a cardiac surgery population. Chest. 1999;116(4):1029–31.
89. Deem S. Limited value of the cuff-leak test. Respir Care. 2005;50(12):1617–8.
90. Riley RW, Powell NB, Guilleminault C, Pelayo R, Troell RJ, Li KK. Obstructive sleep apnea surgery: risk management and complications. Otolaryngol Head Neck Surg. 1997;117(6): 648–52.
91. Johnson JT, Braun TW. Preoperative, intraoperative, and postoperative management of patients with obstructive sleep apnea syndrome. Otolaryngol Clin North Am. 1998;31(6):1025–30.
92. Lamb K, James MF, Janicki PK. The laryngeal mask airway for intraocular surgery: effects on intraocular pressure and stress responses. Br J Anaesth. 1992;69(2):143–7.
93. Brimacombe J. The advantages of the LMA over the tracheal tube or facemask: a meta-analysis. Can J Anaesth. 1995;42(11):1017–23.
94. Nair I, Bailey PM. Use of the laryngeal mask for airway maintenance following tracheal extubation. Anaesthesia. 1995;50(2):174–5.
95. Fujii Y, Toyooka H, Tanaka H. Cardiovascular responses to tracheal extubation or LMA removal in normotensive and hypertensive patients. Can J Anaesth. 1997;44(10):1082–6.
96. Koga K, Asai T, Vaughan RS, Latto IP. Respiratory complications associated with tracheal extubation. Timing of tracheal extubation and use of the laryngeal mask during emergence from anaesthesia. Anaesthesia. 1998;53(6):540–4.
97. Silva LCE, Brimacombe JR. Tracheal tube/laryngeal mask exchange for emergence. Anesthesiology. 1996;85:218.
98. Stix MS, Borromeo CJ, Sciortino GJ, Teague PD. Learning to exchange an endotracheal tube for a laryngeal mask prior to emergence. Can J Anaesth. 2001;48(8):795–9.
99. Dob DP, Shannon CN, Bailey PM. Efficacy and safety of the laryngeal mask airway vs Guedel airway following tracheal extubation. Can J Anaesth. 1999;46(2):179–81.
100. Lee C, Cooper RM, Goldstein D. Management of a patient with tracheomalacia and supraglottic obstruction after thyroid surgery. Can J Anaesth. 2011;58(11):1029–33.
101. Mort TC. Tracheal tube exchange: feasibility of continuous glottic viewing with advanced laryngoscopy assistance. Anesth Analg. 2009;108(4):1228–31.
102. Mort TC. Continuous airway access for the difficult extubation: the efficacy of the airway exchange catheter. Anesth Analg. 2007;105(5):1357–62.
103. Duggan LV, Law JA, Murphy MF. Brief review: supplementing oxygen through an airway exchange catheter: efficacy, complications, and recommendations. Can J Anaesth. 2011;58(6): 560–8.
104. Popat M, Mitchell V, Dravid R, Patel A, Swampillai C, Higgs A. Difficult Airway Society Guidelines for the management of tracheal extubation. Anaesthesia. 2012;67(3):318–40.
105. Ludlow CL, Gracco C, Sasaki CT, et al. Neurogenic and functional disorders of the larynx. In: Ballenger JJ, Snow JB, editors. Otorhinolaryngology: head and neck surgery, vol. 15. Philadelphia: Williams & Wilkins; 1996. p. 556–84.
106. Matioc A, Arndt GA. Intubation using the ProSeal laryngeal mask airway and a Cook airway exchange catheter set. Can J Anesth. 2001;48(9):932.

Index

D.B. Glick et al. (eds.), *The Difficult Airway: An Atlas of Tools and Techniques for Clinical Management*,
DOI 10.1007/978-0-387-92849-4, © Springer Science+Business Media New York 2013